Dr. Patrick Walsh's
GUIDE TO
SURVIVING
PROSTATE CANCER

D0963691

Dr. Patrick Walsh's
GUIDE TO
SURVIVING
PROSTATE CANCER

Fourth Edition

Patrick C. Walsh, M.D.,
and Janet Farrar Worthington

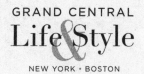

GRAND CENTRAL
Life & Style
NEW YORK · BOSTON

Copyright © 2001, 2007, 2012, 2018 by Patrick C. Walsh and Janet Farrar Worthington
Cover design by Brigid Pearson. Cover copyright © 2018 by Hachette Book Group, Inc.

Grand Central Life & Style
Hachette Book Group
1290 Avenue of the Americas, New York, NY 10104
grandcentrallifeandstyle.com
twitter.com/grandcentralpub

First Edition: June 2001
Revised edition: May 2018

Grand Central Life & Style is an imprint of Grand Central Publishing.
The Grand Central Life & Style name and logo are trademarks of Hachette Book Group, Inc.

The Hachette Speakers Bureau provides a wide range of authors for speaking events. To find out more, go to www.hachettespeakersbureau.com or call (866) 376-6591.

The publisher is not responsible for websites (or their content) that are not owned by the publisher.

LCCN: 2011942040

ISBN: 978-1-5387-2747-8 (trade paperback)

Printed in the United States of America

LSC-C

10 9 8 7 6 5 4 3 2 1

To all the patients, past and present,
who inspired us to write this book, with deep
gratitude for the lessons they have taught us—
which we now share with others

Contents

Acknowledgments

This book would not have been possible without the work and experience of many people, too many to name here. We tried, but the result looked like a telephone book—and had about as much personal meaning. So instead of listing all and inevitably missing one or two of the sources upon which we've drawn to produce this guide, we would simply like to thank those colleagues, patients, friends, and family members who have helped us the very most, including:

For this edition, we recruited Edward Schaeffer and Stacy Loeb, international experts in the diagnosis and management of prostate cancer, to take a leading role in formulating the revision. We were also fortunate to have the assistance of these Johns Hopkins experts: Elizabeth Platz in the epidemiology of prostate cancer; Jeffrey Tosoian on Active Surveillance; Phuoc Tran in radiation oncology; Trinity Bivalacqua in the management of erectile dysfunction; and Michael Carducci in medical oncology. In addition, we relied on the discoveries of other Hopkins experts in updating you on the latest in advances in the field: Jonathan Epstein, H. Ballentine Carter, Daniel Song, Theodore DeWeese, Mario Eisenberger, William Nelson, Martin Pomper, Charles Drake, Janet Walczak, Vicki Sinibaldi, Misop Han, Alan Partin, Ashley Ross, Christian Pavlovich, John Isaacs, William Isaacs, William Nelson, Angelo De Marzo, Tamara Lotan, Paula Hurley, Shawn Lupold, Bruce Trock, Jonathan Jarow, Dan Stoianovici, Daniel Chan, Lori Sokoll, Samuel Denmeade, Emmanuel Antonarakis, Jun Luo, Phillip Pierorazio, Edward Wright, and Kenneth Pienta; and on the work of Charles Drake, Robert Brannigan, and Suzanne Conzen.

We also acknowledge with deep gratitude the valuable contributions of these people: Peg Walsh; Alison Currie; Mark, Andy, and Josh Worthington; Blair and Ted Parrack; Bradley and Carole

Farrar; Sally Worthington; and Ronald Farrar, at twenty years and counting after his successful radical prostatectomy.

We would like to thank the late Leon Schlossberg, for his original illustrations; David Rini, for his superb ability to tell a story with pictures; Channa Taub, our wonderful literary agent and friend; and Katherine Stopa, our excellent editor.

And as always, we would like to honor Tom Worthington, who died of prostate cancer when he was just beginning to live. Every man this book helps is a victory for you, Tom.

Introduction

This is our fourth edition of this book, and our sixth book about prostate disease. With every book Patrick Walsh and I have written since 1993, there has been exponentially more hope, and with this edition, there is so much more good news—especially for those who need it most: men with advanced prostate cancer.

We're not out of the woods yet; men are still dying every day of this heartbreaking disease. In fact, this year, nearly 27,000 American men will die of prostate cancer. *If you are an American man, your lifetime risk of getting prostate cancer is 1 in 8*. But men who are diagnosed early have an excellent chance of being cured, with minimal side effects—particularly incontinence and erectile dysfunction (see chapter 11); in fact, many men with minimal, very slow-growing cancer can be carefully followed without needing treatment for years—or maybe ever. Moreover, men who have advanced prostate cancer are living much longer—some for decades—and a small but growing number of men who in previous years would have succumbed to widely metastatic cancer are not only alive but feeling great, because of unprecedented advances in hormonal therapy, chemotherapy, immunotherapy and radiopharmaceuticals (radionuclides), and new use of surgery and radiation as treatment for men with limited metastases.

From 1993 to 2014, because of early diagnosis—due to the introduction of PSA testing and a growing awareness that this isn't just an "old man's disease," but one that can strike in mid-life, and that prostate cancer screening saves lives—and constantly improving treatment, we have seen a *51 percent decline in deaths* from prostate cancer. Prostate cancer has dropped from the second to the third most common cause of cancer death, after lung and colorectal cancer, in American men.

Who's at higher risk? We know a lot more about that, too. In startling research, scientists have discovered that your risk is not only higher if *prostate* cancer runs in your family; it's higher if you have a family history of breast, ovarian, colon, pancreatic, and some other cancers. It turns out that mutations in the same genes that are involved in these cancers—genes like BRCA1 and BRCA2 and more than a dozen others—can cause prostate cancer, too. This means that the "men at higher risk" group—men who need to start screening for cancer in their forties—just got bigger. It also means that some of the newest gene-targeted drugs (discussed in chapter 13) that work particularly well *against these particular mutations* in breast and ovarian cancer work well in prostate cancer, too.

We know that men of African descent are not only more likely to get prostate cancer, but to have a more aggressive form of the disease. Also sobering: In these men, cancer tends to develop in the part of the prostate that is the most difficult to reach with a needle biopsy. Fortunately, magnetic resonance imaging (MRI) is better than ever, and able to reveal cancer that previously couldn't be detected.

We know that obesity and smoking make it more likely for you to get prostate cancer, and that quitting smoking and losing weight can lower your odds of getting this disease—or, if you already have it, make it less likely that you will die of it (see chapter 3).

We also know, unfortunately, that the U.S. Preventive Services Task Force (USPSTF) did a terrible disservice to all men in 2012 when it recommended against routine screening for prostate cancer for men with no risk factors. One major problem with this decision—made without the advice of a single urologist—is that *a lot of men don't know they are at higher risk*. They might have an African ancestor, or a family history of prostate or other cancer, and not know it—because they've lost touch with their family, or because many men still don't talk about this disease. It is not uncommon for a grown man to find out that his father or grandfather had prostate cancer, got treated for it, and never told the family. What about men who smoke or are overweight, and don't realize that their risk is higher?

Thousands of men who were told by their family doctors that they did not need prostate cancer screening have been diagnosed with the disease when it is more advanced and difficult to kill. This did not need to happen, and we rejoice that in 2017, in response to a huge outcry from urologists, radiation oncologists, medical oncologists, and from patients themselves, the USPSTF has backed off this bad advice.

Maybe you're reading this book because, along with more than 160,000 American men this year, you've been diagnosed with prostate cancer—and have become a member of what many call the reluctant brotherhood, a club nobody wants to join. Or maybe you're in the reluctant sisterhood, and you're reading this so you can help your husband, father, brother, son, or friend. Or maybe you're not yet an official member of the club, but you've received an unwelcome invitation—a change in your PSA, maybe, or a prostate biopsy that turned out to be negative. Maybe prostate cancer runs in your family, and you're interested in learning what you can do now to prevent or delay this disease.

In any case, we're glad you've found your way here.

I wouldn't wish the way I came to this disease on anyone, and I truly hope that you are coming to this book from an entirely different place. Until 1991, it's safe to say that I never thought about the phrase *prostate cancer*, and in fact, I didn't really know much about the prostate at all, except that men had one and women didn't.

That changed dramatically when I watched my fifty-three-year-old father-in-law, Tom Worthington, die of prostate cancer within a year of his initial diagnosis. It's hard to believe now, but in those days, nobody knew about PSA (prostate-specific antigen), nobody got screened, and men who got prostate cancer *really* didn't talk about it. There were few support groups for men with prostate cancer, or for their families. Tom was diagnosed because he went to see the doctor about persistent back pain. That was the cancer, already in his bones. His tumor spread like wildfire. He died in a nursing home, castrated, hooked up to a catheter, in agonizing pain, pitifully thin, his bones so riddled with cancer that his arm shattered when a nurse tried to move him. I thought of him a lot as we wrote chapter 13 of this book. Now, thank goodness, among the many new drugs we discuss are some that target prostate cancer before it has a chance to reach the bones.

Back then, most men who found out they had prostate cancer died of it, and the side effects of treatment were often as frightening as the disease itself. If cancer had spread outside the prostate or had returned after treatment, the philosophy seemed to be to wait until everything else failed before even attempting chemotherapy. That fatalistic worldview has changed. Thanks to research done at Johns Hopkins Hospital and at other great centers, doctors now have means (see the tables in chapter 5) of predicting who's at risk of a cancer recurrence—and instead of waiting for cancer to show up, they go after it much earlier, when it is most susceptible.

One thing you'll learn from this book is that every single case of prostate cancer is different—as individual as a fingerprint. The seriousness of a man's cancer depends on so many things. Some of it's the genetic deck of cards he was dealt. Some of it has to do with what a man eats, how big his waistline is, and whether he smokes. We are still learning how all the seemingly insignificant choices a man makes every day can affect his susceptibility to prostate cancer, and conversely, his ability to fight it off.

It makes sense, then, that the treatment for every man is different, too. Patrick Walsh is a legendary surgeon and one of the most respected prostate disease specialists in the world. In fact, he developed the operation called the anatomic radical retropubic prostatectomy, in which the prostate is removed, but potency and continence are preserved. (This operation is also known as the Walsh nerve-sparing procedure.) He will be the first to tell you that surgery is not ideal for every man. To give you the best possible help, we have asked top pathologists, radiation oncologists, and medical oncologists for their advice and perspective.

When my father-in-law died, I was working at Johns Hopkins as the editor of the medical alumni magazine. I decided to do a story on prostate cancer—mainly with the hope of finding out how this "old man's disease," which men were supposed to die *with*, not *of*, could kill a man in the prime of life.

I made an appointment to see Pat Walsh. So unattuned was I to the world of prostate cancer that I didn't even know who he was, other than that he was the head of urology at Johns Hopkins and his office was right across the street from mine. I had no idea there was a cure for prostate cancer and that Walsh had invented it. I didn't know he had developed the operation after years of intense, meticulous study of the anatomy of the prostate and male urinary and reproductive systems—a bedrock knowledge of the fundamentals, as athletes say. I quickly learned that curing prostate cancer isn't just a job for him, the basis of a successful career that has won him every possible honor and award in the field. It's his life's mission. At Johns Hopkins, Pat Walsh put together a world-class team of oncologists, radiation oncologists, molecular biologists, pathologists, urologists, and geneticists who have been tackling this disease from every angle for the last two decades. The fruits of their labor appear throughout this book. Walsh, along with his longtime research director, a brilliant man named Don Coffey, is the driving force that made much of it happen.

And finally, I had no idea that he would, within a few years, be the reason that prostate cancer was diagnosed early in my own father. What are the odds that this gifted surgeon with whom I would start to write books would one day take out my dad's prostate and cure his cancer? That was twenty years ago; Dad's PSA remains undetectable. I rejoice that for my father, prostate cancer was truly just a blip on the radar screen of his life, and that he is around for me and my brother and his six grandchildren. Dad's was the best example I know of an ideal scenario: prostate cancer detected early, because my mom and I made him get his PSA tested, which he grumbled about but did anyway; treated; and cured. I am so happy for the many men I've met and kept up with over the years who have been treated for prostate cancer and who are doing fine now.

Pat Walsh once told me something that one of his toughest professors in medical school used to tell all his students: "You are not here to make friends. You are here to find the truth." And that's who he is. He doesn't mince words, doesn't gloss over anything, and doesn't pretend all treatments are equal. But if he tells you something, you can trust him.

Today, my husband, Mark, whose family history (on both sides) of prostate cancer first catapulted me into this reluctant sisterhood, continues to have a very low PSA, and we're watching it like a hawk. He had a genetic test (like the one mentioned in chapter 10) to check for the faulty genes we discussed above, and thankfully, it was negative. Are we home free? My husband and I each have a younger brother. What about them? We have two sons. What about them? There is no way we will ever be complacent about prostate cancer.

I'm telling you all this to show that when I welcome you into this reluctant brotherhood and sisterhood, I mean it. I'm in it, too— which means we're in it together. Nobody wants to be in this situation, but believe me: it's infinitely better than it has ever been.

—Janet Farrar Worthington

1

WHAT THE PROSTATE DOES: A CRASH COURSE IN MALE ANATOMY

THE SHORT STORY:
The Highly Abridged Version of This Chapter

Prostate cancer is the last thing most men would ever choose to think about. It's not just a scary subject; it's tough to understand. The disease itself is complicated, and the decisions about what to do next are not always clear-cut. There's a lot to sort through and attempt to make sense of; that's why we have a "Short Story" in every chapter.

If this were a potboiler novel, a real page-turner, you wouldn't need any guidance on how to read it; you'd just get going. If, on the other hand, this were an academic textbook, you might approach it with a highlighter in hand, emphasizing key points and take-home messages in bright yellow marker. This book falls somewhere in between, and people read it in different ways. They kick the tires, in effect—flip through the pages; maybe they head directly to a specific section, such as impotence or biopsy, then backtrack and read about how prostate cancer gets started or jump ahead to chapters on treatment.

With this in mind, in every chapter we've done our best to tell you what you really need to know up front, in a highly abridged form. Consider the Short Story your briefing, or your "headline news."

That said, here's what you need to know about the anatomy of the prostate.

WHAT IS THE PROSTATE?

Like the appendix, the prostate is expendable. Men can live quite comfortably without it. The prostate's biggest job, as far as we know, is to provide part of the fluid that makes up semen. But even this contribution does not appear to be crucial for reproduction—which is why some scientists think the prostate's main role may be to safeguard the reproductive tract from infection in the urinary tract. (In fact, its name in Greek means "protector.") It is not a vital organ. Thus, the major importance of the prostate is not what it does but *what goes wrong with it:* For nearly all men who live long enough, it causes problems. These are:

- Prostate cancer, the most common cancer in men;
- BPH (benign prostatic hyperplasia, also called enlargement of the prostate), one of the most common benign tumors in men and a major source of misery as men get older; and
- Prostatitis, the most common cause of pelvic pain in men.

IF IT'S NOT A VITAL ORGAN, WHY IS IT IMPORTANT?

Although it's only as big as a walnut, the prostate is a miniature Grand Central Station, a busy hub at the crossroads of a man's urinary and reproductive tracts. It has a highly strategic location, right at the outlet to the bladder. Urine and semen cannot leave the body without passing through the prostate. It's also tucked away deep within the pelvis, surrounded by vulnerable structures—the bladder, the rectum, the sphincters responsible for urinary control, major arteries and veins, and a host of delicate nerves, some of them so tiny that we've only recently discovered them. This is why any form of treatment for prostate cancer can produce side effects including incontinence, impotence, and rectal bleeding.

What Else About Prostate Anatomy Do I Need to Know?

The prostate is like a complicated sponge, with five distinct parts called zones (see Fig. 1.3). The two most important for our discussion are the peripheral and transition zones. Located next to the rectum, the peripheral zone is the main site where cancer develops; the transition zone surrounds the urethra and is the principal site where BPH begins. The prostate's growth and function are stimulated by hormones: testosterone is produced in the testicles and converted to another hormone called dihydrotestosterone (DHT, the most active male hormone) in the prostate.

The bottom line: *The prostate is a gland that does much more harm than good and is located in a terrible area that complicates any attempt to treat it.* Despite this, there has never been more hope in the treatment of all prostate disorders—especially cancer.

The Prostate's Strategic Location

Welcome to the prostate—the bustling, walnut-sized hub at the crossroads of a man's urinary and reproductive tracts.

What makes such a small, relatively obscure gland so important to men? The answer is not immediately obvious: the prostate is not, for example, a vital organ like the heart. Its biggest job, as far as we know, is to provide about one-third of the fluid that makes up semen. But even this contribution does not appear to be crucial for reproduction, leading some scientists to suspect that the prostate's main purpose actually may be to safeguard the reproductive tract from infection in the urinary tract. (In fact, its name in Greek means "stands before" or "protector.") The prostate has few other redeeming features, isn't necessary for life or even for sexual function, and is known primarily for the clinical problems it causes to nearly all men who live long enough.

What the prostate *does* have, however, is a highly strategic location right at the outlet to the bladder. Urine cannot leave the body without passing through the prostate via a tube called the urethra. (Think of the urethra as an expressway and the prostate as the Lincoln Tunnel.)

Nothing About the Prostate Is Easy

From a urologist's standpoint, even a routine checkup—to feel for lumps or hardness with a rectal examination—is more complicated and takes more skill than many of our patients realize. (For a detailed discussion of diagnosing prostate problems, see chapter 6.)

The prostate is as tucked away—and as surrounded by booby traps—as any of the prizes sought by Indiana Jones in *Raiders of the Lost Ark* (see fig. 1.1). It lies in the midst of vulnerable structures— the bladder, the rectum, the sphincters responsible for urinary control, major arteries and veins, and a host of delicate nerves, some of them so tiny that nobody knew about them for centuries—that can foil any physician who ventures into the area without exquisitely precise knowledge of the terrain. This is why *any* procedure to treat prostate cancer can produce side effects including incontinence, impotence, and rectal bleeding.

The prostate fits snugly within the pelvis; there isn't much breathing room there. Unfortunately, not only is the prostate packed tightly amid other structures, like pieces of a jigsaw puzzle, it is poorly insulated. The flimsy wall separating the prostate and the seminal vesicles is *thinner than a piece of tissue paper*—not much of a buffer for cancer. Consequently, once cancer reaches a critical size, it can easily penetrate the wall of the prostate and escape into this overcrowded region of the body, spreading to the nearby seminal vesicles or lymph nodes or even farther, into the bloodstream.

This is why, even though treatment for prostate cancer is

improving dramatically, *a man's best protection against this disease is to have it detected as soon as possible.*

Ideally, for an American man at average risk of prostate cancer, *screening should start at age forty with a physical examination and a blood test for prostate-specific antigen (PSA)* (see chapter 5). This first prostate checkup should establish a baseline, an essential comparison point for your doctor to refer to in future visits.

What happens next depends on that first PSA level, but your doctor will probably want you to come back for another exam and PSA test every two to five years. Like a suspicious character—but one on whom the police can pin no actual crime—the prostate is best put under observation at age forty and beyond. This is especially important if you are at higher risk—that is, if you are of African descent or have a family history of prostate cancer (see chapter 3).

To Sum Up the Prostate

It's a gland that does much more harm than good and is located in a terrible area that complicates any attempt to treat it.

Despite this, there has never been more hope in our field. At last, we are finding answers to the toughest questions of prostate cancer: Where exactly does it begin, and why? How does it spread? If we can't cure it, can we contain it—can we make advanced prostate cancer a chronic illness, like diabetes, instead of a fatal one? Can we change our thinking and try drugs that were once considered last-ditch measures sooner? Can we unleash the immune system so it can turn its full force against prostate cancer? Can we try adjuvant therapy, which has proven successful in breast cancer? Can we actually prevent cancer or somehow slow its progress with diet? If PSA comes back after surgery or radiation, what does it mean—and how much time do we have to find a more effective treatment? As for radical prostatectomy and radiation therapy, can we make these treatments even better, with fewer side effects and quicker recovery of potency and continence? How can we help men and their families get their lives back? How can we improve quality of life? Keep reading.

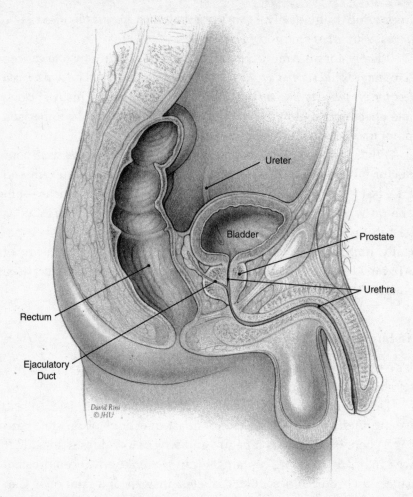

FIGURE 1.1   Crowded Territory

There's the prostate, nestled deep within the male pelvis—at a highly strategic location, right at the outlet to the bladder. The prostate is surrounded by vulnerable structures— the bladder, the rectum, the sphincters responsible for urinary control, major arteries and veins, and a host of delicate nerves.

A Brief Anatomy Lesson

This crash course in anatomy, though brief, still may be more than you ever wanted to know about the prostate and anything even remotely linked to it. But we believe it's essential that you understand where the prostate is and what it does, the two main systems it influences—the reproductive and urinary tracts—and how they can be affected when something goes wrong.

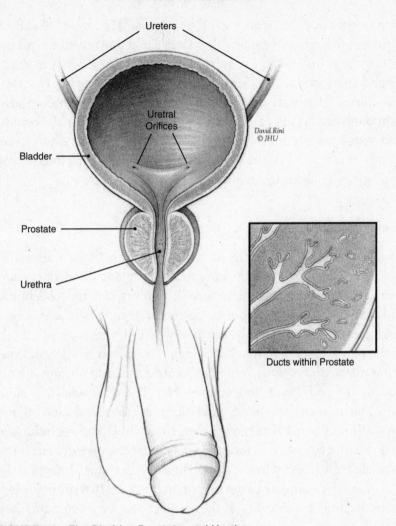

Ureters

Uretral
Orifices

David Rini
© *JHU*

Bladder

Prostate

Urethra

Ducts within Prostate

FIGURE 1.2   The Bladder, Prostate, and Urethra

Urine flows from the bladder via a tube called the urethra, but it can't leave the body without passing through the prostate. Think of the urethra as an expressway and the prostate as the Lincoln Tunnel. *Inset:* Like a sponge, the prostate is made up of tiny glands. These drain into ducts that, in turn, transport secretions to the urethra.

Reproductive Tract

For the reproductive organs, the basic act of sexual intercourse is as highly choreographed and synchronized as a NASA shuttle launch. First, the climate must be just right—in this case, the weather is a chain of coded chemical messages and hormonal signals. The equipment must be working properly, too. The main vessel, of course, is the penis, a remarkable construction that relies on hydraulic principles for erection, requires a delicate balance between arteries and veins, and is orchestrated by many intricate nerves. Orgasm, the climax of sexual intercourse, involves instantaneous, nearly simultaneous firings of fluid from the prostate, seminal vesicles, and testes (which make sperm). Because the prostate is the focus of this book, we'll begin there, although as we'll discuss, sexual potency and intercourse really begin in the brain.

Prostate

The prostate is a complicated, powerful little factory. Its main products, manufactured in numerous tiny glands and ducts, are secretions—components of semen. During orgasm, muscles in the prostate drive these secretions into the urethra (where it is joined by sperm and fluid from the seminal vesicles), which pumps it out of the penis. The prostate's fluid is clear and mildly acidic, and contains many ingredients, most of them designed to sustain sperm outside the body for as long as possible. (These include citric acid, acid phosphatase, spermine, potassium, calcium, and zinc.) Some prostatic secretions also protect the urinary tract and reproductive system from harmful bacteria that may enter the urethra. Here, the prostate truly lives up to its Greek name of "protector." Infections in this area can cause scar tissue to form in the ducts that drain the testicles, leading to infertility. If these infections were common, they would pose a serious threat to procreation—and this may be the major reason that all mammals have a prostate.

After ejaculation, the seminal fluid immediately coagulates—a key part of nature's "safety net" to maximize the odds of reproduction. If semen remained watery, it could not linger in the vagina. (In rats and other rodents, semen actually forms a pellet-like plug that effectively blocks other rats from depositing their semen in the same female.) The semen is gradually broken down again by an important enzyme made by the prostate—prostate-specific antigen (PSA). PSA's other great value is that it can be detected in a simple blood test. (More on PSA in chapter 5.)

Like New York City, the prostate is divided into five zones: anterior, which takes up one-third of the space and consists mainly of smooth muscle; peripheral, the largest segment, which contains three-fourths of the glands in the prostate; central, which holds most of the remaining glands; preprostatic tissue, which plays a key role during ejaculation—muscles here prevent semen from flowing backward, into the bladder; and transition, which surrounds the urethra and is the epicenter of trouble in benign prostatic hyperplasia (BPH).

For reasons not entirely understood, when a man reaches his mid-forties, the prostate tissue in the transition zone tends to enlarge, begins to push nearby tissue for room, and eventually starts to cramp the urethra. With this slow strangulation—think of a man's necktie slowly tightening around his collar—the prostate can make it exceedingly difficult for urine to get from the bladder through the prostate and out of the body. (For more on BPH, see chapter 2.) Most prostate cancer occurs in the peripheral zone. Fortunately, this is the region most likely to be felt during a rectal examination and tapped during a needle biopsy of the prostate (see chapter 6).

On a microscopic level, prostatic tissue is like a squishy sponge, riddled with tiny glands. These are the microfactories that produce the secretions, and they're connected by hundreds of ducts, which transport the fluid into the urethra. When these ducts become obstructed—as they do in BPH—PSA levels begin to rise in the bloodstream. Because prostate cancers don't make any ducts, glands in cancerous tissue become isolated. But these ducts still churn out fluid, which has nowhere to go except into the bloodstream. *That's why, gram for gram, prostate cancer contributes to blood PSA levels ten times more than BPH does.*

Prostate cells come in two basic models: *epithelial cells*, glandular cells that make the secretions, and *stromal cells*, muscular cells that hold the epithelial cells in place. The stromal cells aren't just passive scaffolding; they also help the prostate grow. From the stromal cells, in fact, spring many growth factors. And growth factors play a pivotal role in the development and function of the prostate when it is healthy and when it is cancerous.

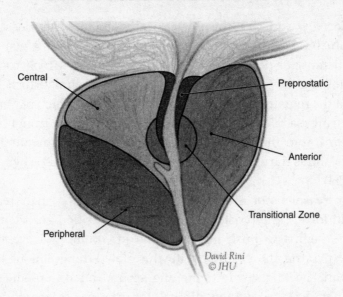

David Rini
© JHU

FIGURE 1.3   The Zones of the Prostate (viewed from the side)

The prostate is divided into five zones: *anterior*, which is mainly smooth muscle tissue; *peripheral*, which contains three-fourths of the glands in the prostate; *central*, which holds most of the remaining glands; *preprostatic* tissue, which plays a key role during ejaculation—muscles here prevent semen from flowing backward, into the bladder; and *transition*, which surrounds the urethra and is the epicenter of trouble in BPH. *Most prostate cancer occurs in the peripheral zone.* Fortunately, this is the region most likely to be felt during a rectal examination and tapped in a needle biopsy of the prostate.

How Do Hormones Affect the Prostate?

The prostate is very sensitive to hormones. In cancer treatment, this is a good thing; cutting off the supply of these male hormones, or androgens, can shrink prostate cancer and delay its progression.

The hormones that control the prostate originate in the brain (see fig. 1.4): the hypothalamus makes a substance called luteinizing hormone-releasing hormone (LHRH), which it transmits using "chemical Morse code," or signal pulses, to the nearby pituitary gland. In response, the pituitary makes its own chemical signal called luteinizing hormone (LH). LH, in turn, controls the testes, which make testosterone.

Among other things, testosterone causes secondary sex characteristics such as body hair and a deep voice, and fertility. Testosterone

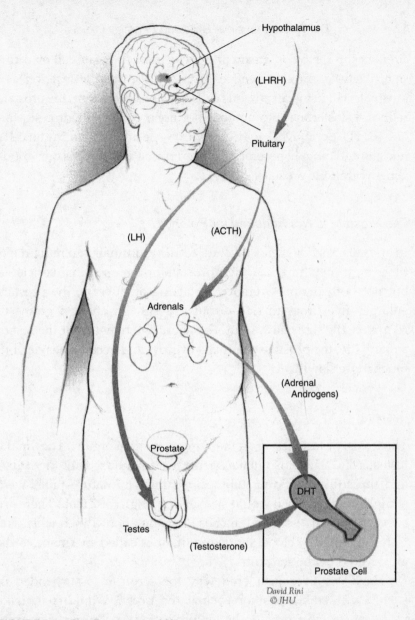

Hypothalamus

(LHRH)

Pituitary

(LH)

(ACTH)

Adrenals

(Adrenal
Androgens)

Prostate

DHT

Testes

(Testosterone)

Prostate Cell

David Rini
© JHU

FIGURE 1.4   The Prostate and Hormones

The hormones that control the prostate originate in the brain: the hypothalamus makes a substance called luteinizing hormone-releasing hormone (LHRH), which it transmits to the nearby pituitary gland. In response, the pituitary makes its own chemical signal, called luteinizing hormone (LH). LH, in turn, controls the testes, which make testosterone—the chief "male" hormone. Testosterone circulates in the bloodstream and seeps into a prostate cell by diffusion, like water through a coffee filter. The prostate, using an enzyme called 5-alpha reductase, refines testosterone into another hormone called dihydrotestosterone (DHT). Soon, DHT joins up with a specific protein in the cell's nucleus that acts like a key, switching on various genes within the prostate.

circulates in the bloodstream and seeps into a prostate cell by diffusion, like water through a coffee filter. To the prostate, testosterone is a raw material: using an enzyme called 5-alpha reductase, the prostate refines testosterone into another hormone called dihydrotestosterone (DHT). Soon, DHT joins up with a specific protein in the cell's nucleus and quickly becomes a powerhouse that switches on various genes within the prostate.

The Prostate Is Not Required for Potency

In animals, it's not even a must for fertility; animals can remain fertile even if they have had their prostate or their seminal vesicles—but not both organs—removed. Starting at puberty, the prostate enlarges five times in size—from a weight of about 4 grams to 20 grams, the size of a walnut—by about age twenty. For the rest of a man's life, the prostate continues to grow and become heavier, but much more slowly.

Testes

The testes, or testicles, are a man's reproductive organs. They make testosterone. They also make sperm inside hundreds of tiny tubes and threadlike, winding tubules. (If these miniature pipes were straightened out, each would stretch to a length of 2 feet.) There are two testes, each less than 2 inches long and about 1 inch wide. The testes, attached to blood-supplying lifelines called spermatic cords, are covered by the scrotum.

Have you ever wondered why the scrotum is suspended in such a vulnerable position, below the body? Wouldn't it make more sense—and provide better protection—if the testicles were inside the body? Yes and no. If the testes were tucked away inside the pelvis, they would indeed be better protected—but there wouldn't be much to protect. The testes are located in the scrotum for the simple but expedient reason that it's a more temperate climate down there, cooler than body temperature by a couple of degrees. Sperm are delicate; they fare poorly when the temperature is too warm. The scrotum, in effect, is nature's cooler. In fact, men who have undescended testicles—which are located inside the abdomen—cannot develop sperm because normal body temperature is just too hot.

Epididymis

The sperm-making tubules in each testis converge to form the epididymis. Compared to the tubules, this is a river as large and serpentine as the Amazon: each tubule (one on each side), though only 1 millimeter wide, could be uncoiled to reach a remarkable length of 15 to 20 feet. It is one continuous tube. Thus, it's easy to see why an infection here could cause scar tissue and blockage that would result in infertility. These tubules are packed side by side, top to bottom, to form the epididymis, an elongated structure about the size of a woman's pinky finger. This is the greenhouse where sperm mature until orgasm, when they shoot from the tail of the epididymis during a series of powerful muscle contractions. The epididymis clings to one side of each testis before turning yet again and heading upward to meet still another tube, called the vas deferens.

Vas Deferens

This impressive tube (again, there is one on each side; together they are called the vasa deferentia), 3 millimeters in diameter, is a hard, muscular cord about 18 inches long. Its job is to pump sperm to the part of the urethra that lies within the prostate (the prostatic urethra). Because it is so thick, it can easily be palpated through the scrotum. (It can also be cut easily in an outpatient procedure called a vasectomy, a form of male birth control. When the cord is cut, sperm cannot exit the penis through ejaculation and instead are reabsorbed by the body.) The vas deferens travels to a space between the bladder and rectum, then courses downward to the base of the prostate, where it meets with the duct of the seminal vesicle to form the ejaculatory duct.

Seminal Vesicles

The lumpy seminal vesicles, each about 2 inches long, sit behind the bladder, next to the rectum, hanging over the prostate like twin bunches of grapes. Arching still higher over them, on either side, are the vasa deferentia, which meet the seminal vesicles at V-shaped angles; these form the ejaculatory ducts, slitlike openings that feed into the prostatic urethra. The seminal vesicles are made up of caves called alveoli, which make sticky secretions that help maintain semen's consistency. (The vesicles got their name because scientists used to believe they stored sperm; they don't.)

Like the prostate, the seminal vesicles depend on hormones for their development and growth and for the secretions they produce. Although the seminal vesicles are strikingly similar to the prostate in many ways, they're almost always free of abnormal growth— benign (as in BPH) as well as malignant. (This is covered in more detail in chapter 3.)

What's the relationship between the prostate and the seminal vesicles? Both produce fluid that makes up semen—yet the prostate is prone to cancer while the seminal vesicle is remarkably free of it. In nature, animals like wolves that are carnivores don't have seminal vesicles. Only veggie-eating animals like cows have both prostates and seminal vesicles. There is only one exception to this rule: men have seminal vesicles, too. In other words, man, a meat lover, has the makeup of an animal that should be a vegetarian.

Penis

The penis—an engineering marvel built of nerves, smooth muscle, and blood vessels—has two main functions: sexual intercourse and urination. (Note: There is no bone in the human penis, although this is not the case in dogs and some other animals.) The penis works like a water balloon. Its basic structure is that of a rounded triangle; all three corners have cylinders of tissue (called the corpora cavernosa and the corpus spongiosum) that fill and become engorged with blood. During an erection, as arteries pump a steady supply of blood into the penis, the veins (which normally drain it back out again) clamp down so the blood can't recirculate, thus keeping the penis "inflated" during sexual activity. All this is made possible by the delicate nerves that lead to and from the penis. For years, these tiny nerves were poorly understood. The sad result was that removal of the prostate almost always meant impotence (see chapter 8). That is no longer the case.

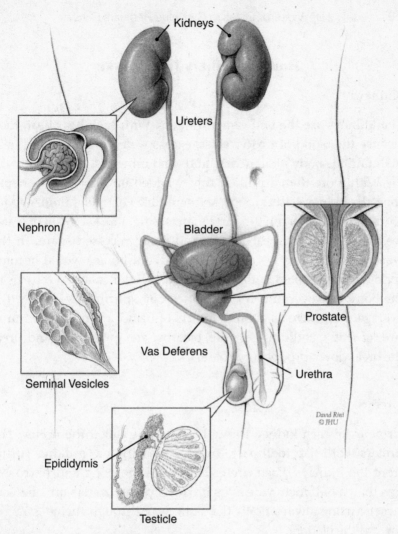

FIGURE 1.5 How Urine Exits the Body

From the top: The kidneys are the body's main filters. With more than a million tiny, wadded-up filters called nephrons, the kidneys sift through an incredible volume of fluid—about 45 gallons a day for a 150-pound man. Every day, the average man excretes about 2 quarts of urine. Urine exits the kidneys through ureters, pipelines that work like toothpaste tubes, squeezing urine downward toward the bladder. The bladder is a big bag. Stretched to its fullest, this muscular tank can hold about a pint of urine. Unlike the kidneys and ureters, the bladder—in normal circumstances—allows us some voluntary control; it generally obeys our decision to eliminate or hold urine. The next stop is the ure-thra, another muscular tube, which begins at the neck of the bladder, then tunnels through the prostate and continues into the penis.

Also seen here are the seminal vesicles, made up of caves called alveoli that make sticky secretions that help maintain semen's consistency, and the testes. The testes are a man's reproductive organs. They make the hormone testosterone; they also make sperm, in hundreds of tiny tubes.

How the Urinary Tract Works

Kidneys

The kidneys are the body's main filters. With each heartbeat, they cleanse the blood of toxic wastes, excess water, and salts and help maintain the body's balance of fluids and minerals.

With more than a million tiny, wadded-up filters called nephrons, the kidneys sift through an incredible volume of fluid—about 45 gallons a day for a 150-pound man (see fig. 1.5). Every sip of water we drink is refined, reabsorbed, and then processed again. (If the water and minerals weren't reabsorbed, our bodies would become seriously dehydrated within hours.) Not all this material returns to the body, however; much of it passes out as urine. Every day, the average man excretes about 2 quarts of urine, a concentrated mixture of water, sodium, chloride, bicarbonate, potassium, and urea, the breakdown product of proteins.

Ureter

Urine exits each kidney through a pipeline called the ureter. The ureters work like toothpaste tubes, squeezing or "milking" urine from the kidneys. Each ureter is about a foot long and narrow—less than a half inch wide at its broadest point. Ureters are one-way streets: urine always flows the same way through them—straight toward the bladder.

Bladder

The bladder is a big bag (see fig. 1.5). Stretched to its fullest, this muscular tank can hold about a pint of urine. Unlike the kidneys and ureters, the bladder, in normal circumstances, allows us some voluntary control; it generally obeys our decision to eliminate or hold urine. With intricately woven layers of muscle and connective tissue, the bladder can collapse or expand depending on the amount of fluid it's asked to hold at a given time. A sophisticated backup system protects the bladder from extreme distention and the risk of rupture: when the bladder is very full, it signals the kidneys to slow down the production of urine. At the neck of the bladder is a gate called the trigone. The purpose of the trigone is to make sure urine flows only one way—downward, away from the ureters and kidneys. The trigone's valve makes a tight seal that prevents urine from backing up into the kidneys, even when the bladder is distended.

Urethra

The next stop on urine's downward passage is the urethra, another muscular tube, about 8 inches long. This one begins at the neck of the bladder, then tunnels through the prostate at a 35-degree angle and continues into the penis. The urethra is divided into three segments—prostatic (the part that runs through the prostate), membranous (in between the prostate and penis—this is where the external sphincter is located), and penile. Like the prostate, it plays a role in both the urinary and reproductive systems; it serves as a conduit not only for urine but also for sexual fluids. The prostatic urethra has its own gate to prevent fluid backup—a ring of smooth muscle located in the preprostatic zone. During ejaculation, this muscle ring contracts along with the bladder neck. This keeps semen from flowing the wrong way—up into the bladder—and directs its course downward, out the urethra.

That's it for the anatomy crash course. Throughout this book, as we describe diagnostic procedures, treatments, and complications, you may need to return to this chapter. That's what it's for—to give you a working familiarity with the territory we'll be covering in the next chapters. If it helps, think of these pages as your Michelin Guide to male anatomy. Now that we've discussed the context of the prostate—a significant gland in both the urinary and reproductive systems—it's time to explain why this tiny gland is so important and what can go wrong.

2

LITTLE GLAND, BIG TROUBLE

THE SHORT STORY:
The Highly Abridged Version of This Chapter

The prostate is a troublesome little gland. In fact, three of the major health problems that affect men are related to the prostate:

- Prostate cancer, the most common cancer in men;
- Benign prostatic hyperplasia (BPH), also known as enlargement of the prostate, one of the most common benign tumors in men; and
- Prostatitis/chronic pelvic pain syndrome (CPPS), a "catchall" diagnosis for symptoms ranging from painful urination to fever and infection in the prostate.

As some men are unlucky enough to endure more than one of these disorders. You need a basic working knowledge of the prostate, and regular checkups to make sure all is well with this small gland. If you are over age 40 and you haven't had your prostate checked in a physical exam, please make it a point to do so, and ask your doctor for a PSA test. This is easy to do: the next time you get your blood drawn, your doctor can simply check a box and get PSA tested along with your cholesterol and lipids. Not that it's a competition, but women are far ahead of men in terms of knowing about their bodies and getting regular checkups. They get regular mammograms and Pap smears; they tend to know whether they have a family history of breast cancer or ovarian cancer. These diseases are on their radar.

The prostate needs to be on your radar, because catching prostate cancer early can save your life, and treating BPH and prostatitis correctly can make a great difference in your quality of life.

What Can Go Wrong with the Prostate: Cancer, BPH, and Prostatitis

For most young men, the prostate falls into the category of "obscure body parts" that includes the spleen—that is, it's in there someplace, it probably does something useful, but it's best dealt with on a need-to-know basis.

Unfortunately, most men *are* going to need to know about the prostate sometime, because three of the major health problems that affect men are prostate-related: prostate cancer, the most common major cancer in men; benign enlargement of the prostate (BPH, or benign prostatic hyperplasia), one of the most common benign tumors in men and a source of urinary problems for most men as they age; and prostatitis/chronic pelvic pain syndrome (CPPS), a catchall diagnosis that ranges from painful urination to actual infection of the prostate. Even worse, some men are unlucky enough to endure more than one of these disorders; for example, men who get BPH may still develop prostate cancer. Although this is a book about prostate cancer, when it comes to making the diagnosis and planning treatment, the other prostate disorders must be considered, too.

Fortunately, effective treatment and relief of symptoms is available for all these prostate disorders. *Even prostate cancer, when caught early, is usually curable*—generally without causing loss of urinary control or sexual function. Better still, for the first time ever, we are very close to understanding how to keep advanced prostate cancer in check, perhaps even for years.

Prostate Cancer

Prostate cancer is the most common major cancer in men and the third-leading cause of cancer death in men. Because prostate cancer is the subject of this entire book, we'll use this space only to make one point: when prostate cancer is small and curable, it is also silent—it produces no symptoms. That's why routine testing is so important to detect cancer as early as possible. If it's caught too late, prostate cancer can be deadly, and if the disease is allowed to run its course, it can produce terrible symptoms and excruciating pain. But *if caught in time,* before the cancer spreads beyond the wall of the prostate, *prostate cancer can be cured* with surgery or radiation. For some men with small, slow-growing tumors, a process called *active surveillance*—following the disease closely—may be a safe option (see chapter 7).

Treatments for prostate cancer are better than ever: we are now able to cure prostate cancer in more men, and with fewer side effects, than ever before. And, for the first time, groundbreaking research and novel methods aimed at stopping advanced prostate cancer in its tracks and unleashing the body's immune system as a powerful cancer-fighting weapon are starting to pay off. At the writing of this book, in five clinical studies around the world, some men with metastatic cancer have achieved results that have astounded doctors and scientists: tumors have melted away; metastases in the liver, lungs, and brain have disappeared; and PSA levels have dropped from the thousands to undetectable. Similarly dramatic results have been achieved with radiopharmaceuticals (radionuclides), molecular, radioactive prostate-targeting agents. Scientists are actively working to understand why some men have been such exceptional responders, and to understand how to help the men who have not yet responded to these agents. And in many men, even though we may not yet be able to cure prostate cancer, we may be able to stop it from growing further or delay its growth for many years.

How can we save lives from prostate cancer? The key is a four-pronged approach:

- Prevention—to ward off prostate cancer entirely, or at least delay its onset for decades;
- Earlier diagnosis—with the help of highly sensitive tests and sophisticated models for analyzing the results, detecting prostate cancer at the earliest and most curable stages yet. *However, this won't work if men don't get screened for prostate cancer;*

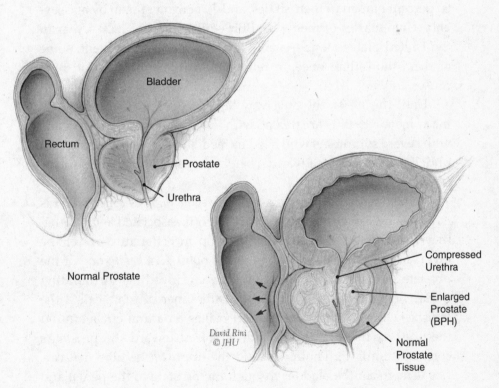

FIGURE 2.1   How BPH Squashes the Urethra

Here are two prostates—one with BPH, one without. What a difference! In the prostate with BPH, lumpy growths of glandular tissue plus tightening smooth muscle tissue act as a "double whammy" to choke the poor urethra and make urination increasingly difficult.

- Better treatment for localized disease—expanding and refining effective treatments, and working to minimize side effects even further; and
- Better strategies to fight advanced disease and resistance to treatment.

Benign Prostatic Hyperplasia (BPH)

Benjamin Franklin reportedly suffered from it; so did Thomas Jefferson. So will most men, if they live long enough. This almost inevitable condition is called benign prostatic hyperplasia (BPH), or enlargement of the prostate. The risk of BPH increases every year after age forty: BPH is present in 20 percent of men in their fifties, 60 percent of men in their sixties, and 70 percent of men by age seventy. One-quarter of men with BPH—more than 350,000 a year in the United States alone—eventually will require treatment, some of them more than once, to relieve the urinary obstruction BPH causes.

Until the 1990s, the only way to treat BPH was surgery; now many men with BPH are treated with medication. However, for men with severe symptoms who need immediate help, or men who wait until the disease is far advanced before they seek treatment, surgery is still the best option.

Remember, *prostate growth is not the same thing as cancer.* BPH is not prostate cancer. Although they're both associated with aging, they are different diseases that develop in different parts of the prostate. Prostate cancer begins in the outer *peripheral* zone of the prostate (see fig. 1.3) and grows *outward*, invading surrounding tissue. BPH begins in a tiny area of the inner prostate called the *transition* zone, a ring of tissue that makes a natural circle around the urethra. In BPH, the growth is *inward* toward the prostate's core, constantly tightening around the urethra (the tube that carries urine from the bladder through the prostate to the penis) and interfering with urination (see fig. 2.1). This is why BPH produces such annoying, difficult-to-ignore symptoms—and why prostate cancer is often "silent," producing no symptoms for months or even years. The key word here is *benign*. (The word *hyperplasia* simply means an increase in the number of cells in the prostate, which causes it to become enlarged.) By itself, an enlarged prostate causes no symptoms and does no harm. If it weren't for the fact that the prostate encircles the urethra, BPH might never require treatment.

What Causes It?

The quick answer is, we don't know. Like wrinkles and gray hair, BPH just seems to come with the territory of aging. Beginning at around age forty—in some men more than others—the inner zone of the prostate begins to grow. But even this is more complicated than it sounds. BPH involves two different kinds of tissue: glandular, made up of epithelial cells (which make the prostate's secretions); and smooth muscle cells (which contract to squeeze the secretions into the urethra). Somehow, BPH sets these two types of tissue at odds; the epithelial tissue forms lumpy lobes (see page 24), and the smooth muscle tissue reacts to this buildup by tightening around the urethra.

Hormones? It may be that with age, the prostate becomes more sensitive to testosterone. As men age, testosterone production starts to fall, but levels of estrogen (which normally are very low) remain about the same. Even a slight amount of estrogen can make testosterone more powerful; it may be that this imbalance in androgen (male hormone) and estrogen levels contributes to the disease.

Cell longevity? In any tissue, there is a finely tuned balance between the number of new cells and the number of cells that are dying. The population boom in BPH isn't due to an increase in cell birth, but to a decrease in cell *death*. For some reason, the cells in BPH live much longer. Some process—perhaps an increase in growth factors—alters their normal life span, creating a "fountain of youth" for prostate cells. Although the growth is not malignant, the process is similar to what's happening in prostate cancer—which suggests that once we understand the factors that control cell death in BPH, we may have a better approach for controlling it in cancer as well.

Is BPH Hereditary?

Several studies at Johns Hopkins suggest that it can be. Hopkins scientists believe that for a small number of men, about 7 percent, age isn't the only major risk factor. These men probably have inherited one or more genes that somehow make them prone to BPH. In one investigation, scientists studied men aged sixty-four and younger with notable prostate enlargement. They also studied their relatives and family histories. They found that the male relatives of these men were four times as likely as other men to require a prostatectomy (surgical removal of excess prostate tissue) to treat BPH. And brothers of these men were six times as likely as other men to need surgery to treat BPH. Understanding how the disease works in these men—specifically, identifying the genes involved—may provide major insight into the far more common form of BPH, and one day may even help us prevent it. If you have a strong family history of BPH, scientists at Johns Hopkins would be very interested in hearing from you. (Send inquiries to the Hereditary Prostate Disease Study, James Buchanan Brady Urological Institute, Johns Hopkins Hospital, Baltimore, MD 21287–2101, Attention: Dr. Patrick Walsh.)

What Does BPH Feel Like?

How does what's happening on the inside translate to the outside—into urinary symptoms? It varies; BPH is a different disease in every man, depending on a delicate interplay of factors, including the shape of the growth, the specific tissue involved, and how these variables affect the bladder. As the cell growth progresses, the tissue becomes lumpy (you can see the difference between a normal prostate and one with BPH in Figure 2.1). Bulbous nodules begin sprouting like mushrooms, forming characteristic clusters, or lobes.

These lobes tend to arrange themselves in one of three basic configurations. *Lateral lobe enlargement* features big knobs that sandwich the urethra, one on either side. When a man urinates, these lobes can swing open and shut like double doors (think of a saloon in a cowboy movie), so despite their size, they may not produce much urinary obstruction. In *middle lobe enlargement*, the lobe sticks up, plugging the bladder neck like a cork in a bottle and causing great difficulty with urination. (Because this form of BPH is much harder to ignore than lateral lobe enlargement, men who have it are far more likely to seek medical relief for their symptoms.) And in *trilobar enlargement*, both areas are affected; there can be obstruction at the bladder neck as well as in the urethra.

As the prostate squeezes the urethra, it impedes urine flow. This may manifest itself as *frequent urination*, needing to go to the bathroom several times an hour; *hesitancy*, or having to wait for the urinary stream to start; *urgency*, or the sudden sensation of needing to urinate, which may culminate in involuntary urine leakage before you reach the bathroom; *repeatedly awakening* in the night to urinate; *starting and stopping* during urination; and a *constant feeling of fullness* in the bladder. BPH can also lead to urinary tract infections and, rarely, can cause damage to the bladder or kidneys. It is often frustrating, annoying, and disruptive.

Think of a man's necktie slowly starting to tighten around his collar. This is what happens, over time, as the prostate's inward growth toward the urethra takes its toll. At first, or in mild cases, this can mean an irritating but still tolerable change in quality of life. However, when it progresses beyond the nuisance point—when the bladder is never completely empty, or when the kidney or bladder become damaged—it needs to be treated.

At first, BPH is invisible. It causes few symptoms, because the powerful bladder muscle compensates for the narrowed urethra by making more vigorous contractions and forcing urine through the prostate. But over time, this extra effort takes its toll on the bladder, making it less efficient. This is when a man may notice a decreased flow rate and obstructive symptoms. The bladder, after months of heavy duty, also becomes a victim of its own powerful muscles. The muscle-bound bladder wall thickens and loses its elasticity. With all that extra muscle, the bladder can't hold as much as it used to; it becomes unstable and overly reactive. When this happens, a man feels the need to urinate more often—unfortunately, sometimes spontaneously. These are *irritative symptoms*: urge incontinence (when a man knows he has to urinate but can't make it to the bathroom in time) and nocturia (the need to urinate often during the night). These symptoms are worse if a man is unable to empty his bladder completely. If the bladder is always partly full with leftover urine, it doesn't take much—half a glass of water, even—to fill it all the way. Some of our patients joke that they've spent the first half of their lives making money, and they're spending the second half making water. Imagine how disruptive and frustrating it is for a man to have to go to the bathroom twice as often as he normally would.

How Do You Know If You Have It?

Some men go right to a specialist, a urologist, for help with their urinary problems, but most men start out with their family doctor or internist. Most likely, all these doctors will approach your symptoms the same way: there should be a digital rectal examination and a PSA blood test. (These and other diagnostic tests are discussed in chapter 4.) You should be referred to a urologist if your doctor suspects BPH (or, for that matter, prostatitis/CPPS or prostate cancer).

Because other conditions can mimic BPH, your doctor will probably begin by taking a detailed medical history and performing a physical exam. It is very important for your doctor to know your entire medical history, even if you have what appears to be a classic case of BPH. For example, an injury to the urethra (from having a catheter inserted into the bladder during a surgical procedure, perhaps) can create a urethral stricture—scar tissue that narrows the urethra—that has nothing to do with the prostate but does a great impersonation of BPH. Blood in the urine or pain in the bladder or penis could point to a bladder tumor or mean that a stone has developed in the bladder, prostate, or kidney. If you have a history of urologic trouble—recurrent urinary tract infections, for example—it could be that an old problem has returned, but in disguise. BPH symptoms can also be produced by bladder cancer, prostate cancer, and neurogenic bladder (trouble with bladder function caused by a neurological problem, such as Parkinson's disease or stroke).

You will also be asked to score the severity of your symptoms and how much they bother you on a questionnaire called the

International Prostate Symptom Score (IPSS; see page 36). This is a short series of questions that can be answered on a scale from 0 to 5. Briefly, symptoms are considered mild if the score total is 0 to 7, moderate if it's 8 to 19, and severe if it's 20 to 35. The last question is the most important of all: *How much do the symptoms bother you?* This is critical, because BPH is not life-threatening. All of its treatments are directed at relieving symptoms—which means this symptom score will be the main basis for selecting therapy. (Thus, it is essential that you be brutally honest in answering these questions, rather than stoic and long-suffering or overly optimistic that this problem will go away by itself.) The big question your doctor needs answered, and the one only you can decide, is whether you could live the rest of your life this way. Are you changing your life to accommodate BPH—giving up seats to a basketball game, for instance, so you won't have to tough it out in the long lines at the men's room? Are you planning your day around trips to the bathroom? If not, if you can put up with it for now, you may choose to delay treatment. But if this problem is driving you crazy and disrupting your life, you should seek treatment.

The physical examination is discussed in detail in chapter 4. Because BPH affects only the innermost core of the prostate, your doctor may not be able to feel anything out of the ordinary. It's important to keep in mind that the size of the prostate may have nothing to do with the degree of symptoms. Some men with major prostate enlargement have no urinary tract trouble, while other men with seemingly minor enlargement or even a small prostate can suffer terrible problems from obstruction.

You may also need other tests, including:

Uroflowmetry

This test measures the speed of your urinary stream and the amount of urine you pass, and is done as you urinate (while you're alone in a testing room) into an electronic machine. It's a urological version of the radar gun used to measure professional baseball pitchers' throws. To ensure an accurate result, it's important that you urinate at least 5 or 6 ounces. This test can identify men whose maximum flow rate is diminished and who may benefit most from treatment.

The normal peak urinary flow rate is 15 cubic centiliters or more per second.

Ultrasound

This is a painless imaging technique. It creates a picture by bouncing high-frequency sound waves off an object, like sonar on a submarine. It can be performed from the outside, through the abdomen, or transrectally, using a wand inserted into the rectum. Ultrasound can be helpful in diagnosing such problems as obstruction of the kidney, stones, or a hidden tumor in the upper urinary tract; in estimating how well the bladder is emptying; and in determining the size of the prostate.

Residual Urine Measurement

If you're not emptying your bladder completely, this important test will find out. Further, it will show how much urine you're leaving behind. This can be done indirectly by an ultrasound examination of the lower abdomen immediately after you urinate, or directly by inserting a small catheter into the bladder (like a dipstick) and measuring what's there. If it turns out that you have large amounts of residual urine, your doctor will probably suggest that you seek treatment to avoid chronic urinary tract infections or damage to your kidneys.

Urodynamic Studies

Your urologist may want to do these studies if there is evidence that the primary problem is with the bladder, not the prostate. *Cystometry* is a way to measure bladder pressure and function. It's performed by threading a tiny catheter into the penis, through the urethra, and into the bladder to monitor pressure changes as the bladder is filled with water. *Pressure-flow studies* check bladder pressure using a small catheter as you urinate. (Note: Any time a catheter is inserted into the urethra, there is a slight risk of a urinary tract infection developing a few days later. Be sure to tell your doctor if you experience any subsequent fever or discomfort.) In these tests, pressure within the bladder is compared with the rate at which urine is flowing. This can determine whether men with high peak urinary flow rates have obstruction. Imagine squeezing water out of a balloon with a small opening. If you can squeeze hard enough, you can make the water flow, not just trickle. Similarly, some men with significant obstruction can produce reasonable urinary flow rates because they can generate high bladder pressure. These men will have relief of symptoms if their obstruction is treated. However, in some men, low urinary flow rates are caused by diseased bladders that can't produce much pressure. Relieving the obstruction in the prostate won't help these men, because the true problem is the bladder.

Cystoscopy

This test, usually performed in an outpatient setting, is uncomfortable but not painful; it is often used to assess the situation before an invasive procedure. A cystoscope is a slender, lighted tube that works like a small telescope. It is inserted into the tip of the anesthetized penis and threaded through the urethra into the bladder. This allows the urologist to see the bladder, prostate, and urethra and spot anything abnormal—such as a stone, stricture, or enlargement. With cystoscopy, your doctor may also be able to see thickened muscle bands in the bladder. Like rings in a tree trunk, these tell a story—that a condition of bladder obstruction has probably evolved over months or even years. (Note: This test carries a small risk of urinary tract infection. Some men also experience blood in the urine or a temporary inability to urinate afterward. Be sure to tell your doctor if you develop a fever or feel any discomfort.) Cystoscopy can also be used to rule out other conditions, such as the presence of a bladder stone or bladder tumor.

How Is BPH Treated?

The first option is observation, particularly for men with mild symptoms—those who say they can live with it for the time being. The course of BPH is often hard to predict. Your symptoms could stay the same, improve, or get worse. Men who choose observation must make an extra effort to avoid any condition (such as constipation) or medication (including over-the-counter cold remedies) that could aggravate the problem. Beyond observation, there are two basic approaches: medical and surgical.

For men with moderate symptoms, the initial treatment should be medical. Here again, there are several approaches. One class of drugs is called alpha-blockers. Remember the two kinds of tissue involved in BPH? One is glandular, made up of epithelial cells that secrete the prostate's fluids. The other is smooth muscle tissue—stromal cells that contract and squeeze this fluid into the urethra. As the glandular tissue enlarges and begins to narrow the urethra, the smooth muscle tissue tightens around it like a fist. In the normal prostate, there are two stromal cells for every epithelial cell. But in BPH, this ratio shifts. It's five to one, leading some scientists to describe BPH as a "stromal process." In other words, it's a smooth muscle problem. Alpha-blockers (often used to treat high blood pressure) counteract this by causing this muscle tissue to relax. These drugs are helpful in men with small prostates and moderate symptoms.

For men who have a significantly enlarged prostate, it is reasonable to try another class of drugs called 5-alpha reductase inhibitors. A chemical called 5-alpha reductase changes testosterone into dihydrotestosterone (DHT), the active form of male hormone within the prostate. This is important because the trouble in BPH starts *after* testosterone is converted by 5-alpha reductase into DHT. There are two drugs—dutasteride (Avodart) and finasteride (Proscar)—that block the activity of this enzyme. Both work equally well in shrinking the prostate and in decreasing obstructive symptoms. Because finasteride is available in generic form, it is less expensive and, thus, the drug of choice. These drugs may also halt the progression of BPH. They neatly manage to block a hormonal process without affecting a man's levels of testosterone (the hormone responsible for libido and sexual function). However, the problem with these drugs is that their effect is gradual. To some men, the pace of change is agonizingly slow, with significant improvement coming only after several months to a year on the medication. Also, these 5-alpha reductase inhibitors work well only if the prostate is significantly enlarged. If your prostate is small, a prostate-shrinking drug isn't going to solve the problem. And the relief of symptoms lasts only as long as you are taking these drugs.

Testing a Combined Approach

Is it possible that, for some men, two drugs are better than one? This idea was tested in a large clinical study. Indeed, long-term use of both an alpha-blocker and a 5-alpha reductase inhibitor proved safe and reduced the risk of clinical progression (symptoms getting worse) more than either treatment alone. Men taking both drugs had a lower risk of developing acute urinary retention (the inability to urinate) and were less likely to need invasive therapy. However, combined therapy is not the miracle answer for every man with BPH. It's expensive, results are not immediate, and although the outcomes of this study were statistically significant, they amounted to only a few percentage points. Further, there is some concern that long-term use of 5-alpha reductase inhibitors may, by artificially lowering a man's PSA level, delay the diagnosis of prostate cancer until it has progressed into high-grade disease. For this reason, if a man's PSA begins to increase while he is taking a 5-alpha reductase inhibitor, he should see a urologist immediately and undergo a biopsy to rule out cancer.

Surgical Options

For men with severe symptoms or men who do not respond to medical therapy, there are many effective surgical options. The gold standard is a procedure called transurethral resection (TUR) of the prostate (sometimes also referred to as TURP), also described by patients as the "Roto-Rooter" procedure. Performed under anesthesia (usually spinal anesthesia), it is a proven, effective way to improve BPH symptoms quickly and keep them at bay for years. In rare cases, if a man has a very large prostate, an open surgical procedure may be necessary. Most commonly, however, surgeons reach the prostate via the urethra by placing an instrument similar to a cystoscope through the penis. This instrument, called a resectoscope, allows surgeons to view the prostate as they chip away at excess tissue from inside, removing the prostate's core in fragments. These tissue chips are then flushed out, collected, and sent to a pathologist, who examines them and checks for prostate cancer. A TUR can also be done using alternate forms of energy—heat, radio waves, ultrasound, microwaves, and laser—to kill the obstructive cells on the spot. These energy waves are generated, focused,

PROSTATE SYMPTOMS AND WHAT THEY MAY MEAN

Symptoms of urinary obstruction...

Weak flow

Hesitancy in starting urination; a need to push or strain to get urine to flow

Intermittent urinary stream (starts and stops several times)

Difficulty in stopping urination

Dribbling after urination

A sense of not being able to empty the bladder completely

Not being able to urinate at all

...could be caused by

Benign prostatic hyperplasia (BPH)

Urethral stricture

Prostate cancer

Medication

Neurogenic bladder (bladder trouble caused by a neurological problem, such as Parkinson's disease)

Symptoms of irritation...

Pain or burning during urination

Frequent urination, especially at night

A strong sense of urgency in urination; inability to postpone urination

Sleep disrupted by the need to urinate

Urgency incontinence

...could be caused by

Thickened bladder, caused by obstruction from BPH

Infection in the bladder or prostate

Bladder tumor

Stone

Neurogenic bladder

aimed, and fired at the overgrown tissue. Some waves work like a shotgun, blasting holes in the prostate. Other procedures—such as GreenLight laser PVP (photoselective vaporization of the prostate) and holmium laser ablation—are as sensitive as a scalpel, delicately nibbling away at overgrown tissue until the urethra is free of obstruction.

There are also several new surgical options that can be performed under local anesthesia in the urologist's office through a cystoscope. One such option, the UroLift System procedure, involves placement of small implants that hold the enlarged tissue out of the way, like tiebacks on a window curtain. The other is called Rezūm. In this procedure, small quantities of vaporized water are injected directly into the obstructing tissue. The early results for these new options look encouraging, with outcomes similar to TUR with little or no side effects.

To sum up: BPH is a common condition that affects most men. It is not cancerous, but it can mimic cancer. Today, there are many effective ways to treat it, and most of them have few side effects.

Prostatitis: Misdiagnosed and Misunderstood

Imagine you have chest pain. You go to the hospital and the doctor in the emergency room assumes you're having a heart attack but doesn't actually do the right tests to make sure. What if your chest pain is actually severe acid reflux (backup of your stomach acid into the esophagus)? Instead of getting what you really need, a strong acid reducer, you end up in a cardiac care unit getting pumped full of blood thinners and expensive medicine to dissolve a nonexistent blood clot. And you've still got the terrible heartburn! That would be a nightmare, and yet this happens to men with pelvic pain all the time. Every year, thousands of men are diagnosed with prostatitis. *Some men actually have it, but most of them don't,* and yet they all take powerful antibiotics for weeks. This is because most doctors don't understand what prostatitis is. Prostatitis is a catchall diagnosis that stretches to fit a variety of symptoms. Pain in the testicles? Prostatitis. Pain in the penis? Prostatitis. Burning when you urinate or ejaculate? Prostatitis. Pain in the bladder or rectum? You guessed it.

For the vast majority of men, "prostatitis" is just what the symptoms sound like: chronic pelvic pain syndrome (CPPS). But what's causing the miserable symptoms in one man with CPPS might not be what's causing them in another man. Everybody's different, and you need to see a doctor who specializes in this, at a medical center where they see a lot of men with these symptoms.

For example, in some men the cause of pain or tenderness in the scrotum or lower back is actually the *pelvic floor muscles in spasm*—like a hard muscle knot in the neck or back, except close to the rectum. The treatment for that is a pressure point release, which is administered in specialized physical therapy.

Other men have bladder symptoms that are related to muscle spasms from *interstitial cystitis*, a bladder problem. Some men with frequent or burning urination get better with Flomax or another drug in the alpha-blocker category. These drugs relax the muscles in the prostate and bladder and help relieve symptoms. Some men get better by changing their diet, because for them, spicy foods seem to set off the symptoms. Men who have difficulty or pain when urinating are often helped by biofeedback and physical therapy.

Chronic pelvic pain itself is a broad diagnosis. "Prostatitis is one of the diagnoses that can cause pelvic pain—not the other way around," says Sarah Flury, M.D., a urologist at Northwestern University and one of the world's experts on prostatitis. "Prostatitis is completely misunderstood and misused as a diagnosis. There are many different causes, and it is incredibly rare that it's actually a bacterial infection in the prostate."

So, if you have these symptoms, or if you've been told that you have prostatitis, what should you do? First, know that you're not alone. Your symptoms are real; you just need to find out what's causing them. If you are diagnosed with prostatitis, did your doctor get a culture to make sure there's a *bacterial infection in your prostate*? Without taking a culture of your prostatic fluid, there's no way to know if you actually have an infection in there. Note that this is different from getting a culture of your urine; in fact, checking the fluid that is inside the prostate begins with a rectal exam, during which your doctor will push on the prostate, causing prostatic fluid to emerge from the tip of the penis. "We capture this on a slide and look at it under the microscope," says Flury.

Flury is troubled by the number of men who have come to see her after another doctor told them, "You have prostatitis. Try these antibiotics for six weeks and see how you feel." It's not that easy. "There may be ten different causes for these symptoms, and twenty possible treatments." Many of these men never even had a culture to confirm the diagnosis; they just got put on antibiotics. Flury explains, "CPPS is a framework, and men have different symptoms within that framework: urinary symptoms, psychosocial symptoms like depression, muscular problems, neurological symptoms, organ-specific problems—in the penis, testicles, bladder, or prostate. All those things fit into CPPS.

"CPPS is a common condition, but many traditional therapies fail," she says. Undoubtedly, that's because the wrong thing is being treated. *Find a doctor who can figure out what you really have. If you've been given a diagnosis of prostatitis, the first thing to do is make sure you actually have it.* If you have an infection, you need antibiotics, but if you don't, you don't need antibiotics. "Many more men have CPPS than prostatitis," says Flury. She recommends that you start by visiting mappnetwork.org. There is a network of centers, across the country, where physicians and scientists are doing research on the entire spectrum of CPPS. Even if you don't want to participate in a clinical trial, physicians at these centers know how to figure out what's actually causing your symptoms and plan treatment accordingly.

Antibiotics: There Are Risks

In July 2016, the Food and Drug Administration advised restricting the use of fluoroquinolone antibiotics for certain uncomplicated infections—because the "serious side effects…generally outweigh the benefits for patients." People with some conditions such as sinusitis, bronchitis, or a simple urinary tract infection have other options; there are lots of antibiotics that treat those problems. However, men with acute or chronic bacterial prostatitis don't have as

INTERNATIONAL PROSTATE SYMPTOM SCORE (IPSS)

	Not at all	Less than 1 time in 5	Less than half the time	About half the time	More than half the time	Almost Always	Your score
1. Incomplete emptying Over the past month, how often have you had a sensation of not emptying your bladder completely after you finished urinating?	0	1	2	3	4	5	
2. Frequency Over the past month, how often have you had to urinate again less than two hours after you finished urinating?	0	1	2	3	4	5	
3. Intermittency Over the past month, how often have you found you stopped and started again several times when you urinated?	0	1	2	3	4	5	
4. Urgency Over the past month, how often have you found it difficult to postpone urination?	0	1	2	3	4	5	
5. Weak stream Over the past month, how often have you had a weak urinary stream?	0	1	2	3	4	5	
6. Straining Over the past month, how often have you had to push or strain to begin urination?	0	1	2	3	4	5	

	None	1 time	2 times	3 times	4 times	5 times or more
7. Nocturia Over the past month, how many times did you most typically get up to urinate from the time you went to bed at night until the time you got up in the morning?	0	1	2	3	4	5

Total IPSS Score

	Delighted	Pleased	Mostly satisfied	Mixed; about equally satisfied and dissatisfied	Mostly dissatisfied	Unhappy	Terrible
Quality of Life Due to Urinary Symptoms							
If you were to spend the rest of your life with your urinary condition just the way it is now, how would you feel about that?	0	1	2	3	4	5	6

If your total score is:

0 to 7 Your symptoms are considered mild.
8 to 19 Your symptoms are considered moderate.
20 to 35 Your symptoms are severe.

many choices, so for them, the risks of fluoroquinolones are probably worth it.

But you don't want to be taking these drugs if you don't need them—and if you haven't even had a prostatic fluid culture to determine the presence of infection.

According to the FDA: "Fluoroquinolones...are associated with disabling and potentially permanent serious side effects that can occur together." Some of these side effects include tendon, joint and muscle pain, a "pins and needles" tingling or pricking sensation, confusion, and hallucinations.

What Is Truly Prostatitis?

Acute Bacterial Prostatitis. If you have this, you know it, because it's debilitating. You most likely also have a fever, chills, and extreme pain. This is not the time to be a macho man and suffer through it. *You need immediate treatment.* Go to the doctor or, if it's after hours, to an emergency center. This is very important: if you have acute bacterial prostatitis and you don't get help right away, you could develop a life-threatening infection in the blood (called sepsis), not be able to urinate (urinary retention, which requires a temporary catheter), or develop an abscess (an infected area of pus under pressure; as you can imagine, this is very painful) within the prostate.

"Acute bacterial prostatitis is an infection that can have very severe symptoms," says New York University urologist Stacy Loeb, M.D. "It requires immediate treatment with antibiotics. It is also one of the potential risks of a prostate biopsy: this is why all men who undergo a prostate biopsy require antibiotics before and after to reduce the risk of a symptomatic urinary tract infection—and acute bacterial prostatitis is really an acute urinary tract infection. In fact, recent studies show that acute prostatitis after a biopsy can be more severe than other cases."

The good news is that once you start taking antibiotics—usually in the category called fluoroquinolones, such as ciprofloxacin (Cipro)—you will start to feel better fairly quickly. *Important:* You will need to stay on antibiotics much longer than you might expect. If you just take antibiotics for a week to ten days and even a tiny amount of infection remains in the prostate, guess what? It is likely that the prostatitis will come back—this time as a chronic infection, which is harder to get rid of. If you have an episode of acute bacterial prostatitis, then you should stay on antibiotics for about six weeks. Be steadfast with the antibiotics and wipe it out the first time. You don't want to go through this ever again if you can help it.

Chronic Bacterial Prostatitis. Here, too, the treatment is antibiotics. The "chronic" part is that this form of prostatitis can come back every so often for years if an episode of acute bacterial prostatitis is not adequately treated the first time. The treatment is the same: six weeks of antibiotics. The hallmark of chronic bacterial prostatitis is that when the infection returns, it's caused by the same type of bacteria that caused the previous infection.

One explanation for persistent bacterial prostatitis may be lingering infection in tiny stones, called calculi, in the prostate. Prostatic calculi (the prostate's version of gallstones or kidney stones) are harmless and very common; about 75 percent of middle-aged men and 100 percent of elderly men have them.

Can I Do Anything to Make It Better?

Many men with CPPS have found that their symptoms improve when they change their diet—eating a good balance of fruits and vegetables; avoiding spicy foods, alcohol, caffeine, and soft drinks that contain saccharin; and drinking enough water to keep urine running clear. A thirty-minute hot bath or sitz bath (sitting in warm water up to the hips) twice a day can relieve pain and make it easier to urinate. Getting daily exercise (but *not* riding a bike or an exercise bike, which can aggravate symptoms) and resuming normal sexual activity may also improve your symptoms.

3

WHAT CAUSES PROSTATE CANCER, AND CAN I PREVENT IT?

This chapter was written with expert opinion from Elizabeth Platz, Sc.D.

THE SHORT STORY:
The Highly Abridged Version of This Chapter

If you're an American man, or a man from any Western country, prostate cancer is something to worry about, because so many men get it. This year, more than 160,000 American men will be diagnosed with prostate cancer, and more than 26,700 will die from it. An American boy born today has a 12.5 percent risk of developing prostate cancer and a nearly 2.6 percent risk of dying from it.

Although these numbers are high, the picture of prostate cancer today is far brighter than it's ever been—much more hopeful than it was even a generation ago. Consider these statistics: of men diagnosed with prostate cancer in the late 1970s who did not die of other causes, only 70 percent survived five years, and more than half died of prostate cancer within fifteen years. How far we have come since then! Today, thanks to early diagnosis and screening, more than 99 percent of men diagnosed with prostate cancer are alive five years later.

Nevertheless, the best way to deal with prostate cancer is to prevent it! That's why this book is more important now than ever. We hope to teach men and their families as much as we know about what causes prostate cancer, how to prevent it, and how we can better treat it.

Let's start with who gets prostate cancer.

Who Gets Prostate Cancer?

If you are an Asian man who has lived all his life in, say, rural China, you are less likely to need this book. That's because in your part of the world, few men get prostate cancer, and fewer still die of it.

This is not the case in America (or even in urban, increasingly "westernized" Asia). One of the most remarkable things about prostate cancer is that throughout the world, there is a huge variability in the risk of getting it and of dying from it. The risk changes from place to place and, in many ways, from man to man. *The most common risk factor for prostate cancer is older age.* But other factors are of major importance, too, particularly being of African descent, your geographic location—where in the world you live—a family history of prostate cancer, and, as we are just learning, a family history of other kinds of cancer. You may be saying, "I can't do much about my race or family history." This is true. But there are some important lifestyle choices you can make that raise or lower your prostate cancer risk.

As far as prostate cancer goes, rural Asian men are lucky; the disease is not in the constellation of things they need to worry most about. Men in Western countries—Europe and North America—do not have that luxury: prostate cancer remains a menace. The statistics are sobering: This year, more than 160,000 American men will be diagnosed with prostate cancer, and more than 26,700 will die because of it. In men, it's the most common cancer that's diagnosed, and the third most common cause of cancer death after lung and colorectal cancers. As we've said, an American boy born today has a 12.5 percent risk of developing this disease and about a 2.6 percent risk of dying from it.

And yet, many patients are *still* told by their doctors that "most men have prostate cancer, and few men die from it"—and thus, men shouldn't worry about prostate cancer. *It's not that simple.*

On the other hand, we're getting better at spotting prostate cancer early; the average age of diagnosis has dropped from seventy-two to sixty-six. Treatments are better than ever, and for the first time, we have hope of extending the lives of men with advanced disease. How far we have come in just a generation! In the late 1970s, of men diagnosed with prostate cancer who did not die of other causes, only 70 percent survived five years; more than half died of prostate cancer within fifteen years. Today, thanks to early diagnosis and screening, more than 99 percent of men diagnosed with prostate cancer are alive five years later.

And yet, in sheer numbers alone, there's a massive cloud on the horizon. It's the aging baby boom generation, which makes up about 25 percent of the U.S. population. Some 76.4 million men and women were born between 1946 and 1964; by the year 2030, they'll range in age from sixty-six to eighty-four. For prostate cancer, this is "prime time." Prostate cancer has one of the highest age-specific probabilities of diagnosis of any cancer.

Now, if you are an American man or someone who loves him, this doesn't mean you should panic. If you lived in a hurricane-prone coastal area or an earthquake zone, what would you do? You would learn what you could, be vigilant, and remain prepared—because your knowledge and actions could save your life. The same is true for prostate cancer. What you learn from this book, from your doctor, and—if you develop the disease—from other men and their families may save your life, too.

What Causes Cancer?

The answer to this question is just three letters: DNA. We hear about DNA all the time—in TV forensics dramas, for instance. But what is it? DNA is short for deoxyribonucleic acid. It's our genetic blueprint, and it's in every cell in our bodies—the "chemical Morse code" that directs each of our cells to make specific building blocks. These blocks are actually strings of chemicals, which scientists identify with letters. Changing just one letter can change everything. A gene is a particular sequence of DNA that directs the production of a single protein. This genetic code is the body's greatest treasure, the secret to life itself, and the body guards it jealously. Each cell has its own security systems designed to protect the integrity of this code. Every time a cell divides, this genetic code must be replicated perfectly. To guarantee that there are no errors in copying this vital information, every cell has a "spell-checker," which examines the code and repairs any defects it finds. The genes given this particular job are called mismatch repair genes—more on them in a moment.

Cancers Are Caused by Damage to DNA

In this sense, all cancers are genetic. By the way, *genetic* doesn't always mean *inherited*, although some doctors use the terms interchangeably. We'll talk about inherited, or hereditary, prostate cancer later in this chapter. Cancer development—sometimes sparked by minor damage to a single gene—may be hidden deep within cells for years or even decades. Like a pothole that grows from one little crack in the pavement or a brushfire sparked by a lone bolt of lightning, cancer arises from one or a series of mutations in the DNA. Incrementally, these changes create an environment that allows "bad" cells—cancerous or precancerous cells with hostile behavior and a disturbing tendency toward immortality—to flourish.

How does damage to DNA cause cancer? Actually, most of the time, it doesn't; damage to DNA is incredibly common. It happens all the time, often at random, and it's almost always repaired instantaneously by the most efficient fix-it crews in the world. However, when mutations happen to transform a pivotal gene or several sensitive genes within a cell, the damage may overwhelm the body's normal defenses, and cancer may result. Think of an old movie in which a kid—like Mickey Rooney in *Boys Town*—"goes bad." Is there a genetic "Father Flanagan"? Can the errant gene be saved? Yes, it can, sometimes, if the damage is reversible. Other times, the body has systems in place to kill cells that have too much DNA damage. That's a way to keep a damaged cell from becoming a cancer cell. Here are three major types of genes that are involved in cancer:

Oncogenes

Some genes make growth factors, whose job is to help cells grow. They function as chemical switches: *click*—turn on cell growth; *click*—turn it off and let the cells rest. However, when these genes are mutated, they can become oncogenes, and normal cell replication can quickly turn into abnormal growth. Oncogenes speed up cell growth so much that this switch acts like a stuck accelerator in a car. If the switch can't be turned off, cell growth goes out of control.

Tumor Suppressor Genes

These are checkpoint genes, and they, too, are normally present in all cells. Their purpose seems to be to put on the brakes—to control cell division and prevent cancer from developing. Mutations here, too, can result in chaos. When these genes are disabled, oncogenes gain even more momentum, and this allows growth to hurtle along even faster.

DNA Repair Genes

These are quality-control genes—like spell-checkers—that constantly monitor the genetic code as cells divide, and fix any mistakes that crop up. If one or more of these inspector genes is mutated or the repair genes are defective, widespread mutations can occur, with disastrous results.

What Causes DNA Damage?

Every day, our cells fend off countless threats from the outside—environmental factors as simple as ultraviolet light from the sun, which can lead to skin cancer, or as complicated as the chemical cocktail packed into each puff of a cigarette, which can cause lung cancer (and which makes prostate cancer worse; see page 65). The most common cancers of all—lung, prostate, breast, and colon—most likely arise from *oxidative damage*, incremental damage accrued as carcinogens hammer away at our genes like invaders with tiny battering rams. Our bodies can withstand this gradual onslaught for decades, until the oxidative damage reaches a critical point. Even our everyday metabolism of nutrients and other chemicals produces a harmful by-product with a dangerous-sounding name: oxygen radicals, also called *free radicals*. These are highly reactive, unstable, electrically charged molecules that can surge with force enough to destroy tissue, melt membranes, and kill cells in an instant. Free radicals damage DNA. Like many key characters in causing disease, they start out with fine intentions and then go astray. Normally, they appear in small numbers as "hit men" for the immune system, wiping out bacteria and other foreign invaders. And normally, they are neutralized by riot-control police, scavenger enzymes and antioxidant nutrients, within cells. However, if these scavenger enzymes are defective or if they're overloaded by too many free radicals, the free radicals can attack the DNA in cells, causing mutations that lead to cancer.

Molecular Causes of Prostate Cancer: The Double Attack of Oxidative Damage and Inflammation

The diagram in Figure 3.1 shows the decline and fall of a prostate cell—think of Anakin Skywalker in the *Star Wars* saga as he gradually crosses over to the dark side. (You can also compare this with the illustration in chapter 5 showing the modified Gleason grading system, which shows the progression of cancer from "not too bad" to highly malignant, as it appears to a pathologist.)

Normal, healthy prostate tissue shows little round shapes, which are tiny glands. Under the microscope, they appear orderly, harmonious, at peace with the world. The first signs of possible danger are lesions called *focal atrophy*. These lesions are often inflamed, and so they are also known as *proliferative inflammatory atrophy* (PIA). Then comes *prostatic intraepithelial neoplasia* (PIN), in which the glands are more disorderly but are not yet cancerous. In early cancer, the tissue still retains some normal structures. But as the cancer becomes more aggressive—as it begins to spread and ultimately becomes unresponsive to hormones—all order deteriorates, and normal glands are overshadowed by dark, sprawling blobs.

All this starts with oxidative damage. But, as always with prostate cancer, even this simple fact is more complicated than it sounds. Oxidative damage can come from *multiple* sources. One, discussed above, is metabolic—our everyday *metabolism* of what we eat. Another arises from *inflammation.* (We mentioned this very briefly in chapter 2 in our discussion of prostatitis.) Look at those poor prostate cells. They're under attack from both sides. On one side, they're getting torpedoed by the body's generating energy from food. On the other, they're being bombarded by inflammation. The overworked scavenger enzymes are supposed to be everywhere at once, protecting the cells from either kind of assault. One of these scavenger enzymes is called glutathione S-transferase π (pronounced "pie"), or GST-Pi. It serves as a genetic fire extinguisher, rendering free radicals into harmless, water-soluble products and providing toxin cleanup on a cellular level. One of the first official functions of prostate cancer cells is to disable GST-Pi. In effect, it's put into a chemical straitjacket—think of Jack Nicholson in *One Flew Over the Cuckoo's Nest*.

If GST-Pi is a genetic fire extinguisher, then inflammation is just the opposite—the gasoline that fans the flames. The concept that inflammation can cause cancer is not new. Inflammation is known to cause damage to cells and to DNA, and long-term—chronic—inflammation is associated with many kinds of tumors. For example, chronic hepatitis causes cancer of the liver; chronic stomach inflammation, caused by a form of bacteria known as *H. pylori*, causes stomach cancer; reflux esophagitis, over time, can cause cancer of the esophagus. Why is inflammation such a potent cause of cancer? It appears to act in two ways.

The inflammatory cells produce harmful forms of oxygen and nitrogen, which can mutate DNA directly. Inflammatory cells can also injure cells, prompting the body to crank out replacement cells as quickly as it can. This rapid turnover of cells is what we see in focal atrophy (see above), and it proves that "haste makes waste." Sometimes the replacement cells are churned out so fast that the DNA doesn't get copied exactly, and these mistakes can lead to further mutations. It's like the children's game Telephone, where someone whispers a phrase and each child whispers it to the next; if a child doesn't repeat it correctly, the muddled words get passed on down the line.

Either way, inflammation induces mutation in nearby cells, and this can be the beginning of cancer.

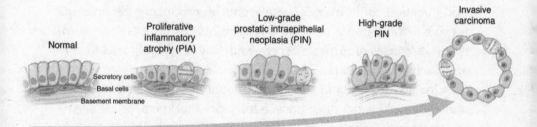

Figure 3.1   Steps in the Malignant Transformation of Prostatic Epithelial Cells

Look at the different kinds of cells a pathologist might see in tissue samples of your prostate. The normal cells, at left, are regular and even, with uniform centers. Things still look fairly normal—just a little shrunken—with proliferative inflammatory atrophy (PIA). Low-grade PIN is still normal-ish. Things start to get weird with high-grade PIN: The cell shapes make no attempt to look the same. They're rounder and more wobbly, without the well-defined walls of the normal cells. Prostate cancer cells are more blobs than rectangles, and instead of lining up in an orderly fashion, they seem to swarm. Adapted from De Marzo AM1, Platz EA, Sutcliffe S, Xu J, Grönberg H, Drake CG, Nakai Y, Isaacs WB, Nelson WG. Inflammation in prostate carcinogenesis. Nat Rev Cancer. 2007 Apr;7 (4):256-69.)

What Causes Inflammation in the Prostate?

This is the $64,000 question, and for now, no one knows. Johns Hopkins molecular geneticist Bill Isaacs and colleagues have been searching for the answer to this question in the genes of families with hereditary prostate cancer. How, they've wondered, do mutations in certain genes stack the deck toward cancer in some men? So far, they have found two genes that appear to be responsible for the development of prostate cancer in small clusters of families. One, located on chromosome 1, is called *RNASEL*. The other, located on the short arm of chromosome 8, is called *MSR1* (macrophage scavenger receptor 1). These genes have something very interesting in common: they're both involved in the body's defense against infection. When animals that lack the *MSR1* gene are infected with bacteria, or animals with a defective *RNASEL* gene catch the herpes simplex virus, 60 percent of them die. And this observation, says Isaacs, "raises the intriguing possibility that *viral or bacterial infections might be the source of the chronic inflammation in some patients*, and that this chronic inflammation might be responsible for the increased risk of prostate cancer." If it's true that some run-of-the-mill infection could trigger these events by producing the immune response of inflammation, "this will profoundly affect future studies of the causes of prostate cancer, and may ultimately lead to new approaches to prevent it."

One last word about this inflammation: If you have prostatitis, don't worry. Doctors have known for years that the prostate seems to attract inflammatory cells. Johns Hopkins pathologists Angelo De Marzo and Jonathan Epstein tell us that pathologists were once taught to ignore them—to consider them an odd quirk of the prostate. What we've been talking about here is not the dramatic type of inflammation that comes with acute bacterial prostatitis or even with the chronic forms of prostatitis. Instead, it falls into the medical category of *asymptomatic*—producing no symptoms—and the current consensus is that we know it's there, but we aren't sure what to do about it.

Supplemental Testosterone, DHEA, and Prostate Cancer Risk

Scientists have known for a long time that prostate cancer is under the control of hormones—that men who are castrated before puberty rarely develop prostate cancer, and that men with advanced prostate cancer can be helped by hormone therapy (shutting off the supply of male hormones to the prostate). Thus, it makes sense that hormones must play a big role in prostate cancer. However, measuring blood levels of testosterone and other hormones in middle and older age has not provided insight into understanding why some men get prostate cancer, some men get aggressive prostate cancer, and other men don't get prostate cancer at all. Blood levels may not be the best indicator of what is going on in the prostate, and later in life may not be the right time to look. Basically, we don't have a clear answer yet.

Given what we know about hormones and the development of prostate cancer, is it okay for a man to pump up his testosterone levels by taking a health food store supplement like dehydroepiandrosterone (DHEA)? Some men do this because DHEA levels drop with age, and the hope is that boosting DHEA will be the proverbial fountain of youth. We don't think this is the right approach. A review of DHEA concluded, "There is no convincing evidence that DHEA has any beneficial effect on aging or any disease. Patients would be well advised not to take it."

What about taking testosterone replacement therapy that is advertised on television?

Maybe you've seen the ads showing men simply rubbing a testosterone-containing gel on their skin. There is no question that as men age and their testosterone levels go down, they have many of the signs and symptoms associated with "low T" in younger men— low sex drive, loss of muscle strength, weakening of the bones, and osteoporosis. But we don't yet know the risks of fanning an incidental prostate cancer against the possible benefits or replacement testosterone. (Testosterone supplementation after radical prostatectomy is discussed in chapter 11.)

What if your testosterone is definitely low and your doctor recommends replacement testosterone?

Well, it could be that the cause of your low testosterone is prostate cancer. Prostate cancer—especially extensive, high-grade cancer—produces a substance that lowers testosterone. When the prostate is removed in these men, their testosterone returns to normal levels. Thus, if your testosterone is low, before you start testosterone replacement, get checked for prostate cancer to make sure it is not the cause.

Known Risk Factors You Can't Do Anything About

Without question, age, race—being of African descent—and family history are risk factors for prostate cancer. No, you can't do anything to change these factors—but knowing you're at higher risk of developing prostate cancer may save your life. It means you should be screened regularly, so that the disease can be detected early and treated as soon as possible.

Older Age

Why is prostate cancer the bane of older men? Because, like many cancers, it takes years to develop. As we discussed earlier, the process of transforming a normal cell into a cancerous cell—one that can divide, grow, escape the prostate, and invade other tissues—requires a number of genetic mutations that alter DNA.

Scientists have estimated that the number of mutations necessary to transform a normal cell into a cancerous one correlates with the number of *decades* it takes, on average, for cancer to develop. For example, there is a highly malignant form of cancer called retinoblastoma that occurs in the eye in infants and children. In those with the inherited form of this disease, only one mutation is necessary for this cancer to begin. In prostate cancer—where most men are not diagnosed until after their mid-sixties—the number of genetic mutations necessary may be seven or eight. These occur gradually, over time, as oxidative damage takes its toll. Even if a boy is born with the deck stacked against him—if he has a family history of the disease, for example, or is of African descent—nothing will happen for many years.

Age is a risk factor for many illnesses because no matter how physically or mentally fit, the body of a seventy-year-old man is different from the body of a twenty-five-year-old man. In men, the incidence of prostate cancer rises dramatically with age, more so than with any other cancer. An American man age seventy or older is almost seven times more likely to develop prostate cancer than is a man fifty to fifty-nine years old. Look at the difference a few decades make: In men aged fifty to fifty-nine, the risk of developing prostate cancer is 1 in 52. In men seventy years or older, it's 1 in 11.

African Ancestry

African Americans, men with African heritage living in the Caribbean, and African men have the highest risk of prostate cancer of any ethnic group in the world. If they get prostate cancer, they are also more likely to die from it. The number of black men per hundred thousand who develop prostate cancer is about 70 percent higher than the number of white men. African American men seem to get more severe forms of prostate cancer and are more likely to have cancer recurrences and die from the disease than white men. And the number of black men per hundred thousand who die of the disease is 2.3 times higher.

Why do black men have a higher risk of the disease and more aggressive disease? There are multiple reasons, some related to socioeconomic status and some to biology. Many studies have shown that people of any race who don't have much money are less likely to undergo preventive health screening and are more likely to delay going to the doctor until the disease is advanced. Then, if they have prostate cancer, they are less likely to be treated with radiation therapy or surgery because without insurance, these treatments are expensive. Hormone therapy is much cheaper. But, as we'll discuss later in the book, *hormone therapy as a first-line attack on prostate cancer is not effective.* There are some differences in *where* the cancer is in these men, too—and this can make it harder to detect early. A recent Johns Hopkins study reported that black men are more likely to have prostate cancers that are toward the front of the prostate, where they are difficult to reach with a biopsy needle. Edward Schaeffer, who led these studies while on the faculty at Hopkins and is now chairman of urology at Northwestern University, uses MRI in addition to biopsy when prostate cancer is suspected in patients of African descent, because it can help show cancer that the needle can't reach.

We believe that prostate cancer kills many African Americans because they didn't get the disease diagnosed in time to cure it. And although there also seems to be an inherent biological aggressiveness in cancers in African Americans, information from "equal-opportunity" health care studies—places such as military clinics or HMOs, where the availability of medical care seems to be equal— suggests that black men seem to fare as well as white men when it comes to prostate cancer *if the cancer is caught and treated early* with surgery or radiation.

WHAT IS HEREDITARY PROSTATE CANCER?

Of all the men who will be diagnosed with prostate cancer this year, about 10 percent will be men born with a head start—one or more bad genes that greatly increase their risk of developing cancer and of developing it at an earlier age.

Although purely hereditary cases of cancer make up only a small percentage of all cases, we believe that understanding hereditary prostate cancer may help us crack the genetic code of how this disease works. The defective gene or mechanisms involved in hereditary cancer are almost certainly the same ones that somehow go wrong in the far more common "sporadic" cancer, which develops over the course of a lifetime.

In most men, cancer probably happens because of an unfortunate chain of events—at least one genetic aberration, plus one or more environmental factors, such as a poor diet. Say it takes three strikes for cancer to begin. Being born with a faulty gene might be worth one or two strikes. Add a lifetime of eating too much food or the wrong foods (or *not* eating the right ones) and other risk behaviors, and bingo—strike three.

We don't know exactly how many American men may carry one of these defective genes, which can be inherited from either parent. While we haven't tested everyone, we estimate that 250,000 men may carry them. But we do know that if your father or brother has prostate cancer, your risk is two times greater than the average American man's, which is about 12.5 percent. It goes up from there; depending on the number of affected relatives you have and the age at which they developed the disease. If you are in a family that meets the criteria for hereditary prostate cancer—if you have at least three close relatives, such as a father and two brothers, affected; or two relatives who were both younger than fifty-five years old when diagnosed; or if your family has disease in three generations (a grandfather, father, and brother)—your risk could be 50 percent. **I recommend that men with a father or brother with prostate cancer should have a yearly digital rectal exam and a yearly serum prostate-specific antigen (PSA) beginning at age forty.** To learn more or to enroll in our hereditary prostate cancer study, visit our website, http://urology.jhu.edu/prostate/hereditary_prostate_cancer.php, email us at kwiley@jhmi.edu, or write to us at Hereditary Prostate Cancer Study, The James Buchanan Brady Urological Institute, Johns Hopkins Hospital, 600 North Wolfe Street, Baltimore, Maryland 21287.

Family History of Prostate Cancer

Does prostate cancer run in the family, or did a lot of men in your family just happen to have it? About 25 percent of men with prostate cancer have a family history of it. But only about 3 or 4 percent of men have hereditary prostate cancer—an inherited, genetic form of the disease (involving mutated genes that can be passed on by either parent) that develops at a younger age. Simply having a family history of prostate cancer raises your own risk of developing the disease, but it doesn't necessarily mean you have this hereditary form of prostate cancer.

How can this be? How can prostate cancer run in families and not be inherited? We see this in other forms of cancer (breast cancer, for example), and the explanation is complicated—or, as scientists put it, "multifactorial." In other words, there are several reasons. One is that there could be shared lifestyle factors—like eating the same foods or living in the same geographic location. Another is that if a man's brother, uncle, or father develops the disease, he may be more likely to get his own PSA tested and begin regular screening.

TABLE 3.1

PROSTATE CANCER RUNS IN MY FAMILY: WHAT'S MY RISK OF DEVELOPING PROSTATE CANCER?

Having a family history of prostate cancer doesn't mean you are definitely going to develop the disease. After all, prostate cancer affects millions of men worldwide, and it may just be coincidence that your father or brother developed the disease. However, the likelihood of this happening goes up if one of your family members develops it at a young age or if several members of your family have prostate cancer. Say your father developed prostate cancer at age seventy and nobody else in your family has the disease. Although your risk is probably somewhat greater than that of someone without a family history of prostate cancer, in this example we'll set your relative risk at 1. (Note: These risks are relative. They are not absolute, but are designed to give you an approximation.) If your father developed prostate cancer at age sixty, your risk would be 1.5 times higher; if he developed it at age fifty, your risk would now be 2 times higher.

What if your father developed prostate cancer at age seventy, but your brother also developed it? Your risk would now be 4. And if your father developed it when he was fifty and your brother has it, your risk would be 7. This is why it's so important to know not only who in your family has had prostate cancer but how old he was when he developed it. And remember, the increased risk of prostate cancer can be passed on by both sides of the family, so it's important to know the health history of your mother's father and brothers, too.

Age at Diagnosis	Additional Relatives	Relative Risk
70	None	1.0
60	None	1.5
50	None	2.0
70	1 or more	4.0
60	1 or more	5.0
50	1 or more	7.0

However, there are some aspects of a family history that make it more likely that a family is dealing with the inherited form. We now understand that men with a hereditary tendency toward prostate cancer actually inherit a mutated gene (possibly one of the same genes that in "regular" prostate cancer mutate over the course of a lifetime). This has two important implications: First, because a man inherited one of these faulty genes, he is more likely to develop prostate cancer and—because he has a head start—to develop it at a younger age. Thus, *men with a family history of prostate cancer need to start yearly screening early.* Second, because prostate cancer *can be inherited from either the mother or the father,* it is crucial that men know as much as they can of the medical history of both sides of their family.

Even though hereditary prostate cancer starts earlier, it is still every bit as curable as "regular," or sporadic, prostate cancer. In a Johns Hopkins investigation, patients with hereditary prostate cancer and those who had no family history of prostate cancer were matched based on the pathology of their cancer (all these terms, signposts for cancer that pathologists look for when they examine the surgically removed tumor, are discussed in chapter 5). The scientists compared the Gleason score, lymph node status (whether cancer had penetrated the lymph nodes), seminal vesicle status, extracapsular penetration (whether cancer had gone beyond the prostate wall), and surgical margins of the men in both groups. They then studied the men's follow-up data for ten years after surgery, looking for a detectable PSA level or any other evidence that cancer had returned. They found no significant difference in either group. Thus, if you have a family history of prostate cancer, you are more likely to develop the disease but are *not more likely to die from it*. The key is to get the jump on it—to realize it's a possibility and to start looking for it.

Scientists didn't always know this much about hereditary prostate cancer. Decades ago, genealogists in Utah noted that prostate cancer seemed to cluster in families. They found that if a man's father died of prostate cancer, his own risk of dying of prostate cancer was two- or threefold greater. This observation was reinforced by a large Scandinavian study of identical twins; researchers found that hereditary factors were highest for prostate cancer, explaining 57 percent of the risk of developing the disease.

In the 1980s, I began to see increasingly younger men with prostate cancer and was struck by how many of them had a family history of the disease. Then, in 1986, I met a forty-nine-year-old man with an unforgettable legacy: Every male in this man's family had died of prostate cancer—his father, his father's three brothers, and his paternal grandfather. These observations led us to launch the first of a series of studies on familial prostate cancer at Johns Hopkins. The first question we asked was: Would the observations that had been pretty much limited to Utah Mormons hold true in a larger, more diverse group of men? A study of 691 patients who had come to Hopkins for radical prostatectomy confirmed that having a family history of prostate cancer did indeed increase a man's risk of developing the disease. When we ruled out nongenetic factors, our results strongly suggested that increased susceptibility to prostate cancer could be inherited from either parent (which we have since proven—see below). We then went on to define and characterize hereditary prostate cancer, showing the clear link between family history and a man's probability of developing prostate cancer (see Table 3.1).

Over the last two decades, there have been many studies on family history and the risk of prostate cancer. This is what they've shown:

- If a first-degree male relative (father or brother) has prostate cancer, your risk is increased two times.
- Your risk is higher if that relative was younger than sixty when diagnosed.
- Your risk is also higher if it's your brother rather than your father (because you can inherit the defective genes involved in prostate cancer from your mother as well as your father).
- If you have two first-degree relatives (brother and father) with prostate cancer, your risk is three and a half times higher.

Family history, however, does not distinguish inherited genetic risk factors from the influence of a shared environment. The most precise way to identify a genetic basis is segregation analysis, which determines if the pattern of transmission between generations is consistent with Mendelian inheritance. We evaluated this in 106 families where there were multiple men with prostate cancer in multiple generations.

This study, which was published in the *Proceedings of the National Academy of Science* in 1992, established for the first time the genetic basis for prostate cancer. The best model that fit all the data predicted inheritance of a rare, "high-penetrance" genetic mutation (discussed on page 58) in families with early age of diagnosis and multiple affected family members. As you will see, it took twenty years to find the first gene that fit this description.

What Can We Learn from Twins?

Another way to distinguish genetic from environmental influences is to study twins. Two boys have exactly the same DNA. They're identical twins, and when they grow up, one eventually gets prostate cancer; the other doesn't. How can this be? The only answer is that *although genetics are important, environment may help turn the tide.* In other words, even if you've been born with the same bad deck of cards as someone who develops prostate cancer, if you play your cards right, you may still win the game.

This is why geneticists love to study identical twins; fraternal, or nonidentical, twins are no more alike than brothers. If being born with the same DNA were the only factor that made a man susceptible to prostate cancer, then we would expect that every time one identical twin developed prostate cancer, his brother would, too. If genetics played no role, identical twins would be as likely to develop prostate cancer as any other brothers who share the same environment but not the exact same DNA. By comparing how often a disease develops in identical twins with how often it occurs in fraternal twins, we can estimate the influence of genetic factors. This is called the heritability index. Studies of twins and prostate cancer, one from Sweden and the other a study of American World War II veterans, found that in the vast majority of cases, both identical twins did not get cancer. The likelihood of both identical twins developing prostate cancer was 19 percent in one study and 27 percent in the other. In both studies, the likelihood of fraternal twins both developing cancer was much lower—only 4 percent in one study and 7 percent in the other. These studies showed that DNA isn't everything: although identical twins were four to five times more likely to develop the same disease, it was by no means inevitable. Other factors, presumably environmental (lifestyle factors), must play a stronger role. Indeed, these studies concluded that the relative role of genetic factors in prostate cancer is 57 percent. In the study from Sweden, investigators also looked at the same question in twins with other cancers and calculated their heritability index. They found that prostate cancer had the highest heritability index (57 percent) of any other common cancer, such as ovarian (39 percent), kidney (38 percent), breast (31 percent), and colon cancer (15 percent). Because genetic mutations responsible for hereditary cancer have been identified in all these other cancers, we were confident that we would be able to have similar success in finding the genes responsible for the development of prostate cancer.

Inherited Risk: Am I Just "More Likely" to Get Cancer, or Is It Already a Done Deal?

Although it's not always clear when scientists talk about genetics, there are two kinds of genetic influences. One of them is what we've been talking about here—true hereditary prostate cancer, which is relatively rare and accounts for only about 3 or 4 percent of all cases of prostate cancer. Hereditary prostate cancer and other inherited diseases are what geneticists call "highly penetrant": if you inherit a specific gene or genes, most men will get the disease if they live long enough.

Highly Penetrant Genetic Mutations

Encouraged by the observations in the twin studies and the study that predicted the presence of highly penetrant genes, my Johns Hopkins colleague William Isaacs looked for these faulty genes in the DNA of people in large families who met the criteria for hereditary prostate cancer.

The genes involved here are genes everybody has. For example, everybody has a *BRCA1* and a *BRCA2* gene, both of which are involved in breast cancer. However, not everyone has the *same sequence* of those genes. The sequences fluctuate from person to person like ingredients in a recipe—just as both bread and salt dough have the same ingredients, depending on the recipe; one is edible and one is not. This is a daunting task, like trying to find one misspelled word in twenty sets of the *Encyclopedia Britannica*—and each set contains twenty volumes! The first job is to try to narrow down the search—to figure out which books are most likely to contain this mistake. That's *linkage*, which involves looking for patterns of association between certain portions of chromosomes and the presence of cancer that couldn't possibly happen just by chance in a family or families. In this way, we can link cancer to a small segment on a chromosome. The next step is to go through those books page by page.

When we first embarked on this task, genome sequencing (looking at the encyclopedia one letter at a time) was so time-consuming and expensive that our ability to search for these genes was limited. However, once next-generation sequencing (NGS) became available, it became possible to study *every letter of every word on each page* to identify potential defective genes. This advance, and the discovery that many men with lethal forms of the disease who had no family history of prostate cancer carried important cancer-causing mutations, transformed our understanding of the field. This story is still unfolding, and we expect major advances in the near future. So, because some of what I am going to tell you will certainly change, look on this material as the first chapter in what will eventually be known about the genetics of prostate cancer.

HOXB13—the first validated prostate cancer susceptibility gene. Our first use of NGS was in collaboration with investigators at the University of Michigan who had reported linkage on chromosome 17. After searching through two hundred genes in a tiny section of that site, we identified one mutation in HOXB13. This gene is known to be prostate-specific, and in mice it plays a critical role in the development and maintenance of normal prostate function. Confirmatory studies involving many thousands of men unequivocally established HOXB13 as the first validated prostate cancer susceptibility gene. It fulfilled the criteria predicted in the segregation analysis twenty years earlier.

The HOXB13 mutation was rare. In European Americans, the average frequency of the mutation is 1.3 percent in prostate cancer cases and 0.3 percent in controls. It is highly penetrant. In men who carry the mutation, 60 percent are diagnosed with prostate cancer by age eighty, which is similar to the findings with BRCA1/BRCA2. In Finland, it is present in 6 percent of early-onset cases.

BRCA1 and BRCA2. These genes repair damaged DNA. Having a bad BRCA1 or BRCA2 gene means that damage might not be fixed, raising the risk for breast cancer, ovarian cancer, prostate cancer, pancreatic cancer, and melanoma. Twenty years ago, studies in Icelandic families implicated BRCA2 as an important gene for prostate cancer. More recently scientists at the Royal Marsden hospital in London showed that prostate cancer in men with defective BRCA2 genes (which represent fewer than 3 percent of cases) may be associated with features of aggressive disease, including a higher Gleason score, higher PSA and higher tumor stage or grade at diagnosis (all of these are discussed in chapter 5). For male carriers of the BRCA2 mutation, prostate cancer risk by age seventy is 8 percent and rises to between 20 and 30 percent by age eighty. The risk for carriers of the BRCA1 mutation is uncertain.

DNA repair genes. Like the BRCA genes, these are molecular "fix-it" specialists that are supposed to correct DNA damage. Recently, we have learned about the consequences of having a faulty DNA repair gene on the development of castration-resistant prostate cancer (CRPC)—cancer that stops responding to hormonal therapy (discussed in chapter 13). The Stand Up to Cancer research group, which carried out the first in-depth sequencing of men with CRPC, showed that 6 percent of men with CRPC had germline (inherited) mutations of BRCA2. When coupled with other genes involved in DNA repair (a gene called ATM, and others discussed in the following paragraphs) the total number of CRPC patients with inherited mutations rose to over 12 percent. In a study at Hopkins, together with our colleagues at NorthShore Research Institute in Chicago, we found that in men who died from prostate cancer before age sixty-five, 10 to 12 percent carried mutations in BRCA2/BRCA1 and ATM.

Lynch syndrome. This form of colorectal cancer is an inherited condition associated with mutations in DNA repair genes including MLH1, MSH2, MSH6, PMS2, and EPCAM. These are "spell-checker" genes, whose job is to prevent mistakes in DNA from being repeated and amplified over time. Mutations in these genes also increase someone's risk of developing cancer in many other organs, including the prostate.

ATM. An estimated 1 percent of us may carry one mutated copy of an ATM gene, which is associated with an increased risk of breast, stomach, bladder, pancreas, lung, ovarian, and prostate cancer.

Clinical implications. Family history is a major risk factor, not only *how many* family members—on your mother's side, your father's side, or both—have had prostate cancer, but *when* these men got the disease. Were they in their forties or fifties, or were they in their late seventies or eighties? A younger age suggests a genetic risk. Factors that suggest a genetic risk include:

- having multiple first-degree relatives with prostate cancer, including three successive generations with prostate cancer (on either your mother's or father's side of the family);
- early-onset prostate cancer (age fifty-five or younger); or
- prostate cancer with a family history of the BRCA1/BRCA2 mutation or other cancers in the family, such as breast, ovarian, or pancreatic cancer.

Should you see a genetic counselor? A good genetic counselor can provide invaluable advice about whether you should get genetic testing, the risk associated with specific mutations, and even whether specific new drugs might be helpful in combating advanced cancer (see chapter 13). If your father, grandfather, or brother has *metastatic* prostate cancer, you should seek genetic counseling as well. Here are some of the latest recommendations regarding genetic testing:

HOXB13: If you are of Nordic descent, you are five to ten times more likely to carry this mutation.

BRCA1/BRCA2: You may carry a BRCA mutation if a close male relative has been diagnosed with prostate cancer that is Gleason Grade group 2 or greater (see chapter 5) at younger than age fifty; if you have a family history of a BRCA1/BRCA2 mutation; if a close relative was diagnosed with ovarian or breast cancer at younger than age fifty; or if two relatives have had breast, ovarian, or pancreatic cancer, or prostate cancer Gleason Grade group 2 or greater at any age.

Other *DNA repair gene mutations*: You may carry one of these mutations if someone in your family has metastatic prostate cancer. A very important reason for this is that new gene-targeted drugs work better in men with specific mutations (see chapter 13), and knowing the genes involved may make a huge difference in treatment. It also means that, if one of these mutated genes runs in your family, you should be screened vigilantly for prostate cancer.

These findings are likely to be changed and expanded as we learn more.

Low-Penetrance Genes Are More Complicated. The second type of hereditary influence is much more common, much more subtle, and leaves the door open to *not* getting cancer. In this case, your genetic makeup may have one or two chinks in it that may have a bearing on whether you get prostate cancer or may make you more susceptible to it—but cancer may not be a predestined conclusion.

One example of this increased susceptibility—scientists call this a *polymorphism*. Scientists have identified changes in "candidate" genes, genes that are suspected of influencing prostate cancer risk. For example, the gene that produces the androgen (male hormone) receptor contains a stretch of DNA with a C followed by an A and then a G. This "CAG" sequence varies in men by race. In men who have fewer CAGs, the androgen receptor signals more strongly—the hormones seem to be more concentrated—than in men who have more CAGs. Black men tend to have fewer CAGs than white men, who have fewer CAGs than Asian men. For more than two decades, scientists at Johns Hopkins and elsewhere have tried to figure out what to make of this difference in CAGs. Is it linked to a higher risk of prostate cancer, particularly in men of African descent? We still don't know what—if anything—it signifies.

In addition to studying candidate genes, investigators from many centers have joined together to look for abnormalities across the entire genome. This type of study is called a genome-wide association study (GWAS), and it's a good way to analyze the genes of vast groups of men with and without prostate cancer. Thus far, we've found genetic irregularities at a hundred places in the genome that are consistently associated with prostate cancer risk. Each variation raises the risk very slightly, and these abnormalities tend to be associated with slower-growing prostate cancer as well as with more aggressive disease, so they don't give us genetic insight as to which men are more likely to develop lethal prostate cancer. It may be that adding these findings together could help us understand more about a man's risk, and whether certain sets of variations may predict the risk of developing prostate cancer in men of different races.

Suspected Risk Factors You Can
Do Something About

What we've talked about so far are risk factors that you can't do anything about. It's not fair, but there are two bits of good news: One, knowledge is power. If you know you're at higher risk and you get regular screening, you have an excellent chance of stopping prostate cancer early. Two, genes are only part of the story. There are some key factors that you *do* have control over.

The best example of the important role environment plays in whether you get prostate cancer is the identical twin studies (see page 57). Genetically, they look exactly the same—and yet one brother gets prostate cancer and the other one doesn't. Their risk varies depending on the choices they make every day. So does yours.

Why doesn't the other brother get prostate cancer? If these men have the same DNA—basically, the same body—why doesn't genetics determine everything? Because *what happens to that body is critical.* This means that if you are an identical twin and your brother gets cancer, you are not necessarily destined to get it, too. If you and your brother have not made *exactly the same* lifestyle choices, then your risk of getting prostate cancer is not exactly the same. This message is extremely important: *your lifestyle can change your risk of developing prostate cancer.* If, in future studies, scientists could determine specifically *how* the twins' lifestyles were different—what good or bad choices these men, or men who inherit the susceptibility genes but don't get cancer, made along the way—we might be able to understand why the disease occurs in the first place.

Until very recently, scientists believed that Asian men who lived their entire lives in Asia developed incidental cancers at the same rate as Western men, and that because of their lifestyle factors, these tumors did not progress to the point where they were detectable. We believed that whatever causes prostate cancer in the first place—the initiating factors or events—happens everywhere, and that the crucial difference is what happens next—whatever promotes these small cancers to grow and become potentially lethal. In the United States, for example, those cells seem to progress into cancer that needs to be treated in 10 to 20 percent of men as they age. In Asia, scientists believed the cancer just sits there like a freckle, as opposed to a cancerous mole. It turns out that we were all wrong. Autopsy studies have found incidental prostate cancer in 30 to 40 percent of American men. But it's in far fewer Asian men—ten times fewer. Also, the inflammation and focal atrophy we talked about earlier are found in the prostates of many Caucasian men—but they occur five times less frequently in Asian men.

Although scientists have recently noted a steep rise in prostate cancer in Japan, there has also been an increase in screening for the disease, so it's not clear whether prostate cancer is actually on the upswing there or whether this is just an artifact of more intensive attempts to diagnose it. It's also important to note that when Asians emigrate to the United States, the increase in the development of prostate cancer doesn't happen overnight; it takes years. This suggests that whatever the lifestyle risk factors are that make a man more prone to cancer, they act late in life—and this, in turn, gives us great hope that once we understand just what these factors are, we may be able to prevent the disease.

Clearly, lifestyle helps determine a man's risk of getting prostate cancer. But *which* lifestyle choices matter the most? What can you do to reduce your risk of getting prostate cancer and dying of it? Two of the most important things you can do are to watch your weight and not smoke.

ENVIRONMENT JUST MEANS DIET, RIGHT? WRONG!

If only it were as simple as a direct cause-and-effect relationship. Then we could say, "Eat this and you'll never get cancer," and "Don't eat this, or else." But it doesn't always work that way. In fact, if it does seem to, we should view that evidence with a healthy dose of caution. For example, for years, scientists assumed that the high incidence of stomach cancer in China was caused by dietary factors—until we learned that many cases were actually caused by bacterial infection with *H. pylori* (which also causes stomach ulcers).

Lose Weight

Go just about anywhere in the United States and see for yourself: As a country, we're hefty. About two-thirds of American adults have too much body fat, and being overweight doesn't just affect your heart, blood pressure, and risk of stroke, diabetes, or premature death. It also makes you more likely to develop certain cancers. Over the last fifteen years, it has become clear that *having too much body fat, especially around your middle, increases a man's risk of developing prostate cancer that is more aggressive and more likely to cause death.* But wait, there's more: Among men who already have prostate cancer and have been treated, evidence is mounting that *being too heavy, having a too big of a waist, and gaining weight* all decrease the chance of surviving their cancer.

If you have a "spare tire," you've probably been told this before by well-meaning family members or your doctor, and maybe you've gotten pretty good at saying, "Yeah, yeah, I know," truly intending to do something about it one of these days and wishing people would find something else to worry about and leave you in peace. Most of us have been in that place for one reason or another, and no one likes a busybody; we get that. But "one of these days" might as well be today if you want to prevent getting lethal prostate cancer or, if you have been treated for prostate cancer, to minimize your odds of having it come back or dying of it.

Don't Smoke

Does cigarette smoking increase a man's risk of getting prostate cancer? The quick answer is yes, men who smoke are more likely to die of prostate cancer, even though smoking doesn't appear to *cause* a man to develop prostate cancer. Evidence is also building that men treated for prostate cancer *who don't quit smoking* are more likely to have a recurrence of cancer and die of it. In a recent study, Johns Hopkins epidemiologists Corinne Joshu and Elizabeth Platz found that men who kept smoking after radical prostatectomy had twice the risk of dying from their prostate cancer.

Once cancer starts to develop in smokers, it's more likely to be a rougher, more aggressive form of the disease that grows more quickly and is less likely to be caught in its early stages. Why is this? Remember GST-Pi (see page 46), which fends off oxidative damage and is inactivated early on in prostate cancer development? This protector enzyme also combats the major carcinogen in cigarettes, a chemical called benzopyrene. Thus, if a man has embarked on the path toward prostate cancer and loses the protection of GSTP, he'll not only suffer greater oxidative damage but also the additional effects of a bunch of toxic chemicals injected into every cell of his body with each puff. So while you may be tired of the message "If you smoke, quit!," if you want to avoid dying of prostate cancer, you should quit. If you are ready to quit smoking ask your doctor, visit https://smokefree.gov/talk-to-an-expert or call 1-800-QUIT-NOW (all U.S. states have Quitlines).

Why Determining Risk Factors Is Not Easy

What raises your risk of getting prostate cancer? What lowers it? We've been asking these questions for decades. It has not been easy. You can probably imagine the difficulty of asking men with prostate cancer what they did and ate in the past, then asking other men who don't have a diagnosis of prostate cancer what they did and ate in the past, and then trying to find key differences. Remember, it takes decades for prostate cancer to develop. Do you remember what you did and ate decades ago? Few of us do.

It made more sense to try a prospective approach: Scientists enrolled large numbers of men *without* a prostate cancer diagnosis into studies and regularly asked them about their diet and lifestyle. They followed these men for years, and eventually, some of them were diagnosed with prostate cancer. The researchers had something to work with: they could compare the two groups and look for notable differences.

Then the PSA test began to be used for screening. As we will discuss later in the book, PSA is prostate-specific, not cancer-specific. It picks up cancers that may never grow enough to cause harm, and it picks up cancers that could be deadly if not treated. We think that some lifestyle choices—smoking is a good example—may affect the risk of getting *lethal* prostate cancer differently from the risk of getting prostate cancer in general. There are other complications, as well; for instance, men who got regular PSA screening might have been more health-conscious in general.

Long story short, what we thought were risk factors back then, before widespread PSA screening, didn't always turn out to be risk factors today. Elizabeth Platz, an epidemiologist at Johns Hopkins and one of the top experts on risk factors, reports that from now on, "investigators have finally decided to look prospectively, where possible, to look specifically for risk factors for lethal disease, and in men already diagnosed and treated for prostate cancer, to identify risk factors for recurrence, progression, and death from this disease."

Over the last two decades, we have reported the latest scientific thinking on risk factors, and the good news, if you like red meat and dairy products and hate tomatoes, is that now—despite promising early studies—we can't definitively say that eating cheeseburgers causes cancer, and that not eating tomato sauce will lead to lethal cancer. In our view, right now we need more evidence to support these as risk factors for lethal prostate cancer: eating a lot of red meat, eating processed meats (like lunch meat and hot dogs), drinking a lot of milk, eating a lot of cheese or otherwise getting a lot of calcium.

Nor can we say for certain that *not* eating very many tomato products and having lower levels of lycopene (a key ingredient in tomatoes), having lower levels of vitamin E, and having lower levels of selenium (found in foods such as root vegetables) will increase your risk of getting prostate cancer.

Still, it is clear that red meat and processed meat are known risk factors for colorectal cancer, and the world's top scientists, including William Nelson of Johns Hopkins, remain concerned about the production of carcinogens (cancer-causing agents) created when meat is fried or charred. And not being deficient in nutrients is important for good health in general.

In sum, your diet and the way you prepare your food do matter, and in fact are very important.

THE COMPLICATED BUSINESS OF FOOD RESEARCH

Think for a moment of the many nutrients you ingest every day—hundreds of them, in varying portions. Look at the labels of prepared foods—your morning cereal, a box of cake mix, a package of frozen lasagna, even a slice of bread—and consider just how many different things you're putting into your body with every meal.

Now imagine you're a scientist exploring the link between diet and prostate cancer, trying to figure out exactly what's wrong with the Western diet or what's right with the Asian diet. Where do you begin? How many Americans eat one-ingredient meals? In the United States, even a pet goldfish consumes more than a dozen nutrients in a single flake of fish food. But even the simplest meal—a plain potato with no butter, salt, or pepper, for example—raises a host of questions: What is it about that potato that might raise or lower cancer risk? Is it selenium, a nutrient found in potatoes and other root vegetables? Or is it something else? Is it something found in all potatoes, or does it vary, depending on the mineral content of the soil in which that particular potato was grown?

Get the picture? Food research is intensely complicated and frustrating because what seems obvious in lab studies—in petri dishes and test tubes—doesn't always pan out when those same tests are attempted in humans. It's also time-consuming. Say the scientist isolates a food or nutrient that actually seems to prevent prostate cancer. What's the dose? How much of it, in other words, does a man need, per day, per week, to achieve the desired effect? When in his life does it matter? Will he have to take it forever? Does it depend on the man's nutrient status? Does he already consume enough of that nutrient, so eating that food source does not increase or decrease his risk of cancer? Is that man deficient in that nutrient such that eating that food source regularly might increase his levels and reduce his cancer risk? These aren't short-term questions and finding the answers to these questions has proven to be difficult. So what should you do?

Eat Smarter

Rather than pinning your hopes on a single nutrient or food as a magic bullet to prevent prostate cancer, it's better to hedge your bets. Eat for good health in general. The *2015–2020 Dietary Guidelines for Americans,* published by the U.S. Department of Health and Human Services and the U.S. Department of Agriculture, offers some good advice. Here's some of it:

Follow a healthy, lifelong eating pattern. Every single food and beverage choice you make matters. Figure out how many calories you need in a day. This will either be less than you're used to, if you need to lose weight, or it will be about the same amount you are getting, so you can maintain your current weight, make sure you're getting adequate nutrition, and reduce the risk of chronic disease.

Focus on variety. Look for "nutrient-dense" foods—in other words, foods that pack a lot of power into each punch. For example, salmon not only has a lot of protein; it also has omega-3 fatty acids, magnesium, potassium, selenium, and B vitamins. Kale has vitamin C, vitamin A, vitamin B_6, potassium, calcium, magnesium, copper, and other nutrients—and it's only 50 calories! Blueberries are chock-full of antioxidants.

Junk food, in contrast, is full of fat, sugar, and salt—none of which is known for its cancer-fighting powers.

What do the guidelines recommend? You could probably write this part yourself. We all could; let's face it, we know what's healthy, and we know what's not—and it's not realistic to tell you to become an ascetic food monk, only eating nuts and berries. Remember, moderation in all things. Have pizza or a hamburger sometimes, and then more often, try to eat the foods listed below:

- **A variety** (this maximizes your chances of getting lots of different vitamins and nutrients) of vegetables from all the subgroups—dark green, red and orange, legumes (beans and peas), starchy, etc.
- Fruits
- Grains; err on the side of whole grains (for instance, brown rice instead of white rice, which is processed)
- Fat-free or low-fat dairy, including milk, yogurt, cheese, and/or fortified soy beverages (almond and cashew beverages are also quite tasty)
- **A variety** of proteins: seafood, lean meats and poultry, eggs, legumes (beans and peas), nuts, seeds, and soy products

For more information, visit https://health.gov/dietaryguidelines /2015/guidelines/executive-summary.

Exercise Is Good, and Being a Couch Potato is Bad

Whether a man's amount of exercise or occupational exertion—or lack of it—has an influence on the development of the disease especially lethal disease, and on outcome of the disease in men treated for prostate cancer, are still open questions. But scientists suspect that exercise helps protect your body from getting prostate cancer and helps men do better at every stage of prostate cancer—so strongly that investigators are studying exercise in patients with prostate cancer, breast cancer, and colorectal cancer to see whether physical activity helps them do better. And then they hope to figure out some specifics—such as, what kind of exercise helps? Hard-core aerobics and heavy weights, or, as many suspect, is there a benefit even to moderate activity, such as walking the dog? And when does it help? Before diagnosis, before treatment, after treatment? In the meantime, we can tell you that not being active and, specifically, being sedentary—sitting for hours at work or at home—is bad for your health in general. Also, if you are taking in more calories than you are burning, you are going to gain weight. So, if you are inactive, get moving!

Does Drinking Alcohol Affect My Risk?

A huge number of studies—we've lost count—together indicate that drinking alcohol *does not* appear to be an important factor in prostate cancer. However, alcohol drinking does cause other cancers and health problems. The best approach here is "moderation in all things."

Sexual Activity, Vasectomy, Prostatitis, Alcohol, and Agent Orange

A few studies have found that more frequent sexual activity may somewhat lower your risk of getting prostate cancer, but this is far from certain. Scientists suspect that sexually transmitted infections may indirectly raise the risk of prostate cancer by causing inflammation.

What about a vasectomy?

You may have heard in the news that men who have had a vasectomy seem to be more likely to be diagnosed with prostate cancer. There is no scientific evidence of this; more likely is that having a vasectomy might give a man a better shot at having prostate cancer detected early, simply because he has a urologist and may be more likely to go see that urologist for checkups.

What about prostatitis?

Several studies have suggested a weak link between prostatitis and prostate cancer. This may be similar to the explanation for the increased risk in men who undergo vasectomy: men who go to a urologist for prostate symptoms are more likely to have a biopsy. However, as we noted earlier, asymptomatic inflammatory prostatitis—the kind you know about only if your prostate is biopsied—does appear to be weakly associated with the development of prostate cancer. Johns Hopkins scientists are actively looking for factors that could reduce inflammation in the prostate as a strategy to reduce the risk of prostate cancer.

And what about benign prostatic hyperplasia (BPH)?

There is no evidence that having BPH increases or decreases the risk of prostate cancer—but if a man undergoes surgical treatment, because tissue samples may be examined by a pathologist, there may be a slightly higher chance that cancer will be found. Again, because BPH starts in the prostate's transition zone and cancer begins in the peripheral zone, the two conditions are probably not related.

Exposure to Agent Orange

There is a known connection between exposure to Agent Orange, a toxic defoliant used during the Vietnam War, and prostate cancer. The U.S. government provides service-connected disability to any Vietnam veteran who develops prostate cancer. If you were exposed to Agent Orange, this website has helpful information: www.benefits.va.gov/compensation/claims-postservice-agent _orange.asp.

What About Factors That Might Prevent Prostate Cancer Altogether?

In the not-too-distant future, we hope to look back on the era of cancer just as we now reflect on the eras of polio and smallpox—as a plague of the past. It sounds like wishful thinking—an ideal right up there with eliminating poverty and crime, and having world peace. And yet scientists firmly believe that one day this will happen for cancer, including prostate cancer. This is the public health approach: prevent disease before it starts! Prevention is usually the simplest, most effective, and least costly solution. If we could prevent prostate cancer or significantly lower men's risk of developing it, we wouldn't have to worry so much about what's called secondary prevention—treating the disease as soon as possible after early detection. Prevention could spare us this worrisome game of catch-up; it could also lower the chances that we'll find prostate cancer when it's too advanced to be cured. Prevention could save men the cost of expensive procedures and eliminate all the worry about the side effects that go with various treatments.

One good thing about prostate cancer's timing—coming, as it often does, later in life—is that for many men, it may be enough simply to delay the progression of the disease. This is also a kind of prevention—it's not keeping prostate cancer from developing in the first place—but if it means that a man can live *with* his cancer without even knowing it is there, and that it won't progress, this tactic will still save lives. Imagine that you're watching a pretty good program on TV when, suddenly, it's interrupted by a very unwelcome message. That's how, if you'll forgive the TV analogy, prostate cancer blasts into men's lives today. But imagine that you can reduce this disruptive message to a crawl across the bottom of the screen; you can even hit the mute button. It's still there, but it can't hurt you; you're okay. Wouldn't that be wonderful?

Ideally, of course, prevention means forestalling prostate cancer, nipping it in the bud. There are two ways to do this: One way is to *stop* doing something that you've been doing for years; that's what we discussed above. The other way is to *start* doing something new.

We talked about losing weight and quitting smoking as strategies to reduce the risk of developing prostate cancer, and in men treated for prostate cancer, to reduce the risk of recurrence or dying of their disease. It would be a lot easier if we simply had a pill to prevent prostate cancer, whether a nutrient or a drug—this is *chemoprevention*. Well, there is no magic pill. *Your best strategies for now: don't smoke and quit if you do; maintain a healthy weight and lose weight if you are overweight or obese; be active and, even if you are already active, decrease your time spent just sitting around; eat a wide array of fruits and vegetables, eat less red meat and more fruits and vegetables; and don't overdo your consumption of alcohol.*

Many organizations offer such recommendations, including the American Cancer Society and the American Institute for Cancer Research. If you would like to read more, see the National Cancer Institute's recommendations for preventing cancer.

Chemoprevention: There's No "Baby Aspirin" for Prostate Cancer Yet

Cancer has three basic phases: initiation, promotion, and progression. Chemoprevention—adding a drug or dietary agent to your usual regime—can be used as a weapon in any of these phases. The idea is either to keep cancer from forming or to delay or stop its growth. Chemoprevention is what you're doing when you use a fluoride toothpaste to keep cavities at bay. It's the daily baby aspirin you might be taking to prevent heart disease. Or it's the cholesterol-lowering drugs or blood pressure medication you might be taking to lower your risk of a stroke or heart attack. It's the chemical idea of "an apple a day," and it has had great success in many areas of medicine.

In prostate cancer, however, for the most part, chemoprevention has not worked. Here we will briefly describe the drugs and nutrients that have been formally tested as chemopreventive agents against prostate cancer in large, randomized intervention trials. The thing is, intervention trials are experiments. Participants are enrolled and randomized (assigned by a flip of the coin) to receive the agent or a placebo (a lookalike pill that has no active ingredients). Then they are followed for years to see whether they develop prostate cancer. Here, then, is a brief look at some of the chemoprevention research:

5-Alpha Reductase Inhibitors (Finasteride and Dutasteride)

The active form of the male hormone in the prostate is not testosterone but dihydrotestosterone (DHT; see chapter 1 for more details). It is the job of two enzymes called 5-alpha reductase 1 and 2, toiling away in the prostate (type 2) or elsewhere (type 1)—like Rumpelstiltskin, transforming straw into gold—to turn testosterone into DHT.

But this process can be stopped short. Two drugs, finasteride (Proscar) and dutasteride (Avodart), can block this process. Finasteride inhibits the type 2 enzyme and dutasteride blocks both type 1 and 2 enzymes. As a result, the amount of DHT in the bloodstream and in prostate tissue drops. Both of these drugs, called 5-alpha reductase inhibitors, are already in use for BPH. They shrink the prostate, especially the tissue surrounding the urethra, and ease the urinary symptoms of benign prostatic enlargement. Because testosterone is not affected, impotence is generally not a side effect. (Note: Blocking both enzymes doesn't really make a big difference, and doesn't make dutasteride work any better. There is little or no type 1 enzyme in the prostate, and a randomized trial demonstrated that finasteride and dutasteride worked equally well in the treatment of men with BPH. Also, because finasteride is available in a generic form, it is much less expensive.)

In the Prostate Cancer Prevention Trial (PCPT), which was conducted by SWOG (formerly the Southwest Oncology Group) and funded by the National Cancer Institute, nearly nineteen thousand men were randomly assigned to take either finasteride (5 milligrams a day) or a placebo for seven years. The men underwent a prostate biopsy if they had an abnormal rectal examination or elevated PSA level, and when the study was over, about one-third of the men also underwent biopsies. The study's authors first reported that there were 25 percent fewer cases of prostate cancer in the men who received finasteride, but there was also a worrisome

65 percent *increase* in the number of men who developed high-grade (Gleason 7–10; see chapter 5) disease. Another trial, called Reduction by Dutasteride of Prostate Cancer Events (REDUCE), tested the effect of dutasteride in eight thousand men over four years. Results were similar to those in the PCPT, including more Gleason 8–10 cases among men taking dutasteride. Although the drug makers requested changes to the labels for these drugs, they are not approved by the FDA for the prevention of prostate cancer, and I don't recommend that you take them for this purpose. However, they are still approved for treating the symptoms of benign enlargement of the prostate.

If you are taking one of these agents for the treatment of an enlarged prostate, you need to know two important things: These drugs lower the production of PSA arising from the benign tissue (not cancer). For this reason, to estimate your true PSA—that is, what it would be without the drug—you need to multiply it by two for the first two years you are on it, then by 2.3 for the next five years, and after seven years, by 2.5. Next, and most important, once you are on the drug, your PSA should continue to decline slowly and *never increase*. If it begins to increase while you are taking the drug, you should see a urologist, because this is a strong indication that you have cancer, and it may be a very aggressive form.

Selenium and Vitamin E

As we discussed earlier in this chapter, oxidative damage plays a key role in initiating and promoting prostate cancer. It makes perfect sense, then, that counteracting this damage with antioxidants should be effective in helping to prevent the disease. Until recently, selenium and vitamin E appeared to be perfect candidates for the job...but then the SELECT trial published its disastrous findings (see page 78).

Selenium

Selenium is one of nature's defenses against oxidative damage. A mineral found in the soil, it appears in fruits and vegetables, and also in meats and fish. The average American probably eats about

70 mcg (micrograms) of selenium a day. However, this can vary depending on where we live and, more important, where the food we eat was grown, because some soils are far richer in selenium than others.

How does it work? It turns out that selenium is an essential component of an antioxidant: glutathione peroxidase, an enzyme like GST-Pi (see page 46) that helps the body fight off potentially toxic substances. Several years ago, people who had been treated for skin cancer who lived in parts of the United States where the soil doesn't have much selenium took part in a large study. They were given selenium supplements in hopes of preventing that cancer from coming back. During the course of the study, the researchers noticed that the patients taking selenium developed fewer other cancers—prostate, lung, colon—than patients in the placebo group did. In fact, the incidence of prostate cancer in these men was *two-thirds less* than that of the men in the placebo group. This was the first suggestion that selenium may be effective in preventing prostate cancer. A subsequent analysis of the data from the trial suggested that the men who benefited from the selenium supplement were the ones who had the lowest blood levels of selenium in the first place.

Vitamin E

In laboratory studies, vitamin E—an antioxidant, or free-radical fighter—has been shown to slow down cancer growth; it also may help boost the body's immune system to help it battle cancer more effectively. The Alpha-Tocopherol Beta-Carotene (ATBC) trials, conducted in Finland, enrolled more than 29,000 men—all of whom smoked—and randomized them either to supplements of vitamin E alone, beta-carotene alone, to both compounds, or to a placebo for five to eight years. The primary endpoint of the study was to see whether one or both of these supplements could reduce the number of men who developed and died of lung and other cancers. The men in both vitamin E groups (with or without beta-carotene) had a death rate from prostate cancer that was 41 percent lower than that of the other men. Remember, all the men in the trials were smokers. Beta-carotene had no effect on prostate cancer risk.

THE FIZZLE OF BETA-CAROTENE

Identifying beta-carotene as a possible cancer preventer was a milestone in dietary research, and it's important for you to know about it for the simple fact that here was a substance, extracted from vegetables, that sounded good, seemed promising in every way, but shocked everyone. It turned out to be a dud when used as a high-dose supplement for chemoprevention of cancer. This stunning reversal of promise has had a profound impact on scientists who study diet and cancer, whose great fear is ending up with "another beta-carotene."

Some years ago, in several case-control studies, scientists noticed that smokers who ate a lot of fruits and vegetables seemed to be protected against lung cancer. What was it about fruits and vegetables that warded off cancer? The scientists homed in on beta-carotene, which is related to vitamin A and is abundant in vegetables. They hypothesized that people who consumed lots of beta-carotene from foods and supplements and had higher levels of beta-carotene in their blood would have a lower risk of lung cancer. Sure enough, in early studies with lab animals, beta-carotene performed like a champ, seeming to protect against several kinds of cancers.

Suddenly, beta-carotene was the hot new scientific flavor of the month, the focus of three separate cancer prevention trials. In those trials, participants were randomized to receive a supplement with high levels of beta-carotene—much higher than typically could be consumed from food—or a similar-looking "supplement" that did not contain beta-carotene. But then look what happened: "All of them showed not only that beta-carotene did not do what it was predicted to do and prevent lung cancer development—in two of the trials, it actually made things worse," explains Johns Hopkins scientist William Nelson. In one trial, men who received beta-carotene had an 18 percent *increase* in the incidence of lung cancer. Also, their rate of prostate cancer was 23 percent higher, and the death rate in these men was 15 percent higher than in men who did not receive the beta-carotene.

Beta-carotene turned out to be a cautionary tale that confirmed the perils of leaping before looking—and onto the wrong bandwagon, no less. We still don't know why long-term use of high-dose beta-carotene supplements increases lung cancer risk in smokers. In any event, the story of beta-carotene highlights yet again the trouble of trying to pinpoint an element of diet and determine whether it has the power to prevent cancer. By the way, a 2017 review that included these and other beta-carotene trials concluded that when given alone and in high amounts, beta-carotene is associated with an increased risk of death in general (ref: Schwingshackl L et al. Dietary Supplements and Risk of Cause-Specific Death, Cardiovascular Disease, and Cancer: A Systematic Review and Meta-Analysis of Primary Prevention Trials. Adv Nutr. 2017 Jan 17;8(1):27-39. doi: 10.3945/an.116.013516. Review. PubMed PMID: 28096125; PubMed Central PMCID: PMC5227980).

The beta-carotene story is not unique. We've learned along the way that taking single nutrients may not reduce your cancer risk or make you live longer while being healthier. Remember the SELECT trial? Neither selenium nor vitamin E protected men against developing prostate cancer. In fact, men who were given the vitamin E supplement by itself had a higher risk of prostate cancer than men who were given the placebo. Most Americans already have sufficient intake of key nutrients. Getting more—in big doses from supplements—is not better and could be harmful. Your best bet is to get these nutrients from food, including fruits and vegetables, rather than from high-dose supplements.

The SELECT Trial

Based on these encouraging observations that selenium and vitamin E may prevent prostate cancer, the National Cancer Institute funded a trial conducted by SWOG (formerly the Southwest Oncology Group) called the Selenium and Vitamin E Cancer Prevention Trial (SELECT), in which 32,000 men were given either vitamin E alone, selenium alone, both vitamin E and selenium, or a placebo. The scientists in this study looked to see which of these men developed prostate cancer and which of these supplements, if any, seemed to have a protective effect. This trial began recruiting participants in 2001 and was originally scheduled to last for twelve years—but it was ended early in 2008, because of a slight increase in prostate cancer risk among the men who received the vitamin E supplement, and a small increase in the risk of diabetes among men who received the selenium supplement. The investigators continued following the men who had been in the trial. At seven years of follow-up, there was a significant *increase*—17 percent—in the number of cases of prostate cancer found in those men who were taking vitamin E.

Sadly, selenium and vitamin E supplementation do not prevent prostate cancer. But why not? If prostate cancer is caused by oxidative damage to DNA, why didn't these antioxidants work? Well, we don't know. There is no question that the results were disappointing, and we are still trying to figure it out. One reason may be timing. Maybe the oxidative damage that starts the ball rolling has already occurred. Remember, by the time a man has been diagnosed with cancer, *the tumor has been there for, on average, twelve years.* If that's the case, we may need to rethink strategies for prevention and begin treatment a decade earlier. Or, maybe these agents are only effective in men who have a nutritional deficiency. In the original Nutritional Prevention of Cancer trial that showed a beneficial effect of selenium in reducing the risk of prostate cancer, the effect was pretty much restricted to the men who had the lowest baseline levels of selenium. The same could be true for vitamin E. Smokers have a higher oxidant burden, so they may be functionally deficient in antioxidants—and this may explain why vitamin E appeared to be effective in these men (in ATBC), not men overall (in SELECT).

You should also know that taking high-dose nutrient supplements might not be harmless. Sometimes it can be harmful. For example, in the ATBC, men randomized to take a high-dose beta-carotene supplement had a higher risk of lung cancer than those not randomized to beta-carotene. And a meta-analysis published in 2005 documented a significant dose-dependent *increase* in death from all causes when men took 400 IU or more vitamin E daily. (*Dose-dependent* means that the increase went up as more vitamin E was taken.)

Do I Need a Daily Multivitamin?

Given the worries about mega-doses of nutrients tested in prior trials, the Physician's Health Study II provided some insight into the benefits of long-term use of a standard daily multivitamin. The trial, which began in 1997, randomly assigned more than 14,000 men, all physicians age fifty and older, to either a multivitamin or placebo. Then it followed them through 2011. At the study's beginning, 1,300 of the men already had been diagnosed with some form of cancer. By 2011, 2,669 men had been diagnosed with cancer, and 1,373 of them had prostate cancer. The men who were taking a multivitamin had a very small reduction in risk of cancer overall, but not in their risk of getting prostate cancer.

So there's no magic pill for preventing prostate cancer. But here is some promising research that might lead to new preventive treatment one day:

Nonsteroidal Anti-Inflammatory Drugs (NSAIDs)

Earlier, we talked about inflammation's role in the development of prostate cancer. This inflammation is usually so subtle that it causes no symptoms; men don't even know they have it. But within the prostate, it's a different story. Imagine how uncomfortable your face feels when it's sunburned; this is inflammation, and when it's persistent, it can create a situation of chronic stress. Over time, explains Johns Hopkins epidemiologist Elizabeth Platz, "it may create an environment that is conducive to cancer." This begs the question: If inflammation can cause prostate cancer, could anti-inflammatory agents help prevent it?

Scientists are very interested in finding this answer, and they have a ready-made population in which to start looking—men taking aspirin or other nonsteroidal anti-inflammatory drugs (NSAIDs, including acetaminophen and ibuprofen). These drugs block the cyclooxygenase enzymes, which play a key role in the body's inflammatory response. Observational studies in which men who don't have prostate cancer are asked about their use of aspirin and non-aspirin NSAIDs and then followed to see whether they develop prostate cancer suggest that these drugs might help prevent prostate cancer—but the benefit is likely modest and requires long-term regular use.

In 2016, the U.S. Preventive Services Task Force recommended beginning "low-dose aspirin use for the primary prevention of cardiovascular disease (CVD) and colorectal cancer in adults aged 50 to 59 years who have a 10 percent or greater 10-year CVD risk, are not at increased risk for bleeding, have a life expectancy of at least 10 years, and are willing to take low-dose aspirin daily for at least

10 years." But the recommendations didn't say anything about taking aspirin or other NSAIDS as chemoprevention of prostate cancer. Note: Although these are OTC drugs, they can still have side effects. Aspirin can increase the risk of bleeding and stroke (as it inhibits clotting) and other NSAIDs can interfere with the cardiovascular benefits of aspirin. But scientists are actively investigating whether these drugs do indeed reduce inflammation in the prostate.

Statin Drugs

Statins are prescription drugs that lower cholesterol and reduce the risk of a heart attack or stroke by blocking an enzyme called HMG-coenzyme A (CoA) reductase. Can they also lower the risk of prostate cancer? So far, their effect on prostate cancer, has been somewhat inconsistent. But several recent studies suggest that long-term use of statins may reduce the risk of the most deadly kinds of prostate cancer—advanced and metastatic disease.

My colleague Johns Hopkins epidemiologist Elizabeth Platz led a large investigation of nearly 35,000 men as part of the Health Professionals Follow-Up study. The men, ages forty-four to seventy-nine, did not have prostate cancer when the study started in 1990. Ten years later, 2,074 men from the entire study group (those taking statins and those not taking them) had developed prostate cancer. Platz and colleagues found that men who took the cholesterol-lowering drugs had no difference in the risk of early, curable prostate cancer. However, they were 50 to 60 percent less likely to have advanced and metastatic prostate cancer than other men. Interestingly, the longer the men used these drugs, the lower their risk of having advanced prostate cancer became. Several other studies have observed this, as well.

Was it the actual cholesterol-lowering drugs that protected these men, or did the protection stem from having lower cholesterol? To find out, Platz and colleagues looked at men's cholesterol levels, and found that men who had low cholesterol in general—whether they were taking cholesterol-lowering drugs or were lucky enough not to need them—were less likely to be diagnosed with high-grade prostate cancer. "Having low cholesterol or getting rid of the cholesterol may interrupt the communication of some proteins that act in prostate cancer," says Platz. One of these, called the hedgehog protein, is active in high-grade cancers. (Note: Statins can have side effects in some people, and they are not currently recommended as a means of preventing prostate cancer. However, because of the promising results of these studies, they are being investigated in this light.)

Vitamin D

About ten years ago, evidence seemed to be building that avoiding low blood levels of vitamin D might protect against cancer, including prostate cancer. Scientists aren't so certain anymore that keeping vitamin D levels up is enough to stave off prostate cancer. Nevertheless, vitamin D is so important for health in general that it makes sense to talk to your doctor about whether you need to have your vitamin D level checked (this can be done as part of regular blood work). If it turns out that you have too little vitamin D, one easy way to help your body make more naturally is to spend some time—ten to fifteen minutes—outside in the sunlight every day. Another way is by taking a vitamin D supplement. But, as for most things in life, moderation, whether in amount of sun exposure or in the amount of a vitamin D supplement, is a good way to live.

Now What Do I Do?

If you want to lower your risk of developing prostate cancer and dying from it, and want to be healthy in general, the first thing you should do is quit smoking, if you smoke. The second thing is to *eat fewer calories* and exercise more, so you can lose weight or maintain a healthy weight. There is no downside to this—and it will help men at risk for prostate cancer, as well as men who have been treated for prostate cancer.

After that, just think about your health, in general:

- If you must drink alcohol, do not have more than two drinks per day.
- If you can't give up red meat, then eat less of it, and try hard to minimize or eliminate processed meats—salted, cured, smoked,

or preserved meats such as bacon, sausage, ham, hot dogs, and deli and lunch meat.

- Don't get all your protein from animals: plenty of vegetables and legumes—pinto beans, for example—are packed with protein, too.
- Beware of charred food. Those grill marks contain carcinogens.
- Don't take finasteride or dutasteride, selenium, vitamin E, or any of the myriad pills advertised in magazines, on the Internet, or sold in health-food stores that have "Pros" (for prostate) in the name to prevent prostate cancer. The benefits do not outweigh the harms, and many of these supplements are not regulated by the FDA.
- If you are on a statin or NSAID for other reasons, you should keep taking it, under your doctor's care. However, because these drugs can have side effects, you should not *start* taking them purely with the hope of preventing prostate cancer.

4

DO I HAVE PROSTATE CANCER? SCREENING AND DETECTION

This chapter was written with expert opinion from Stacy Loeb, M.D.

THE SHORT STORY:
The Highly Abridged Version of This Chapter

At its earliest stages, prostate cancer is silent. There are no early-warning signals—no symptoms at all—until the cancer grows outside the prostate and progresses to the point where it's rarely curable. Thus, if a man wants to maximize his odds of surviving prostate cancer, he needs to find out that he has it when the disease is easiest to cure. Men who are healthy and can expect to live another ten to fifteen years should get regular screening.

Although scientists are working hard to prevent prostate cancer, we're not there yet. The best we can do now is catch it early, and if it needs to be treated, to go after it with curative therapy. The last two decades have seen great breakthroughs in prostate cancer detection and treatment that have saved thousands of lives.

Prostate Cancer Screening: What Should I Do?

Here is what the National Comprehensive Cancer Network (NCCN) recommends:

You should consider a digital rectal exam and PSA test in your forties to determine a baseline level, and also to gauge your risk for developing the disease.

Regardless of when you start, if your PSA level is lower than 1 ng/ml, come back in two to four years for your next examination.

If your PSA level is between 1 and 3, begin screening every one to two years.

If your PSA level is above 3 or you have a prostate exam with a suspicious lump or hard spot, you need additional testing. You can proceed directly to a biopsy or consider a "second-line" test to help determine if a biopsy is really necessary.

One second-line option is the "free PSA" test. This works best in men with PSA levels between 4 and 10, and less well in men with PSA levels lower than 4. If your free PSA is less than 10 percent, you should undergo a biopsy. (Confusingly, with free PSA, the lower numbers are the ones to watch, whereas with regular PSA, the lower the number, the better.) If your free PSA is greater than 25 percent, you are more likely to have benign disease (BPH, discussed in chapter 2). Levels between 10 and 25 percent are considered intermediate;

they don't mean cancer is present, but they don't rule it out, either. Two other second-line blood tests that can be used to help decide whether you need a biopsy are the Prostate Health Index (PHI) and the 4Kscore.

Why You Should Be Tested

Nobody wants to think about prostate cancer. Nobody wants to get screened, and especially, nobody wants to even think about getting a rectal exam to check for prostate cancer (even though it takes less than two minutes of your life). But the fact remains that an estimated one in eight American men will be diagnosed with prostate cancer at some point in his life.

You may be one of the lucky seven out of those eight who is destined not to get it. But you may not. If you are in your forties or older, you need to get screened for prostate cancer. If you are at higher risk—if you have a family history of prostate cancer, or if you are of African ancestry—then you *really* need it, because not only are you more likely to get it, you're more likely to get a kind that needs to be treated.

A disturbing trend: Since 2012, millions of American men stopped getting prostate-specific antigen (PSA, an enzyme made by the prostate) screening. Many of these men have prostate cancer, and it was not being diagnosed when it should have been. A big reason for this is a policy-setting group called the U.S. Preventive Services Task Force (USPSTF). In 2012, this group, which did not include a single urologist, recommended against screening "average risk" men for prostate cancer. This USPSTF recommendation has done a disservice to men and their doctors; at least, that's the consensus of many urologists and cancer specialists.

The good news: Just recently, the USPSTF reversed its recommendations! After reviewing the available data on PSA screening, the USPSTF now states, "The decision about whether to be screened for prostate cancer should be an individual one. The USPSTF recommends that clinicians inform men ages 55 to 69 years about the potential benefits and harms of prostate-specific antigen (PSA)–based screening for prostate cancer." This is a major change in the language and policy of the USPSTF—and a major step back in the right direction for men.

"Hindsight is 20/20, and upon reflection there's no question that when PSA screening first became available, many men were over-diagnosed," says Edward Schaeffer, M.D., Ph.D., and chairman of urology at Northwestern University. Indeed, when the PSA blood test first came into widespread use in the 1990s, it was not clear what a "safe" PSA level was. Scientists have learned a lot about PSA over the last two and a half decades. Tens of thousands of lives have been saved—because cancer can be found years before it grows large enough to be felt or to cause symptoms—by the highly effective combination of the PSA test and the digital rectal examination. ("Digital" here doesn't mean some high-tech test; indeed, it's just the opposite. It simply means that this exam is performed using the doctor's gloved finger, or digit.)

We have also figured out many ways to fine-tune PSA to help determine if cancer seems to be aggressive or slow-growing. We have developed other biomarker tests, too, to help show who needs to be treated and who can safely take part in active surveillance. This is a huge improvement in care. Thousands of men with prostate cancer don't need to be treated at all, and over the last decade we have gotten a lot better at safely determining who these men are.

So one of the basic assumptions made by the USPSTF—that many men are treated needlessly—is not universally true anymore. Yes, some men are overtreated, but not nearly so many as there used to be, and those numbers keep getting better.

The new USPSTF recommendations also acknowledge that all men are not the same. Some men are a lot more likely to develop prostate cancer, and to develop the bad kind of cancer that really needs to be treated. These are men with a family history of cancer, including prostate cancer—on either their mother's or father's side of the family—and men of African descent. *But many men don't know their family medical history; they may be at high risk and not know it.*

"Even among men of average risk, there's a gradient," says Schaeffer. "Some men are more likely to develop prostate cancer than other men," for a host of reasons, including cigarette smoking, obesity, and other environmental factors scientists are still working to understand.

In recent years, Schaeffer, who studies the molecular biology of lethal prostate cancer, has seen a disturbing trend in his patients. They're not getting diagnosed as early as men in the 1990s did. Many have been told by their family doctor that they don't need PSA screening.

Concerned, Schaeffer and colleagues at Northwestern decided to "look at the landscape of men who are newly diagnosed with prostate cancer in the United States." They looked at all men diagnosed with prostate cancer in the National Cancer Database from 2004 to 2013 at nearly 1,100 different medical centers in the United States. They found something other scientists had noted: declining rates in the diagnosis of low-grade, localized prostate cancer (after the bubble in the 1990s when PSA screening was introduced, and thousands of men were diagnosed with cancer that was never diagnosable before). But they also found something unexpected: "We saw that there was a *sharp increase in the number of men newly diagnosed with metastatic prostate cancer.*" The results of their study were published in the journal *Prostate Cancer and Prostatic Diseases.* This observation has also been supported by work analyzing advanced, more aggressive prostate cancers among men in another national cancer registry called SEER. Dr. Jim Hu, a urologist from Cornell, also noted that over the last several years—a time when PSA screening dropped—more men were being diagnosed with aggressive and advanced cancers.

"Now we are seeing the number of men being diagnosed with metastatic prostate cancers rising," says Schaeffer. The findings can't be explained completely by the USPSTF recommendations alone, he notes. Environmental factors may be responsible for the general rise in metastatic disease. For example, we now know that being overweight makes men more likely to develop aggressive prostate cancer, and to die of it. Smoking and diet play important roles here, as well.

But clearly, not detecting prostate cancer early—a tactic proven to save lives in European studies—is taking a toll, Schaeffer says. "We need nationwide refinements in prostate cancer screening and treatment to prevent men from being diagnosed with metastatic prostate cancer, as this cancer is not curable. We don't want to diagnose low-grade cancers," which may never need to be treated. "But we really need to pick up the disease before it becomes metastatic. I am very pleased that the USPSTF has changed its recommendations. I believe that all men should be allowed to participate in their health, and screening for prostate cancer is a key part of it." (Screening men after age seventy-five is discussed later in this chapter.)

Some background: When PSA screening was first introduced in the late 1980s, many doctors and scientists truly agonized over it. They worried that the test would open a diagnostic can of worms by finding cancer in every man—and then what would happen? This is because, at autopsy, about 50 percent of men are found to have a small amount of prostate cancer that doesn't do a whole lot—it never causes symptoms, is very slow growing, does not spread, and may never need treatment. Would the PSA test do more harm than good? Would it take these heretofore happy men, put the fear of cancer in them, force them to choose a course of treatment—which, nearly two decades ago, often had unpleasant side effects and did not always cure the cancer—and otherwise generally ruin their lives?

Fortunately, over the years, we have learned enough about PSA to identify these men with slow-growing, indolent cancer—"good" cancer, if there is such a thing—and manage their disease conservatively without subjecting them to premature, aggressive treatment.

In the early days of PSA screening, there was also great concern, and for good reason, that the test was not cancer-specific, but merely prostate-specific. And because not every man with an elevated PSA level had cancer, this screening forced some men to undergo unnecessary biopsy, sometimes multiple times.

For perspective, let's look at the accuracy of mammography. Which test do you think is more of a bull's-eye for cancer? Say a fifty-year-old woman learns that her mammogram is positive, and on the same day her fifty-year-old husband finds out he has a PSA level greater than 4 ng/ml. Who's more likely to harbor cancer? The husband. In the United States, the odds that a woman with a positive mammogram will have cancer vary with her age. The likelihood of having cancer is 19 percent for women over age seventy, 17 percent for women in their sixties, 9 percent for women in their fifties, 4 percent for women in their forties, and 3 percent for women in their thirties. For a man in his fifties with a PSA greater than 4, the likelihood of having prostate cancer is 25 percent.

Screening Is Saving Lives

In the world of prostate cancer, the introduction of PSA testing in the late 1980s was the equivalent of an earthquake. The number of new cases diagnosed increased sharply—by a staggering 83 percent—between 1988 and 1992. This was no sudden epidemic of prostate cancer; the number of men with the disease was the same then as it is now. It's just that, for the first time, we could catch it earlier, in men who had not yet developed symptoms. And there were a lot of them—ticking time bombs, in effect. After this "bubble" of not-yet-symptomatic men was diagnosed, the number of new cases has fallen steadily.

By and large, the cancers diagnosed with PSA testing have proven to be significant, not harmless. In the United States between 1994 and 2003, the death rate from prostate cancer dropped by 40 percent, and today the death rate is 51 percent lower than before PSA began. Even more exciting: There has been a decrease in the detection of advanced cancers at the rate of 18 percent a year since 1991—and today, fortunately, fewer than 4 percent of men are diagnosed with prostate cancer that has metastasized, although that number may have risen slightly since 2012 with the USPSTF recommendation.

Simply put, it's an unbelievable improvement from the pre-PSA era: In 1988, 20 percent of American men had metastatic disease by the time it was diagnosed. In 1995, the American Cancer Society estimated that 35,000 men died of prostate cancer; by the mid-2000s, the number was down to 29,000. In short, what was supposed to happen with screening has happened. In 1997, researchers at the National Cancer Institute found that the number of men between the ages of sixty and seventy-nine who died from prostate cancer was lower than in any year since 1950. This study's senior author, for years an outspoken critic of PSA testing, told the *New York Times*, "We are starting to have evidence that there may be a positive to prostate cancer screening and treatment." Another large study found that *men who died of prostate cancer were 62 percent less likely to have undergone regular screening with a PSA test and digital rectal exam than men who did not die of it.* More recently, the ProtecT trial from the UK showed that men diagnosed through screening had a very low risk of prostate cancer death within ten years, irrespective of the treatment they received.

Clearly, we're doing something right. What is it? Back in the 1980s, men were not diagnosed with cancer until they had symptoms—or, if they were lucky, a cancer that was large enough to be felt. Back then, few men—only 7 percent—underwent surgery, and radiation treatment was not strong enough to provide a cure. Essentially no one was being treated with curative intent. By 1990, with the advent of a better, safer surgical procedure (see chapter 8) and an increase in the number of men being diagnosed with localized disease through screening, 70 percent of men in their fifties and 50 percent of men in their sixties chose surgery, and in 1992 more than one hundred thousand men in the United States had a radical prostatectomy. Critics originally pointed to this rise in radical prostatectomy as a troubling trend. However, it may well prove that this, too, is something we were doing right. For the first time, men with prostate cancer were being treated aggressively, by surgeons aiming for a cure, in large numbers. We're still not where we need to be, however. Unfortunately, the number of deaths from prostate cancer remains significantly higher in men with less education, and in men who do not have access to early diagnosis and high-quality treatment.

In the European Randomized Study of Screening for Prostate Cancer, men were randomly assigned either to be screened or not screened for prostate cancer. After thirteen years, PSA testing led to a 27 percent reduction in deaths from prostate cancer and a 42 percent reduction in metastatic disease in the men who underwent screening.

Another large study in the United States called the Prostate, Lung, Colorectal and Ovarian (PLCO) Cancer Screening Trial also randomly assigned men to screening and control groups. However, unlike the men in the European study, most men in the American study—in both groups—had already undergone PSA testing, and *more than 90 percent of men in the control group continued to get screened anyway*. Also muddying the water was the fact that *only 30 percent of the men who had an abnormal screening test underwent a prompt prostate biopsy*. Thus, it is not surprising that the study found no difference in mortality between the screening and control groups.

Finally, the investigators from one of the European Study centers in Sweden found a 44 percent reduction in prostate cancer deaths in the screening group compared to the control group at fourteen years.

In summary, many well-done studies have clearly demonstrated that checking for prostate cancer with PSA testing saves lives. PSA is a powerful tool that can help diagnose prostate cancer and reduce deaths. The most important message here is that we are on a winning streak. Prostate cancer is being diagnosed earlier and treated at a more curable stage, and fewer men are dying from the disease.

How Do You Know If You Have Prostate Cancer?

No Early-Warning Signs

If prostate cancer happened primarily in the same area of the prostate as benign prostatic hyperplasia (BPH) does—right around the urethra—then the disease would almost announce itself: "Something's wrong; I'm having trouble urinating! I need to get this checked out!" But it doesn't. Instead, the disease begins in a different part of the prostate, relatively far away from the urethra, in the peripheral zone (see fig. 1.3), and grows silently for years. As a result, there really aren't any clear-cut, telltale symptoms of early prostate cancer—signs that men notice and worry about; signs that make a doctor say, "Aha! This must be prostate cancer!"

Every Single Symptom of Advanced Prostate Cancer Can Be Attributed to Another Cause

Say a tumor becomes large enough to encroach on the urethra and block the urinary tract. It produces classic symptoms of BPH: frequent or urgent urination, hesitancy, interrupted or weakened flow, dribbling, trouble urinating at all, or even blood in the urine. A less common symptom is the development of impotence or of less rigid erections, which can happen with advanced tumors as cancer invades the nearby nerves involved in erection. But this, too, may be blamed on something else—a normal sign of aging. In fact, men may be so used to seeing the ads for treatments of erectile dysfunction that they may be more likely to discount this symptom as nothing out of the ordinary.

Similarly, a decrease in the amount of fluid ejaculated, a problem that results when the ejaculatory ducts become blocked by the tumor (this blockage can also cause blood in the semen), can be written off as normal aging. Still other manifestations, such as severe pain in the back, pelvis, hips, or thighs, which can develop if the cancer spreads to the bone, also might be mistaken for other problems, such as arthritis.

Obviously, if you have any of these symptoms, see a urologist right away. But better yet, don't wait until you have any symptoms to get tested for prostate cancer. Men can have palpable cancer—a tumor big enough to be felt during a rectal exam—and never even feel a twinge or experience the slightest change to suggest that something is wrong. Look at it this way: if you haven't had a PSA test and a digital rectal exam, how do you know you're *not* harboring a potentially lethal cancer?

Why You Need the Rectal Exam

Why do men over forty need a rectal exam? Why not get the PSA test by itself and then have a rectal exam if the blood test suggests cancer? *Because the PSA test is not foolproof.* About 25 percent of men *with prostate cancer* have a low PSA level—one that doesn't

THE RECTAL EXAM: AN INSIDER'S GUIDE

This is the test men dread. In fact, some men hate the idea of a rectal examination so much that they jeopardize their health by avoiding it like the plague. The rectal exam is certainly not fun; in fact, it's downright awkward and uncomfortable. But it shouldn't hurt, it's generally brief, and—most important of all—this little exam can provide essential information that simply can't be gotten any other way. (Note: If what you feel during the exam goes beyond the obvious discomfort of having someone's finger in your rectum and is clearly pain, don't be stoic—tell your doctor. This could be an important signal of another problem, such as prostatitis or inflammation.)

Unfortunately, many men hate this test for another reason—their doctor's bedside manner, or lack of it. It turns out, a soft touch can detect areas of suspicious firmness much better than a rough hand. If your doctor's unfortunate bedside manner or technique is keeping you away from this exam, find another doctor. There are plenty of good ones out there.

Now, from your standpoint, what can you do to make the rectal examination as painless and productive as possible? First and foremost is how you "assume the position." The best way for the doctor to feel the prostate is for you to bend over the edge of the examining table. (Some doctors perform the examination by having the patient lie on his side. This is not as good. At best, the doctor can feel only the lower edge of the prostate.) For most men, the worst part of the exam is the introduction of the doctor's finger through the anal sphincter and past the muscles in the pelvic floor. Although the examining finger is gloved and well lubricated, if these muscles are tense (a very normal reaction, especially in men who are undergoing this exam for the first time), the doctor must exert more pressure—which adds to the discomfort, which then makes the man even more tense.

How can you relax these muscles? Don't even try; let your position do it for you. First, don't rest your elbows on the examining table—even though it feels more comfortable. Instead, put all your weight on your upper torso. Bend your knees. Your feet should not be supporting any weight. This way, your buttocks muscles will be completely relaxed, permitting the doctor's finger to be introduced easily—and ideally slowly, giving the muscles a chance to relax ahead of time.

To understand what the doctor is looking for, feel your hand. The normal prostate usually feels like the soft tissue in your palm—the fleshy part at the base of your thumb. Now slide your fingers around to the other side and feel the knuckle of your thumb: this is how cancer often feels—like a knot or hard lump.

get flagged as suspicious. For this and other reasons (including the way some tumors make PSA), the PSA test does not detect every cancer early. Then again, neither does the digital rectal exam. In many men with prostate cancer, the tumor may be growing in an inopportune spot, just out of finger's reach, where it simply cannot be felt by a doctor. In other men, the cancer is multifocal—there are several patches of cancer, not just one—and the prostate feels uniform in consistency. It's a deceptive feeling, but the doctor's finger doesn't have a microscope on it and doesn't always know when it's being fooled. Even a firm prostate doesn't necessarily mean cancer; although most normal prostates feel soft, some don't—so this alone might not call attention to itself as something that warrants further investigation. Similarly, not all prostates feel smooth; in some men, the balance between muscular (stromal) and the smoother, glandular (epithelial) tissue tilts toward muscle; these men have small, dense prostates. Finally, the cancer may simply be too small to feel yet, even though it's growing and dangerous.

Also, the PSA test may spot *different* cancers than the digital rectal exam—another reason doctors can't rely on an either-or approach for early detection. (It's like using breast exams and mammograms together to find breast cancer in women.) This was confirmed in one study of 2,634 men; investigators found that the PSA test and the digital rectal exam were nearly equal in cancer-detecting ability but that they didn't always find the same tumors—that if only one technique had been used, some cancers would have been missed. Together, these two tests make a formidable team.

BEFORE THE PSA TEST

Don't ejaculate for at least two days before you have your blood drawn (this can raise your PSA level) and don't get the test if you are in the middle of a urinary tract infection or recently underwent surgery inside your urinary tract.

Be sure to have this test *before* your digital rectal exam (the physical exam can raise PSA levels, too).

Remind your doctor if you are taking finasteride (Proscar) or dutasteride (Avodart) for BPH, or finasteride (Propecia) for hair loss; all three of these drugs lower PSA. To correct for this, if you have been on one of these drugs for 2 years your PSA level should be multiplied by 2.0, then by 2.3 for the next five years, and after seven years, by 2.5. Fortunately, these drugs do not affect free PSA measurements. Also, report any history of prior prostate surgery. A transurethral resection (TUR) or laser procedure for BPH can make your PSA much lower, giving the false impression that everything is okay. If your PSA begins to increase steadily, even if this increase is very small, you should see a urologist.

If the PSA reading indicates a borderline elevation or a significant increase since the last reading, *repeat the test in the same laboratory.* In 25 percent of such cases, the reading will be back down to its former level.

Why is it so important to use the same laboratory if you need a repeat PSA test? Because there's more than one lab assay to measure PSA, and the results may vary slightly between them. In one study of more than 1,900 men, New York University urologist Stacy Loeb and colleagues tested the same blood sample using two different PSA assays. They found a 17 percent difference in the average PSA level. If you got back-to-back PSA tests at Lab A and Lab B, and they were markedly different, you might easily think something important was going on, when in fact there was no change.

Many urologists used to routinely prescribe antibiotics to men with an elevated PSA, but this is no longer recommended. You should only take antibiotics if you are found to have a urinary tract infection that is also causing the elevated PSA.

If you are an American man, you should have a baseline screening for prostate cancer in your forties. With PSA tests, earlier is better; younger men don't have BPH to muddy the waters, so this makes the PSA test more accurate. If you are African American or you have a strong family history of prostate cancer, it's all the more important to begin testing at age forty, because in high-risk men—this means you—these cancers are diagnosed at an earlier age. As for the rectal examination, just bite the bullet. This exam can tell an astute clinician many things about the prostate itself (for example, whether it is unusually tender or enlarged) and about prostate cancer—whether it encompasses part of one lobe, an entire lobe, or both lobes of the prostate; and whether it has spread outside the prostate, into the pelvic side wall or seminal vesicles. (For a description of the prostate's anatomy, see chapter 1.) But as good as this exam can be, frankly, it is only as good as the doctor performing it. It is a subjective test. In this area, urologists probably have some advantage over general practitioners simply because diagnosing prostate cancer is a major part of this specialty. In some cases, a general practitioner has felt a suspicious area on a rectal exam but has not pursued it because the PSA level was in the normal range (less than 2.5 ng/ml)—not realizing that one-quarter of men with prostate cancer have a low PSA level.

Why You Need the PSA Test

No other cancer is diagnosed strictly by trying to feel it. Why? Just think how much a cancer must grow—how many times those early cancer cells must divide, what a tremendous head start this gives the tumor—before it becomes big enough to be felt. This is why for years, doctors searched for a man's version of the Pap smear—an early-warning cancer detector that could spot a tumor long before it is clinically evident—and why the PSA test was such a major development.

Although our knowledge of PSA has grown exponentially over the last decade, doctors are still figuring out how best to use the test and how to make sense of the information it provides. An American man's lifetime risk of death from prostate cancer is 3 percent, but his lifetime risk of being *diagnosed* with prostate cancer is 12.5 percent. Inevitably, until we have surefire markers that can accurately identify which men have life-threatening cancers, screening is going to result in the overdiagnosis of some men.

Remember, PSA is *prostate-specific*, not *cancer-specific*. This is why this test alone isn't enough, why a rectal exam is important along with it, and why many new tests are being developed to give more information. *Having a high PSA level does not necessarily mean you have prostate cancer*—many men with high PSA levels don't. And *you can have prostate cancer and still have a low PSA level*. Fifteen percent of men who turn out to have prostate cancer have a very low PSA level, less than 4 ng/ml. About 25 percent of men with a PSA level between 4 and 10 turn out to have cancer. In men with a PSA level over 10, about 65 percent are found to have cancer. Finally, many conditions can cause PSA to rise (see page 98).

Gram for gram, cancerous tissue results in PSA levels in the blood that are about ten times higher than levels in benign tissue. This is because normally, PSA is an enzyme that is secreted and disposed of through tiny ducts in the prostate. But prostate cancer doesn't have a working ductal system; its ducts are "blind"—dead-end streets. So instead of draining into the urethra, PSA builds up, leaks out of the prostate, and shows up in the bloodstream. That's why it has proven to be such a good marker for cancer.

MY PSA IS ELEVATED: WHAT ELSE COULD IT BE?

Just as having a low PSA doesn't mean you *don't* have prostate cancer, having a high PSA doesn't automatically mean you *do*. If your PSA is high, you have some form of prostate disease—trauma, enlargement, infection, or cancer—and you need to see a urologist to figure out what it is.

For example, trauma, even a particularly vigorous rectal exam, can make a man's PSA levels shoot up temporarily. (To illustrate how complicated PSA is, consider this. In one study, French scientists found that the rise in PSA after a rectal exam is mainly in free PSA; still, the number went up, and the result could be misleading.) This means that, ideally, your blood should be drawn before you have a rectal exam or any other procedure, such as catheterization, cystoscopy, or prostate biopsy, that could affect the prostate and falsely elevate PSA. For this reason, it makes sense to wait six to eight weeks after you have a needle biopsy before having your PSA taken if you are planning to use the results to make treatment decisions. And even then, it can still be higher than it was before your biopsy—so if this happens, don't panic, thinking your PSA is shooting up uncontrollably.

BPH itself can elevate PSA. A mild case of prostatitis can raise PSA, too, and an acute infection, such as bacterial prostatitis, can cause it to skyrocket. Sexual activity can elevate PSA as well: PSA levels can increase by as much as 41 percent in less than an hour after ejaculation. (Thus, it is wise to abstain from sex for two days before you are due to have your PSA tested.)

An episode of urinary retention (from BPH or urinary tract infection) can also cause an abrupt elevation in PSA, which takes as long as a week to return to normal. In rare cases, BPH can block blood supply to areas of the prostate. This is called a prostate infarction, and the cutoff of blood is much like that in a myocardial infarction, or heart attack. An episode of prostate infarction can trigger urinary retention and cause a temporary jump in PSA, sometimes to startling levels—as high as 100 to 200 ng/ml.

Finally, a mistake in the medical laboratory can cause a wrong PSA reading and create needless anxiety in the process. This happens more often than you might think. For all these reasons, *no management decision should be made based on a lone PSA reading, and you should repeat the test to make sure before having a biopsy.* (For more on confirming a diagnosis of prostate cancer, see chapter 5.)

Note: One activity that *does not* raise PSA levels is bicycling. In one study, published in the *Archives of Family Medicine*, scientists studied twenty men who were members of a cycling club and found that even long-distance cycling (although it did seem to cause numbness in the perineum, the area between the scrotum and rectum) did not raise blood levels of PSA.

New Approaches to PSA Testing

As good as the PSA test is, there is still room for improvement. Many scientists are working to make it more meaningful and specific. Some of the most promising approaches include:

Bound and Free PSA

Chemically speaking, a PSA molecule is like a tiny pair of sharp scissors (the main function of PSA is to break down coagulated semen after intercourse; see chapter 1). Now imagine millions of these tiny scissors clanking around in the bloodstream, each pointed blade slicing tissue to ribbons. Normally, PSA is packed in a protective case—a chemical straitjacket that keeps it from harming innocent tissue. In this form, PSA is bound—tied to other proteins and rendered harmless. But sometimes, PSA inactivates itself. Imagine a pair of scissors with one broken blade. These scissors don't fit in the case anymore, but they don't need it; they are chemically passive. This form is called free PSA. It circulates freely in the bloodstream on its own.

In a regular, or total, PSA blood test, both of these forms are lumped together—the dangerous scissors in the case and the scissors with the broken blade. But scientists have developed tests to measure both the bound and free forms of PSA, which can help men in two important ways: It can make the PSA test more specific, for one thing. It can also help determine how aggressive a man's cancer is.

A More Specific Test: The Free PSA Test

Having an elevated PSA level does not automatically mean that you have prostate cancer. What it means is that you have prostate trouble—which could mean cancer, enlargement, infection, or even recent trauma—and you need to see a urologist to figure out exactly what's going on in there. The most common reason for a higher-than-normal PSA level is prostate enlargement, or BPH. It is common for a man's PSA to be as high as 10 percent of his prostate weight; for example, if a man has an enlarged prostate that weighs 60 grams, he may well have a PSA of 6 ng/ml—but not have cancer.

Free PSA Comes Almost Exclusively from BPH Tissue

An easy way to remember this is "The higher the *free* PSA, the more likely that you are *free* of cancer." Men with prostate cancer are more likely to have low levels of free PSA (also known as percent-free PSA). Thus, if a man has an elevated PSA and most of it is free, it's probably coming from BPH; if it's mostly bound, the PSA elevation is probably coming from cancer. This is where measuring free PSA is especially useful.

Can the free PSA test reduce your risk of an unnecessary biopsy? Probably. Can overreliance on the free PSA test mean your prostate cancer might be missed? Possibly. In one study, researchers used a free PSA cutoff of 19 percent in men with total PSA levels between 3 and 4 and detected 90 percent of all cancers. Another study, of men with PSA levels between 2.6 and 4, had a higher cutoff—27 percent free PSA—but also detected 90 percent of cancers. This study found that 18 percent of unnecessary biopsies could be avoided by using this cutoff. (Note: Again, because men with low free PSA levels are more likely to have aggressive cancers and more advanced disease found at the time of radical prostatectomy, even if the needle biopsy is inconclusive or shows little cancer, if the percent-free PSA is lower than 10 percent, a man is likely to be harboring more tumor than a man with a higher level of free PSA.)

Another study of men with higher PSA levels (between 4 and 10 ng/ml) found that using the free PSA test—and performing biopsies only on men with less than 25 percent free PSA—could diagnose 95 percent of the cancers and reduce unnecessary biopsies by 20 percent. However, some scientists, worried about diagnosing that remaining 5 percent of cancers, object to this cutoff number, because it means that some cancers will be missed.

Should You Get Your Free PSA Tested?

There are several points to consider. One drawback to the free PSA test is that it's more expensive, because two blood components must be measured—the total amount and the free amount, from which the percent-free number is calculated. Some urologists recommend biopsy only when the percentage of free to total PSA is lower than 10 percent. This is good, in that it reduces the number of unnecessary biopsies, but it also means that 5 to 10 percent of cancers may be missed. It may come down to what bothers you most—the thought of missing cancer at the earliest possible diagnosis or having an unnecessary biopsy because of a false alarm.

However, there are two situations in which percent-free PSA can be particularly useful. Say a man has had multiple biopsies because his total PSA is higher than normal. Every biopsy is negative, yet the worry remains. Here, if the free PSA is high, the man and his doctor can relax. If it's very low, it means he will need further biopsies. The second situation is the man with a strong family history of prostate cancer who worries that he is headed down the same pathway as his father, brother, or other male relatives, even though his PSA is low for his age. Here again, knowing the free PSA percentage can be reassuring. If it's high, this man can relax. If it's very low, this is a good reason to have a biopsy.

How Aggressive Is the Cancer?

If a man has prostate cancer, his doctor can't tell just by looking at the total PSA level how much of the PSA is coming from the cancer and how much is everyday PSA from benign prostate tissue. For example, in many men with small amounts of early-stage cancer, most of the PSA is actually coming from noncancerous tissue in the rest of the prostate. However, *if the free PSA is less than 10 percent, it's more likely that most of that PSA is coming from cancer, that the cancer is significant in size, and that it will prove aggressive.* The differences in PSA illustrate once again that not all prostate cancers are created equal. Some are very slow-growing and never need treatment. Others can be fatal within a matter of years after they are diagnosed. So for scientists, just as important as finding cancer early is knowing which kind of cancer—the "good" or the "bad"—we're dealing with.

Evidence shows that free PSA can predict which tumors will be aggressive—and need to be treated as soon as possible—several years before regular PSA tests can even spot cancer. In one Johns Hopkins study using the large database of the Baltimore Longitudinal Study of Aging, urologist H. Ballentine Carter compared blood samples from men who developed prostate cancer with those from men who did not and found that *fifteen years before cancer was diagnosed*, all the men who turned out to have aggressive prostate tumors had levels of free PSA that were lower than 15 percent. Men with slower-growing, nonaggressive cancer all had free PSA levels greater than 15 percent. This landmark study suggests that free PSA percentage may be an excellent predictor of aggressive tumors that will need to be treated.

PSA Velocity

Another promising diagnostic approach using PSA testing is to look at PSA velocity—its rate of change from year to year. The supposition is this: if cells double at a much faster rate in prostate cancer than in BPH, and if prostate cancer produces more PSA than BPH does, it's likely that PSA's yearly rate of change will be much greater in a man with prostate cancer than in a man with BPH.

However, for this technique to be accurate, multiple PSA measurements taken in the same laboratory are needed over at least one to two years. It is not helpful for a man to have two PSA tests in a short span of time—a couple of months apart, for example—because there is a natural fluctuation in PSA readings of as much as 15 to 30 percent. Say you have a PSA test result of 4.1 ng/ml; two months later, your PSA level is 4.7. This could be a normal variation, yet it could well spark panic if you believed you had cancer and it was growing fast. PSA velocity is also not useful if you only have two PSA values separated by more than four years.

In a study using twenty years' worth of stored blood samples from the Baltimore Longitudinal Study of Aging, investigators looked at three groups of men—those with BPH, those with prostate cancer, and a control group of men with no prostate disease. They found that PSA velocity can be a veritable crystal ball at predicting prostate cancer. The men who turned out to develop prostate cancer had "significantly greater rates of change in PSA levels than those without prostate cancer *up to ten years before diagnosis.*" In other words, by tracking changes in PSA levels, they were able to detect prostate cancer years before it could be diagnosed by other means. For example, at five years before diagnosis—when PSA levels weren't appreciably different between men with BPH and men with prostate cancer—there was already a big difference in PSA velocity in men who turned out to have prostate cancer versus men who had BPH and the control group.

The idea with PSA velocity is that it's a fluid continuum, not a cut-and-dried, one-shot reading. It's like having a prostate barometer, so your doctor doesn't have to wait for the PSA level to reach a magic number (such as 2.5 ng/ml) before acting. With PSA velocity, what matters is a significant change over time, and this varies, depending on the level of PSA. *For men with PSAs greater than 4, an average, consistent increase of more than 0.75 ng/ml over the course of three tests is considered significant.* Say that over eighteen months, a man's PSA level went up from 4.0 to 4.6 to 5.8 ng/ml. Clearly, something's going on here. With PSA velocity, we can make a more accurate diagnosis of prostate cancer at even lower levels than the raw cutoff of 4. Because we now realize that men with PSA levels as low as 1.0 may have cancer, guidelines have been established for PSA velocity in men with PSA levels between 1 and 4. In fact, work by Carter and colleagues suggests that *any consistent increase in PSA is alarming,* even an increase as small as 0.35 ng/ml a year. Their research found that even many years before a man's prostate cancer was diagnosed, when his total PSA levels were still low, a PSA velocity of greater than 0.35 ng/ml a year predicted who would later die from prostate cancer. *If you have a PSA level between 1 and 4 and it is consistently rising faster than approximately 0.4 ng/ml a year, you should get a biopsy.*

Also, PSA velocity is more specific. For example, among men with PSA levels greater than 4, about 40 percent turn out to have only BPH and undergo unnecessary biopsies. But with PSA velocity, this number is reduced so that only 10 percent of men with BPH would undergo an unnecessary biopsy.

MY PSA IS LOW—AM I OKAY?

Taking a 5-alpha reductase inhibitor, such as finasteride (Proscar) or dutasteride (Avodart), to treat BPH can artificially lower the PSA reading by as much as half. The drug Propecia, used to deter hair loss, is a low-dose form of finasteride, and it lowers PSA as well. To account for this, if you have been taking one of these drugs for two years, your PSA should be doubled, then by 2.3 for the next five years, and after seven years, by 2.5. (Fortunately, these drugs do not appear to affect free PSA percentage.)

What else can affect your PSA? Quite a few things. For example, being very overweight can artificially lower your PSA. This is thought to occur due to a greater amount of circulating water, diluting the PSA in the bloodstream. Certain other medications, such as statins (commonly used to lower cholesterol), thiazide diuretics, and NSAIDs may also lower PSA levels. However, although scientists have worried that these factors could mask prostate cancer from being diagnosed as early as possible, the changes involved seem to be relatively small.

If you have had a surgical procedure to treat BPH (such as a TUR), your PSA should fall to a new lower baseline and stay there. If your PSA begins to rise after that, even if it's still considered low, this should be investigated.

A major change in PSA can also be a sign that something is very wrong—that there is significant cancer, and that it may be difficult to cure. Several large studies showed that men who had a PSA velocity of 2 within the year before diagnosis were much more likely to have an aggressive form of cancer and more likely to die from prostate cancer within ten years. Thus, if you have a sudden jump in your PSA level and it is confirmed in a repeat measurement at the same laboratory, you may have significant disease that needs treatment immediately, and that may require more than surgery or radiation therapy alone to cure. (For more on this, see chapter 10.)

Although PSA velocity is a big improvement over looking at a raw PSA score and trying to figure out what it means, even this isn't a perfect system. Paradoxically, in men who already have prostate cancer but have not yet received treatment, following changes in PSA during the first two years after diagnosis is less helpful. (For more on this, see chapter 7.)

PSA Density

This technique begins with a theory—that most men in the age group for prostate cancer also have at least some BPH, which can elevate the PSA concentration and make diagnosis more difficult. One way to distinguish between BPH and cancer, some doctors believe, is PSA density—the blood PSA score divided by the volume of the prostate, as determined by transrectal ultrasound. Basically, if you have BPH, your PSA should be approximately 10 percent, and no higher than 15 percent, of the weight of your prostate (which translates to a PSA density of 0.1 to 0.15). For example, if you have a PSA of 8 ng/ml and your prostate weighs 80 grams, most of the PSA is probably coming from BPH. But if your prostate weighs only 30 to 40 grams, your PSA level is too high to be explained by BPH alone.

TABLE 4.1

HOW MANY MEN MY AGE HAVE MY PSA LEVEL?

Age	50–59	60–69	70 or above	Total
PSA Level				
2.5 or lower	88%	75%	61%	78%
2.6–4.0	8%	14%	18%	12%
4.1–9.9	3%	9%	16%	8%
10 or higher	1%	2%	5%	2%

Data adapted from the *Journal of the American Medical Association*.

The next question you might have is, "How do we measure the size of my prostate?" Well, there's the problem. Although doctors frequently attempt to estimate prostate size based on the digital rectal exam, these estimates are highly inaccurate. It is impossible to estimate a man's prostate size accurately without transrectal ultrasound or MRI. For men who have had one of these tests, PSA density can be helpful to predict the risk of cancer and its aggressiveness.

PSA Thresholds

First, there was the number 4. When PSA testing first came out, the general consensus was that a PSA greater than 4 ng/ml was considered abnormal. Then we learned about the need to lower the threshold to 2.5 for men in their forties. At that point, some experts suggested that 2.5 should be used for everyone. That way, they argued, we wouldn't miss anybody by delaying biopsies until the PSA rises above 4. Far better, they said, to strike cancer sooner, while men have lower PSA levels. They do have a point. But the counter-argument to this is that prostate cancers detected at lower PSA levels are more likely to be small in volume and low in grade, and thus more likely to represent clinically insignificant disease—and may not need to be treated right away, if ever. True, any approach to prostate cancer screening that finds more cancers without telling us how dangerous they are will only increase overdiagnosis and over-treatment. In an article published in the *Journal of the National Cancer Institute*, some scientists have estimated that lowering the threshold for biopsies from 4 to 2.5 ng/ml in the United States would double the number of men defined as abnormal—up to six million. This could be disastrous.

And then, in the midst of this 2.5 vs. 4.0 debate, a bombshell exploded. In a study published in the *New England Journal of Medicine*, based on biopsies of three thousand men with PSAs lower than 4, investigators found that 15 percent of these men had cancer. And of the men diagnosed with cancer, 15 percent had Gleason scores (see chapter 5) of 7 or higher. This study left a number of unanswered questions—specifically, how many of those men had small-volume cancers—but it removed all complacency with using absolute PSA thresholds as a means to distinguish men with and without cancer.

It should be noted that in the European study discussed earlier in this chapter, PSA screening was shown to save lives using a threshold of 3 ng/ml at most centers. This suggests that setting a threshold in the range of 2.5 to 3 may strike a reasonable balance between early detection and overdiagnosis. But really, the only absolute PSA threshold that we can use to rule out cancer entirely is 1. Although some men with a PSA this low may harbor prostate cancer, it is unlikely to be the life-threatening, high-grade kind. For this reason, many investigators now believe that what matters more is *what happens to this PSA level—whether it rises over time, and how fast—and the context of the patient, his general health, and his risk factors.*

TABLE 4.2

WILL MY BIOPSY SHOW CANCER?
WHAT ABOUT HIGH-GRADE DISEASE?

PSA	Odds that the biopsy will be positive for cancer	Odds of high-grade disease (Gleason 7–10)
Less than 0.5	7 percent	0.8 percent
0.6–1.0	10 percent	1.0 percent
1.1–2.0	21 percent	2.6 percent
2.1–3.0	27 percent	5.7 percent
3.1–4.0	30 percent	9.4 percent
4.1–10	23–38 percent	5–15 percent
Greater than 10	65 percent	–

Data adapted from the *New England Journal of Medicine.*

BPH Makes It More Confusing

The presence of BPH clouds the crystal ball of PSA, making a man's levels harder to interpret—causing higher PSA levels that usually have nothing to do with cancer. Because of this, the PSA test is better at finding cancer in men who don't have BPH; these men generally have lower PSA levels anyway, are younger, and have more to gain from an early diagnosis of cancer. It may be that we should rethink the emphasis on absolute PSA thresholds, explore in depth the patterns of increase in PSA when it is less than 4 ng/ml, and identify any factors that can help us predict life-threatening disease at a time when the disease is most curable. As the Johns Hopkins urologist H. Ballentine Carter discovered, men with PSAs between 1 and 4 who had a PSA velocity greater than 0.35 ng/ml per year were more likely to die of their prostate cancer. Overall, a man's baseline PSA level in his forties and how it changes gives valuable information about his risk of developing life-threatening prostate cancer.

PSA and Race

Studies show that black men without prostate cancer have higher PSA levels than their counterparts of other races. This might suggest that there should be a higher PSA cutoff for African Americans. However, the other side of the coin is that black men also have a greater risk of developing cancer (see chapter 3) and, when they are tested with the same PSA cutoff level as white men, are more likely to be harboring a cancer. In one study using a PSA cutoff of 4 ng/ml, 38 percent of white men were found to have prostate cancer, but 52 percent of black men turned out to have cancer. One reason for this may be the recent observation by Johns Hopkins pathologist Jonathan Epstein that prostate cancers in African American men make less PSA per gram of tissue than white men.

More research is needed to determine the guidelines for PSA testing of black men. However, because African American men are more likely to develop the disease—and to have a more advanced, lethal form of it—they need to be followed carefully. It may be that combining PSA with additional tests, such as free PSA or other new markers, will prove to be most useful for these men.

Other PSA-Based Blood Tests

The more we discover about PSA and its subtleties, the more we're learning about the chemistry of the prostate and the many biochemical signals it sends out all the time. If we can only figure out how to read them! Several sophisticated tests look at other PSA-based markers in the blood.

Prostate Health Index (PHI)

This blood test combines total PSA and free PSA with another form of PSA called pro-PSA. The PHI test can predict who is likely to have significant prostate cancer on biopsy.

4K Score

This is another new test combining different forms of PSA along with other information about the patient into an algorithm that predicts your risk of having high-grade cancer on biopsy. Similar to PHI, studies show that the 4K score is more specific than regular PSA.

A Urine Test for Prostate Cancer?

A completely different approach to diagnosing prostate cancer is based on the molecular detection of prostate cancer cells in the urine after a vigorous digital rectal examination.

PCA3 (DD3)

The *DD3* gene, discovered at Johns Hopkins, is one of the most prostate cancer–specific genes known, making it a promising marker for the early diagnosis of prostate cancer. A commercial test called PCA3 was developed and shown to help predict the results of biopsy. This test can help guide the decision for repeat biopsy in men with a PSA that's higher than it should be, but who have had negative biopsies.

Who Needs Screening?

Most men with curable prostate cancer feel perfectly fine. Men who do not feel fine—who have symptoms of prostate cancer—probably do not have curable disease. And this leads to the philosophy of screening: men who can expect to live ten to twenty more years and who don't want to die from prostate cancer should be screened. This is especially true for the men who are at highest risk of developing the disease—men of African descent and men with a strong family history of prostate cancer.

What does that mean? Simply that if a man's age or health suggests that he won't live longer than ten years, there is no reason to make an early diagnosis of prostate cancer. If a man who is very old or very ill has early, localized prostate cancer now, it is unlikely that he will live long enough for the cancer to become a problem. If the cancer progresses, there are many ways to control the disease and keep symptoms at bay for years. Creating anxiety about what to do—what treatment decisions to make—is not helpful for these men. One of the major missing pieces here, especially as the average life span lengthens—is determining how long a man is going to live. Scientists have created computer models to help urologists predict life expectancy as a way to pilot these difficult decisions—but even then, they are only guidelines, not guarantees.

Obviously, nobody wants to die from prostate cancer—or heart disease, or any ailment, for that matter. For many men, however, this is much more than an abstract concept; it is a great fear. These men have seen death from prostate cancer, watched the suffering of their father, brother, or friend, and prayed it wouldn't happen to them, too. But other men don't understand this. They know only what they read in the newspapers and hear on television—that the treatment of prostate cancer is associated with a lot of side effects and is a thing to be avoided at all costs. If you have not seen a family member or friend die of prostate cancer, it's hard to imagine it. The disease progresses relentlessly, ultimately culminating in death from metastases to bone, which are agonizing to experience and tough even to witness. Because prostate cancer rarely interferes with any normal bodily functions, patients die a painful death, with their body's defenses usually broken down to the point at which they succumb to pneumonia. Watching this terrible thing happen to someone you love makes you feel helpless and angry. You think, "With all of the wonders of modern medicine, shouldn't we be able to do something? Shouldn't we be past suffering like this by now?" We aren't past it yet, although there are bright new rays of hope— some men with metastatic disease are seeing their disease go into remission in clinical trials—and this may change someday soon. This is the side of prostate cancer that you rarely hear about. It's the side of prostate cancer that critics of screening avoid talking about. Instead, they emphasize the side effects of treatment.

The thing is, today—thank goodness—all forms of treatment for prostate cancer have fewer side effects, especially if men are diagnosed when they are young. As we have discussed, there is now hard evidence that both screening and effective treatment have reduced the rates of metastatic disease and death from prostate cancer. Thus, the man who's going to live long enough to need to be cured should have the opportunity to be cured. Conversely, men who are diagnosed with low-risk cancers may not ever need to be treated. Screening is the first step to finding out what you have while all doors are still open, so you can make informed decisions about treatment.

You Should Start Screening at Age Forty

When prostate cancer is discovered in younger men, it is more likely to be curable. Recognizing this fact, Johns Hopkins urologist H. Ballentine Carter and colleagues began looking for a way to improve prostate cancer screening. They used an approach that has worked well to answer questions about screening in cervical and breast cancer—a highly sophisticated computer model that mathematically simulates the progression of a disease in a group of people.

WHY SHOULD I BEGIN IN MY FORTIES?

Three reasons: First, many men whose prostate cancers go undetected before they're in their fifties eventually die of the disease. Most of these men have no particular reason to worry about prostate cancer—they don't have a strong family history, and they're not African American. But it is possible that the men between ages fifty and sixty-four who die of prostate cancer could have been saved if the disease had been caught when they were in their forties. Second, younger men are more likely than older men to have curable disease and have fewer side effects from treatment. And finally, PSA is a better, more specific test in younger men who—unlike older men—don't tend to have BPH, which can falsely raise the PSA level. PSA measurements taken when a man is in his forties also provide a baseline to be followed over time.

The results, published in the *Journal of the American Medical Association*, were unexpected: For men who are not at higher risk of developing prostate cancer, beginning screening at age fifty was *not* the best strategy. Instead, they found a more effective strategy was to give PSA tests at age forty and at age forty-five, and then at age fifty (or earlier, if PSA was 2 ng/ml or above), start testing every other year instead of every year. "That was the only strategy that did three things: it reduced the death rate of prostate cancer, reduced the overall number of PSA tests, and reduced the overall number of prostate biopsies for each cancer detected," says Carter.

But many scientists, including Carter, are very troubled by the recent finding that 15 percent of men with a PSA level lower than 4 ng/ml have cancer, and 15 percent of these men with cancer have high-grade cancer. Remember, *there is no safe, absolute cutoff above a PSA level of 1.0* at which a man can rest assured that he is not at risk of harboring a high-grade cancer. Thus, what probably is going to matter the most in the future is your PSA history. Getting your first PSA test and digital rectal examination at age forty, when you are unlikely to have BPH, will give you a valuable baseline for every other PSA measurement you'll ever need; the results of these baseline PSA tests have been shown to predict a man's risk of being diagnosed with prostate cancer over the next twenty-five years. After this, depending on the baseline level—specifically, whether you are above or below the fiftieth percentile for your age—all you need to do is take a repeat PSA test every two to five years. Men in their forties who have a PSA level greater than 0.6 ng/ml are in this group, as are men in their fifties who have a PSA level greater than 0.7. (In a study of a larger group of men, urologists Stacy Loeb of New York University and William Catalona of Northwestern University found the comparable numbers to be 0.7 for men in their forties and 0.9 for men in their fifties.) If you are in this group, you should have your PSA measured at least every two years during your forties. If your PSA is below this percentile, you may be able to wait as long as five years for the next test.

SHOULD I THINK ABOUT GENETIC TESTING?

One of the most powerful predictors of prostate cancer risk is a strong family history. Johns Hopkins scientists have shown that men with a family history have double the risk of prostate cancer. At even higher risk are men with two or more relatives who developed prostate cancer at a young age. If one of your relatives has had metastatic prostate cancer, you should undergo genetic testing.

But wait—there's more. The risk of lethal prostate cancer is tied to the risk of other cancers, too—and to genes that nobody ever connected with prostate cancer before. These discoveries are very new. For the last two decades, molecular geneticists such as William Isaacs of Johns Hopkins have been looking for genes that are linked to a family history of prostate cancer, and they have found a few, but these only account for a small percentage of cases of prostate cancer. The major reason for this is that much of this work has been done looking at the removed prostate specimens of men diagnosed with *early-stage cancer* that is confined to the prostate and curable with surgery.

But in new work by Isaacs and research groups around the world, scientists looked at the genes of men who were diagnosed with the most aggressive prostate cancer, and they hit pay dirt. It turns out that there is a short list, a genetic "who's who" of very bad genes that appear in lethal prostate cancers; these mutated genes are also involved in the worst cancers of the breast, colon, ovaries, and pancreas and in melanoma. They can be inherited by men and women.

The job description for these genes is "DNA damage repair," and normally, they are supposed to protect the body against the genetic mistakes that can lead to cancer. Imagine a car factory where someone in charge of quality control breaks his eyeglasses: he misses delicate mistakes in the machinery he's supposed to inspect; those faulty parts then get put into bigger sections, and before you know it, a defective engine is on its way out the door.

Many men have slow-growing prostate cancer, and chances are, those men *do not* have one of these damaged genes. In fact, "in many studies of men with less aggressive disease, we have been unable to detect genes linked to lethal prostate cancer," Isaacs says. He should know; he has identified many genetic variants called single-nucleotide polymorphisms (SNPs) that raise a man's risk of getting prostate cancer. But these bad stretches of DNA raise the risk by a very small amount, and just because a man inherits one of them doesn't necessarily mean he will get prostate cancer, or that it will be the aggressive kind that really needs to be treated.

In the first study of its kind, Isaacs and colleagues including Jian-feng Xu at NorthShore Research Institute in Chicago recently completed a detailed genetic analysis of 96 men who died of prostate cancer at an early age, younger than sixty-five. "We sequenced all regions on each chromosome that code for proteins," Isaacs explains. "Surprisingly, we found that *more than 20 percent of these patients carry inherited mutations which inactivate a class of genes responsible for repairing damaged DNA.*"

Two of these genetic culprits are BRCA1 and BRCA2, genes most famous for their role in inherited breast and ovarian cancer. "We found the highest frequency of mutations in BRCA2," says Isaacs. "Studies are under way worldwide to understand the role of this *heretofore breast cancer gene* in inherited prostate cancer. Family history is a powerful tool, but we need to characterize *what kind of family history* is most meaningful. While much work remains to be done to fully understand these results, we are very excited about these new findings and how they may translate into better ways to identify a man's risk for aggressive prostate cancer before the cancer even begins."

Another study, led by Peter Nelson of the Fred Hutchinson Cancer Center, published in the *New England Journal of Medicine*, looked at inherited mutations in twenty damage repair genes in 692 men with metastatic prostate cancer at institutions in the United States and United Kingdom, and found mutations in sixteen of them. Because of this work, Nelson and colleagues estimate that *one in nine—12 percent—of men with metastatic cancer have them*, even if they have no family history of prostate, breast, or ovarian cancer.

Note: Cancer is not inevitable if you carry one of these mutations. It may well be that if you live your life doing some things we know help prevent or delay prostate cancer—such as not eating a lot of red meat and dairy products, eating foods like broccoli and tomatoes, not smoking, not drinking an excessive amount of alcohol, and not being overweight, which stresses your cells and makes them less resistant to cancer—you will never develop prostate cancer. And if you start getting screened for prostate cancer at age forty, and if you are then screened every year to look for changes in your PSA and other markers, if you do develop cancer, it will be caught early and you will be cured.

There is a Latin proverb: *Praemonitus, praemunitus* ("Forewarned is forearmed"). If one of these genes runs in your family, doctors will look more carefully for cancer in you, your children, and your grandchildren, and if it's found, they will be more aggressive about treating it right away.

This news also offers new hope for treatment. There are entirely new kinds of drugs that target specific genes. For example, PARP inhibitors such as olaparib (Lynparza) are being used to treat women with BRCA mutations in ovarian cancer. Olaparib has now been approved as a treatment for advanced prostate cancer in some men.

If a family member has high-risk or metastatic prostate cancer, or if you have a strong family history of prostate, breast, or other cancers, ask your doctor about cascade genetic screening. You may also want to talk to a genetic counselor (see chapter 3).

What If You Don't Have a Baseline?

What if this is your first PSA test? If you are in your forties, fifties, or sixties and have never had a PSA test, if your level is greater than 2.5 ng/ml and you are otherwise healthy and can expect to live at least another fifteen to twenty years, you should consider a biopsy. If you are not sure, ask your doctor about having one of the other second-line tests described on pages 108–109 to help with the decision. If your biopsy finds no cancer, you should have your PSA level rechecked at regular intervals, using both the total PSA level and the speed at which it rises over time to determine whether and when you need to have a repeat biopsy. MRI can also be used to check for any suspicious areas that can be targeted on the next biopsy.

When Should You Stop Screening?

This decision depends entirely on you. The USPSTF recommends against screening for men over seventy-five. And it may be that screening could be discontinued earlier in life if you have maintained PSA levels consistent with a low risk of developing prostate cancer. In other words, if your PSA track record is good, you can probably retire earlier from PSA screening. Johns Hopkins urologist H. Ballentine Carter showed that if PSA testing were discontinued at age sixty-five in men who had PSA levels below 0.5 to 1.0 ng/ml, it would be unlikely that prostate cancer would be missed later in life. A more recent study suggested that it is safe to discontinue PSA testing for men aged seventy-five to eighty years with PSA levels lower than 3 ng/ml (none of the men in this study later died from prostate cancer); however, the men aged seventy-five to eighty who had PSA levels greater than 3 remained at risk of developing life-threatening disease.

That said, results of a recent Johns Hopkins study suggest that *healthy men over age seventy-five should not stop PSA screening.* We are living longer, and seventy-five is not the ripe old age it used to be. Continuing to use age seventy-five as a blanket cutoff age for PSA screening is missing cancer in men who really need to be treated. In fact, there is increasing evidence that this age-based approach is significantly flawed. Population studies have shown that men *diagnosed at seventy-five years or older* account for *48 percent of metastatic cancers and 53 percent of prostate cancer deaths*, despite representing only 26 percent of the overall population.

Why are older men more likely to die from prostate cancer? To find out, the Hopkins team studied 274 men over age seventy-five who underwent radiation therapy for prostate cancer. They found that men who underwent PSA testing were significantly less likely to be diagnosed with high-risk prostate cancer, and that men with either no PSA testing or incomplete testing—either a change in PSA was not followed up, or a biopsy was not performed when it was indicated—had more than a threefold higher risk of having high-risk disease at diagnosis, when adjusted for other clinical risk factors. Also, many of these men who had a low PSA were found to have cancers that were palpable on rectal exam, indicating that *older men need both a PSA and a digital rectal examination.* Although this was a small study and more research is needed, we believe that PSA screening should be considered in very healthy older men.

5

DIAGNOSIS AND STAGING

Optional Imaging Tests for Staging Prostate Cancer	**Lymphadenectomy**
PET Scan	Who Should Get It
Chest X-ray	**To Sum Up**

This chapter was written with expert opinion from Stacy Loeb, M.D.

THE SHORT STORY:
The Highly Abridged Version of This Chapter

Do you have prostate cancer? Maybe your prostate-specific antigen (PSA) level was high, or higher than it was last year and the year before that. Maybe your doctor felt something suspicious during the rectal exam. What happens now? The next step is to determine whether you have cancer, and the only way to do that is with a biopsy.

But before we go on, we should note that *if it is cancer, there is no need to panic and make any hasty decisions.* If you do have cancer, it didn't start today, this month, or even this year; it's been in there a long time—most likely at least ten years—growing very slowly. Taking a few more weeks—to be absolutely certain of the diagnosis, to determine the extent of the disease, to decide on the right treatment, and to find the best doctor to administer that treatment—won't mean that you'll miss your window of opportunity to be cured. Instead, taking a few weeks or even several months to be sure you have enough information to make the right decision may be the best investment in your health, and your life, that you'll ever make.

For most men, the diagnosis of prostate cancer is unexpected—like a sudden punch in the stomach. As with any other unexpected calamity in your life, you've got to face it square on and collect all the facts. At your fingertips are three facts you will probably come to know as well as your Social Security number—your PSA, Gleason score, and clinical stage. With just these three facts, almost immediately you will have a good idea of where you stand. The cancer either appears to be clinically localized to the prostate—the most common scenario in the United States today because of screening—or the cancer has spread locally but does not appear to be present at distant sites; or rarely, less than 10 percent of the time, the cancer has been caught later and has spread to either the lymph nodes or bone. Once you know where you stand, your next move is to examine the options for treatment and find the one that you feel is best for you. *Whatever the finding, don't become discouraged. There is more hope now than ever.*

Diagnosis and Staging

Do you have prostate cancer? Maybe your PSA level was high, or it's higher than it was last year and the year before that. Maybe your doctor felt something suspicious during the rectal exam. What happens now? The next step is to determine whether you indeed have cancer, and the only way to do that is with a biopsy.

But before we go on, we should note several things. Think of this as the "take a deep breath" section of the chapter. First of all, the chances are good that the biopsy will be negative. Only 15 percent of men with a PSA level lower than 4 ng/ml and 25 percent of men with a PSA level between 4 and 10 will turn out to have cancer. And even if it is cancer, *there is no need to panic and make any hasty decisions.* Nothing has to happen today. If you have cancer, it didn't start today, this month, or even this year; it's been in there a long time—most likely at least ten years—growing very slowly. Taking a few more weeks or months—to be absolutely certain of the diagnosis, to determine the extent of the disease, to decide on the right treatment, and to find the best doctor to administer that treatment—won't mean you'll miss your window of opportunity to be cured. Instead, taking a little time to be sure you make the right decisions may be the best investment in your health, and your life, that you'll ever make. How do you make any wise investment? By learning as much as you can before you commit to a plan of action.

One more thing: "Just because you have a PSA test doesn't mean you have to have a biopsy, and just because you are diagnosed with cancer doesn't mean you need treatment," notes New York University urologist Stacy Loeb. "At each decision point, there should be a discussion with your doctor about the pros and cons of taking the next step."

Now let's move ahead with this crash course on biopsy.

IF YOU ARE OF AFRICAN DESCENT, HERE'S WHAT YOU REALLY NEED TO KNOW

PSA Can Be Unreliable

In a man of, say, European descent, the way PSA and other biomarkers work is pretty well understood: a certain PSA number correlates with a certain risk of having a cancer. But new research suggests that *those numbers aren't always the same in men of African descent.*

"Our work has shown that prostate cancers in black men can make *less PSA per gram of cancer* compared to prostate cancers in Caucasian men," says Edward Schaeffer, Chairman of Urology at Northwestern. Thus the ideal values for a "safe PSA" in an African American man are not well established. More troubling: "Some of the most aggressive prostate cancers never produce PSA at a high level."

It is important to get regular prostate exams in addition to PSA tests, and if you are of African descent, Schaeffer says, "it is important to understand your numbers" and to find a urologist "who appreciates that your PSA score needs special attention."

Biopsies Miss the Cancer

"When men of African descent get a biopsy, their cancer can be missed because it can hide in the region of the prostate that is hardest to reach with a biopsy needle." Schaeffer tells his patients to imagine the prostate as a house. The biopsy comes in underneath the basement—through the rectum, which sits just below the prostate. "In most Caucasians, tumors occur in the basement. If you are directly underneath that area, you can get a good sampling with the biopsy needles, and you're more likely to pick up a cancer." But in men of African ancestry, "There's a higher chance that the tumor will be in the attic of the house—what we call an anterior tumor." It is easy to miss a tumor in this out-of-the-way spot with the needle in a standard biopsy.

To be extra cautious, Schaeffer gets MRI images of his patients who are at highest risk of prostate cancer—men with a strong family history of prostate cancer and African American men—and does an MRI-guided biopsy (see page 127).

Prostate Cancer Needs to Be on Your Radar

Of all the men in the world, African American men are in the group prostate cancer hits hardest. You are not only more likely to be diagnosed with prostate cancer, but also to have a more aggressive form that needs to be treated. *You are twice as likely to die of prostate cancer as a man of a different heritage.* So if you are a man of African ancestry and you are diagnosed with prostate cancer, you will more likely need to go after it with curative treatment—surgery or radiation. Active surveillance may not be the best option for you. And you need to get a baseline PSA and prostate exam starting at age forty.

"African American men have a one-third higher chance of having more aggressive cancer than the biopsy suggests," says Schaeffer. This means that if you are diagnosed with cancer and have surgery to remove it, when the pathologist looks at the cancer under the microscope, it very well might turn out to be of a higher grade, or there may be more of it than expected. More worrisome: "When these men need surgery, they are more likely to need additional adjuvant treatment, or to experience a recurrence of cancer, compared to Caucasian men. *Biologically, their cancers are different.*" Schaeffer is a pioneer in this area, and what he has learned, and is actively continuing to study, may save your life.

"Almost everything we understand about prostate cancer is based on data from Caucasians," he says. "Our understanding of the presentation, natural history and biology of prostate cancer is based predominantly on research done on the cancer of Caucasian men." Many of the assumptions that scientists made about prostate cancer—and even some of the markers developed to test for prostate cancer—don't hold up in black men.

To begin to unravel this important problem, Schaeffer teamed up with Kosj Yamoah, a radiation oncologist at Moffitt Cancer Center in Tampa. They looked at how twenty different established molecular markers for prostate cancer performed in African American men compared to Caucasian men. "Surprisingly, we found that only about one-third of them were the same between whites and blacks."

But in a striking development, "We also found that about one-third of these markers behaved in *inverse fashion* in black men compared to Caucasians." This means that a marker that *goes up* in white men to signal cancer actually *goes down* in men of African ancestry when cancer or aggressive cancer is present. "In men of African ancestry, a lot of established biomarkers are not the same as the established markers in Caucasians. The clinical implications for the behaviors of biomarkers and how they differ are unknown. We can certainly extrapolate that *how we follow cancer in white patients may not be the best way to do it in men of African ancestry.*"

Biopsy

Until the early 1990s, biopsy of the prostate was done "blind"—doctors couldn't see what they were doing—and often, the biopsy wasn't actually taken from the part of the prostate doctors thought they were reaching. Today, using transrectal ultrasound as a guide, urologists can see what they're doing in real time, and magnetic resonance imaging (MRI) can help target specific areas of concern in the prostate. So a biopsy of the prostate is more accurate than ever—and, because the needle is smaller, it's less painful, and complications are usually minimal.

Imagine the prostate as a large strawberry—except this strawberry has just a few seeds, maybe seven little black dots in all. These seeds are tumors, and *three to seven is the average number of separate cancers found in a radical prostatectomy specimen*. The development of several cancerous spots happens because prostate cancer is *multifocal*. It causes a "field change," in which the entire prostate undergoes a transformation. Multiple tumors pop up like dandelions, all at about the same time. Each spot can be millimeters in size.

This is the challenge facing urologists, for whom the prostate biopsy is a critical scouting mission. Our tactical weapon in this search for cancer is the spring-loaded biopsy gun, a tiny device attached to the ultrasound machine. It's a sophisticated needle, hollow in the center, designed to capture tiny cores, or glands—each about a millimeter thick—of tissue, which pathologists will then analyze under a microscope.

Before the biopsy, you will be asked to have an enema and take some antibiotics to minimize the risk of infection. (For more information, see page 129.) A biopsy is usually done with you wide awake, lying on your side. The urologist inserts the ultrasound probe through the rectum and uses the ultrasound image to inject local anesthetic and then direct the needle to strategic sites in the prostate.

Although needle biopsies are much better than they used to be, they don't always provide indisputable answers. Sometimes what's under the microscope is almost impossible to label definitively as cancer. Just as often, the needle misses the cancer, because it's just plain tricky to hit a tiny seed inside a strawberry—especially one you can't see.

Thus, we hedge our bets. It used to be that urologists took just four measly samples of tissue, one from each quadrant of the prostate. Then, the number increased to six (one from the top, middle, and bottom of the gland on the right and left sides). Now it's clear that taking ten or twelve samples is better still. We have also become much more strategic in where we fish for cancer. We know, for instance, where the cancer is most likely to be hiding—in the prostate's peripheral zone, extending along its sides like a shallow horseshoe (see fig. 5.1). We also know that it's likely to spread laterally—like a thin sheet—and that it's easy to stick the needle in too deep and overshoot the target area. We know to guide the needle so it catches the edge of the prostate for a higher yield of cancer cells. And in men with very large prostates—the size of an orange, say, instead of a large strawberry—we know we may need to sample even more tissue. An option is for some men to undergo an MRI before the prostate biopsy, which might show specific areas of concern that can be targeted with the biopsy. Note: Insurance companies have been reluctant to pay for an MRI in men who have never had a biopsy, but they will usually approve MRI if the initial biopsy was negative and a repeat biopsy is indicated. We expect this to change, and for MRI fusion biopsy (see page 127) to become standard practice in the future.

"Breast or lung cancer makes a solid nodule, just like a fist, that you usually can detect by palpation or imaging," says Johns Hopkins pathologist Jonathan Epstein. But prostate cancer tends to infiltrate normal tissue, meandering around normal cells. Or, as Johns Hopkins scientist Don Coffey described, it spreads out like a hand whose fingers flow into nearby tissue "like a river flooding a valley." This means that there can be a significant amount of cancer, even if it's not in the form of an obvious lump that's easy to feel or see on ultrasound. An MRI-guided biopsy is much better than ultrasound at identifying prostate cancers, but it still may miss some small tumors.

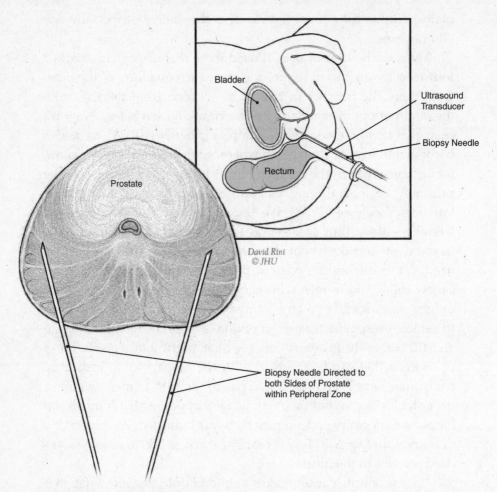

Bladder

Ultrasound
Transducer

Biopsy Needle

Rectum

Prostate

David Rini
© JHU

Biopsy Needle Directed to
both Sides of Prostate
within Peripheral Zone

FIGURE 5.1   Fishing for Cancer

Cancer is most likely to be hiding in the prostate's peripheral zone, extending along its
sides like a shallow horseshoe. Because prostate cancer tends to spread laterally—like a
thin sheet—it's easy to stick the needle in too deep and overshoot the target area. Urologists are learning to guide the needle so it catches the edge of the prostate, rather than
sampling tissue from the center, for a higher yield of cancer cells.

TRANSRECTAL ULTRASOUND: BEAUTIFUL PICTURE, LIMITED VALUE BY ITSELF

Like sonar on a submarine, ultrasound creates pictures using sound
waves. Transrectal ultrasound can sometimes detect differences

between cancerous and normal tissue in the prostate by means of a probe inserted in the rectum (that's what *transrectal* means—literally, "through the rectum").

A decade ago, many doctors believed transrectal ultrasound could be a "male mammogram," another means of screening for and detecting prostate cancer early. That hasn't happened, and the quality of the images often depends on the skill of the doctor using the ultrasound equipment. But the biggest drawback is that even though ultrasound can produce spectacular images of the prostate, these are often misleading.

Hit or Miss: Just as prostate cancer can feel different to a doctor's finger based on many factors (see chapter 5), it can also *sound* different from man to man. Transrectal ultrasound misses about half of prostate cancers greater than 1 centimeter in size because they sound just like regular prostate tissue. And, because some normal tissue sounds just like cancer, ultrasound also mistakes many benign lesions for cancer. *Thus, most cancers are not seen on ultrasound, and most lesions that are seen on ultrasound are not cancer.* The main role for transrectal ultrasound is in guiding the needle biopsy to make sure that the prostate is systematically sampled. Ultrasound can also be useful in determining the size of a man's prostate, which can, in turn, be used to determine PSA density.

The bottom line: Ultrasound can neither diagnose cancer nor rule it out. *Beware of the doctor who wants to do an ultrasound "just to see if there's cancer there" because, again, ultrasound is not a diagnostic technique.* Its only purpose is in helping the urologist aim the biopsy needle. MRI is much more accurate for localizing and staging prostate cancer than ultrasound.

BEFORE AND AFTER THE BIOPSY: WHAT TO DO AND WHAT TO EXPECT

The specifics vary from hospital to hospital, but here are some basic guidelines.

Before

No dietary restrictions. Eat breakfast or lunch before you go to the hospital. Drink plenty of fluids—juice, coffee, or water.

Give yourself an enema (such as Fleet) the morning of the biopsy.

Continue taking your regularly scheduled medications, but *do not take* aspirin, arthritis medication, high doses of vitamin E, ibuprofen, or any blood-thinning medications, such as warfarin (Coumadin) or heparin, unless your doctor has given specific permission. If you have pain, take acetaminophen (Tylenol).

If you are taking a daily dose of aspirin for prevention only, *stop taking it ten days before the biopsy.* If you take aspirin for a medical issue such as a heart condition, the biopsy can be performed without stopping the aspirin, but be sure to tell your urologist that you have not discontinued its use.

Do not urinate or empty your bladder just before the procedure. Your bladder should be partially full (this makes it easier for the ultrasound to get a good image).

Take antibiotics ahead of time. You should receive antibiotic tablets to minimize the risk of infection. The most common antibiotic used for this is a fluoroquinolone, such as levofloxacin (Levaquin) or ciprofloxacin (Cipro). If you have ever had ciprofloxacin—for example, if your doctor suspected that you had an infection in your prostate—you may be resistant to it. Talk to your doctor about using an alternative antibiotic or checking a rectal swab culture. You should be given antibiotics to take before the biopsy and for up to twenty-four hours after the biopsy.

During

The biopsy will take about fifteen minutes.

You will be asked to lie on your side. The procedure itself is uncomfortable but usually not painful.

Afterward

Your urine will probably be tinged with blood; you may even pass a few blood clots during urination and see blood when you have a bowel movement. This is normal; do not be alarmed. The bleeding should stop the same day or the next morning.

Force fluids—basically, this means drink a lot—for the rest of the day. This is to dilute your urine to prevent the formation of blood clots in the bladder.

Resume any prescription medications except blood-thinning agents such as warfarin (Coumadin) or heparin (don't start taking these again until your urologist gives you the go-ahead).

Do not do any heavy lifting or straining for five days after the biopsy.

You may see blood in your ejaculate for several months after the biopsy; this is normal.

Call Your Doctor Immediately If…

You have a fever or chills. Because of a recent increase in antibiotic-resistant bacteria, serious infection is possible, so if you experience these symptoms, you should proceed directly to the emergency room for evaluation.

Your bladder feels very full and you are unable to urinate (this is serious; if you experience these symptoms, go directly to the emergency room).

You have blood in your urine or rectal bleeding (usually with a bowel movement) that is significant or lasts more than a few weeks.

WHAT IS AN MRI FUSION BIOPSY?

Ultrasound is not a magic cancer finder; it mainly just makes sure that we systematically sample the prostate in the areas where cancers are most likely to be located. An *MRI fusion biopsy* is different. If we find a suspicious lesion on a multiparametric MRI (mpMRI), this image can be electronically transferred to a sophisticated ultrasound machine located where the biopsy is going to be performed. Suspicious areas of the prostate are fused with live, real-time ultrasound to provide a detailed 3-D ultrasound/MRI view showing us precisely where they are. Then we can guide our biopsy needles to the areas that really need to be sampled.

Multiparametric MRI looks at the prostate in several ways. One part of the scan uses a contrast dye injected in the blood. By looking at how much of the dye is taken up or washed out of the prostate, doctors can see cancer, and may also be able to determine whether it's aggressive. Note: Some people can be allergic to the contrast material. Your doctor may ask you to have a creatinine test (a blood test) ahead of time.

The scan itself lasts about an hour. It is done using a lubricated probe, inserted into the rectum. You lie on your back and are moved into the MRI machine, which is like a big tube. You will need to lie still and not fidget; if you move too much, the results might be difficult or impossible for the radiologist to interpret—which means you just wasted money and an hour of your life. Not everyone can lie still for this period of time, so make sure you talk to your doctor ahead of time if you have any special concerns.

What Complications Can I Expect from My Biopsy?

Prostate biopsy is an invasive procedure—a minor one, but invasive all the same—and there is a minor risk of complications.

Pain

Although nobody would describe a biopsy as fun, for most men the experience is more in the category of discomfort than significant pain. However, in some men, particularly those who have twelve or more tissue samples taken, the biopsy can really hurt. What's hurting is not, as you may think, the rectum (there are no pain fibers in the tissue lining the rectum); the pain is from the needle traveling through the prostate itself. How can you make the biopsy less painful?

One choice is *conscious sedation*. This is what doctors use in procedures such as colonoscopies. Patients feel no pain and remain awake throughout the procedure—but don't remember anything that happened during it. (So be aware that even though you may carry on a full conversation with your urologist during the biopsy, afterward you will almost certainly ask the same questions all over again because you won't remember asking them the first time.) Note: Sedation of any kind increases the cost of a procedure and also introduces the rare but serious risk that there will be complications from the sedation itself.

Another solution is the use of a *prostatic block*, a local anesthetic similar to the kind your dentist uses to numb your gums before you have a cavity filled. This block is injected into the tissues surrounding the seminal vesicles on both sides of the prostate. The same nerves that are responsible for erections (called the neurovascular bundles, discussed in chapter 8) also carry pain fibers that run to the prostate. Simply blocking these fibers can reduce pain markedly. Injecting the local anesthetic in other sites around the prostate may help decrease pain, as well. Alternatively, some urologists believe that the procedure is less painful if an anesthetic jelly is used to lubricate the probe.

Biopsy can also be done in the operating room under general anesthesia. If a more extensive biopsy is needed, it can be done through the perineum (the area of skin under the scrotum) instead of through the rectum.

Infection

Despite the fact that the biopsy is done through the rectum, infection is hardly ever a problem if its risk is kept to a minimum—if a cleansing enema is administered beforehand and antibiotics are given. In most patients, this means getting an oral dose of an antibiotic (such as a fluoroquinolone) an hour or so before the biopsy and then taking it for up to twenty-four hours afterward. In some men, however, this may not be enough.

Some options to reduce the risk of infection are to use more than one antibiotic for extra coverage, or to have a "rectal swab culture" done before your biopsy to check for antibiotic-resistant bacteria. "Usually, fluoroquinolones are used for prostate biopsy," says New York University urologist Stacy Loeb, "but if the patient's rectal culture shows bacteria that are resistant, he can be given a different antibiotic. Another option is to have your biopsy done through the perineum, which has a lower risk of infection."

Not all hospitals offer a rectal swab test. Another option is to ask your doctor to check with the hospital's infectious diseases doctors for antibiograms. An *antibiogram* is the result of lab tests for antibiotic sensitivity. Resistance to antibiotics can vary, not just from person to person, but in groups and places. For instance, "fluoroquinolone resistance varies a lot," says Loeb. "Some regions have much higher rates of resistance to this type of antibiotic than others. If you're in an area where there's higher resistance to one type of antibiotic but low resistance to another that may be a much better choice." Loeb practices at three hospitals affiliated with NYU, and "All three of them have different antibiograms." In other words, antibiotics that work well at one hospital may not work nearly as well at another.

Who's at higher risk of infection?

Men with a chronic illness such as diabetes, men with prostatitis, urinary tract infection, or men who use a urinary catheter. Men at higher risk may need a longer course of antibiotics or different antibiotics.

Also, *if you have been on antibiotics recently, or if you have taken antibiotics for a long time,* tell your doctor. You may need different antibiotics. "Patients are not necessarily asked about certain things, such as if they have recently taken antibiotics for another problem," Loeb says. Just because your doctor doesn't ask doesn't mean the answer doesn't matter.

Very important: If you don't feel well after the biopsy, go to the emergency room. "The main reason why complications after a biopsy can really escalate is a delay in treatment," says Loeb. *If you have any fever or chills after biopsy, go to the ER.* Don't be stoic. Don't call and leave a message on the doctor's answering machine and sit home and wait until the next day for someone to call you back. "You don't want to do that. A biopsy infection has the potential to be serious, so go to the ER, tell them about your procedure, about recent exposure to antibiotics, and if you've been hospitalized recently or had another medical procedure. These are the kinds of situations where you may have been exposed to other bacteria." *If you are unable to urinate, you should also go to the ER. Although it is common to have a few drops of blood or even to pass a blood clot in the urine (see page 127), if you have significant bleeding (see below), go to the ER.* But be assured: In the vast majority of men, infection never happens, and complications are minimal.

Bleeding

The urethra, the tube that carries urine from the bladder out of the body, runs right through the prostate (see fig. 1.2). It is very common for a man who has had his prostate biopsied to notice a little bit of blood in his urine immediately afterward. You also may notice traces of blood in the ejaculate, sometimes for several months after the biopsy. Don't let this scare you. The prostate is like a sponge, riddled with tiny ducts, and any bleeding caused by the biopsy can seep into its many nooks and crannies. This blood turns brown with age, and although it's unpleasant, it is no cause for concern, and it absolutely does not signal some turn for the worse in your cancer. It's just old, dried-up blood.

There's a different type of bleeding that can occur during the biopsy, and although this, too, is rare, it can also be serious and require immediate attention. If a man has large hemorrhoids and the biopsy needle inadvertently punctures one of these veins, it can cause significant rectal bleeding and may necessitate another procedure on the spot—sewing up or tying off the broken vein to stop the bleeding. After the procedure, you may have a few spots of blood in the stool, but this is usually not serious and will go away on its own.

Temporary Erectile Dysfunction (ED)

A much rarer complication after biopsy is erectile dysfunction (ED). Some men have reported that after their biopsy, their erections are not as strong as they were before the procedure; rarely, a man will even experience impotence. If this happens, it is most likely because the biopsy led to some inflammation around the neurovascular bundles (for more on these, see chapter 8). *This is temporary, because the nerves are still there and still intact, and there should be a full recovery of sexual function once the bruised nerves heal.* Again, this is extremely rare—and most important, you should never let the fear of temporary ED keep you away from a biopsy. Urologists don't schedule biopsies lightly, and you wouldn't be getting one if your doctor didn't think you needed it.

If I Have Cancer, Will the Biopsy Spread It?

This is a very common fear. It just makes sense, doesn't it, that if you poke a hole in a wall that's holding back cancer, the cancer might escape? Doctors have worried about this, too, in many forms of cancer. But the good news is that there is no evidence this has ever happened or that it could ever happen. Think about it: Almost every cancer you can think of—breast, lung, prostate—is diagnosed by biopsy. If the biopsy itself could spread cancer, the whole concept of early diagnosis and treatment wouldn't work. But many thousands of people—all of whom had initial biopsies to confirm what they had—have been cured of cancer.

But What If Some Cancer Cells Escape into My Bloodstream?

Well, they may. In fact, the more we learn about cancer in the prostate and elsewhere, the more we understand that the circulation of cancer cells in the blood is probably a fairly common event, even in cancers that are curable. And it's not unreasonable to assume that a few more cancer cells may find their way to the bloodstream when the tumor is manipulated, as it is during a biopsy. The key is the stage of your cancer. When cancer is confined to the prostate, even if a few cells escape into the blood, they won't survive. This is because they haven't yet gotten the hang of living outside the area where they developed. But over time, cancer cells change. They get more aggressive with age, and they become, in many ways, smarter. They not only move to distant sites but have the wherewithal to thrive in these new locations as well. So there are two different issues: one is the presence of cancer cells in the blood; the other is the *survival* of these cells in distant locations. Prostate cancer cells are simply unable to live outside their normal environment until they develop this ability, called metastatic capability.

They Didn't Find Cancer: Am I Off the Hook?

Does a negative finding truly mean there's no cancer there—and if so, then why did your PSA level go up, or what was that hard lump your urologist felt during the rectal exam? No easy answers here. If something suspicious prompted the biopsy in the first place, that something is still there. Each needle biopsy samples only 1/1,000th of the prostate; if there is no nodule to aim at, it's easy to see how a tumor could be missed. One explanation for a no-show of cancer is that if a doctor can feel a tumor, that means it's hard—and sometimes, when a needle hits this hard tissue head-on, it just glances off the edge of it without actually penetrating the tumor, so no sample is taken. Alternatively, the area that felt suspicious may have been inflammation rather than cancer.

Similarly, if your PSA level is significantly higher than it should be for your age or if it's been going up more rapidly than it should, or if your free PSA level is low (see chapter 4 for PSA guidelines), it's possible that the needle biopsy simply missed the cancer. It's not uncommon for a needle biopsy to be negative *even though cancer is present*. This is called a false negative, and it can give both the urologist and the patient "a false optimism that the cancer isn't there," says Johns Hopkins pathologist Jonathan Epstein. Imagine the difficulty of trying to capture this elusive tissue in a biopsy using only a tiny needle. In some cases, it's like looking *with* a needle in a haystack.

Several tests are now available to help men decide whether and when to have a repeat biopsy. These include additional blood and urine tests (discussed in chapter 4) that can help determine your risk of having cancer. Ask your doctor about tissue tests (Confirm-MDx; see page 136) and MRI (see page 161); these can provide extra information on where a tumor might be hiding.

HOW HELPFUL ARE REPEAT BIOPSIES?

There is definitely a point of diminishing returns here. In a large study from Europe, men with PSA levels between 4 and 10 ng/ml underwent eight-core biopsies, and if cancer was not found but still suspected, they had repeat biopsies. Cancer was present in 22 percent of the men on the first attempt, in 10 percent on the second attempt, and in 5 and 4 percent, respectively, on the third and fourth attempts. Looking at the cancers discovered on the first and second biopsies, the pathologists found the tumors to be similar in volume, grade, and extent. But the cancers detected on the third and fourth go-rounds had lower stages, grades, and cancer volumes—cancers that may not have cried out for urgent detection. The biggest reason to avoid unnecessary biopsies? Your risk of experiencing a complication goes up a little bit with every biopsy. The researchers felt that a second biopsy was justified in all cases when the initial biopsy was negative. But they felt third and fourth biopsies should be done sparingly—only in men in whom there is a high suspicion of cancer.

In a repeat biopsy, more samples should be taken, and the search for elusive cancer should broaden to include out-of-the-way locations, such as the transition zone, where BPH occurs, and up near the top of the prostate (in the anterior or lateral part; see fig. 1.3), where a needle would not normally go. The American Urological Association and Society of Abdominal Radiology both recommend that MRI should be considered before any repeat biopsy. This can provide more specific guidance on where to look for cancer and improve the chances of finding a significant prostate cancer.

Interpreting the Biopsy Findings

What "Atypical" Means

Is a biopsy ever just negative? Yes, often the pathologist will state that no cancer is seen, that everything that was biopsied was benign. That's called a negative biopsy (although you should still seek a second opinion; see page 145). However, there are two other diagnoses that sound like cancer is not present, but that can be misleading. The first is a word that pathologists love: *atypical*. Atypical means the cells can't definitely be called cancerous, but then again, cancer can't be ruled out with certainty. In other words, *atypical* means "maybe." (This finding is also known as ASAP, for "atypical small acinar proliferation," or as "atypical glands suspicious for carcinoma.") It also means two other things: You should have your slides reviewed by a pathologist who is an expert in prostate cancer to be sure that cancer isn't present. And if that pathologist concurs that it is atypical, you need a repeat biopsy within six months. (For more on getting a second opinion from a pathologist, see page 145.)

What If It's PIN?

As any pathologist will tell you, diagnosing prostate cancer is like trying not to fail a particularly tough multiple-choice test—the kind with bewildering answer options like "All of the above" and "Other." This brings us to another wrinkle in the ambiguous world of needle biopsies: *prostatic intraepithelial neoplasia* (PIN). If you have it, you're not alone: every year, an estimated fifty to seventy thousand men are told their biopsy shows this finding.

What *is* PIN? That's a good question, and the answer has just changed. PIN is so often found along with cancer that, just a few years ago, we believed that if PIN was found on a needle biopsy, a man needed another biopsy because the cancer was just missed—that the needle had found Tweedledee but somehow missed Tweedledum. Like cancer itself, PIN has its own distinct patterns—low-grade and high-grade. It is generally believed that low-grade PIN is insignificant. High-grade PIN, however, may not be. Some men with high-grade PIN develop prostate cancer, and some do not.

"For many years, we thought high-grade PIN represented a precursor of prostate cancer," says William G. Nelson, director of the Sidney Kimmel Comprehensive Cancer Center at Johns Hopkins. "Thus, a diagnosis of high-grade PIN was unsettling for both the patient and the physician." Just to make sure cancer wasn't there, "often men with high-grade PIN were subjected to a second biopsy, and some of the men were indeed found to have cancer."

Because nobody really knew what PIN was, and with the hope that it might be reversible, over the last decade several clinical trials were undertaken to see "whether PIN could be intercepted and prevented from progressing to cancer." Scientists, including Nelson, studied dietary components including green tea catechins, lycopene from tomatoes and other fruits and vegetables, selenium, and vitamins. "Unfortunately, the numbers of men ultimately found to have prostate cancer were unaffected by any intervention."

If your biopsy shows the presence of extensive amounts of high-grade PIN, your urologist will probably want to do a repeat biopsy—although, as Johns Hopkins urologic pathologist Angelo De Marzo notes, "other considerations such as prostate imaging, urine tests, and PSA and related blood tests should be taken into account," as well.

The current National Comprehensive Cancer Center (NCCN) guidelines are that men who have PIN in more than two biopsy specimens should have a repeat biopsy within six months. Men with only one or two spots of PIN should continue to have close monitoring with PSA and prostate exams.

ON THE HORIZON: MORE ACCURATE BIOPSY

Thanks to multiparametric MRI and the ability to fuse the images obtained with ultrasound imaging, doctors have an unprecedented look inside the prostate. It's not as good as it needs to be yet, but it's much better than it was.

"If you think about breast cancer," says Johns Hopkins urologic pathologist Angelo De Marzo, "you never make the diagnosis other than by *sticking a needle into a lesion that somebody felt or saw by imaging*. But in prostate cancer, most diagnoses are made by sticking a needle *blindly* into something we can't see or feel. Prostate cancer is the only cancer where you are systematically making the diagnosis in a blinded way. That's not done with any other cancer: every other cancer, you can see or feel."

No one wants unnecessary biopsies. They are painful and costly, and the risk of infection increases with each one. Thus, De Marzo suggests, "After an inconclusive biopsy, the next step may be to do a multiparametric MRI first and then do another biopsy based on whether the imaging is suspicious or if it's warranted by other clinical tests such as PSA, PCA3, or some of the newer PSA tests such as PHI or 4K."

Next, we need molecular tests, and some of those are already here.

For example, the ConfirmMDx test uses leftover tissue in negative biopsy cores to help determine whether a repeat biopsy is needed. Studies done so far "look promising as a way of reducing unnecessary repeat biopsies," says De Marzo.

If there is a diagnosis of cancer, certain molecular markers can be used on prostate tissue samples to help predict "upgrading"–the presence of higher-grade cancer. These include:

PTEN

PTEN is a type of gene whose job description is "tumor suppressor." It helps prevent the out-of-control cell growth that can lead to cancer. "It acts like the brakes on a car for cancer cells," says De Marzo, whose laboratory has been studying this gene's loss in prostate cancer for a decade. But cancer doesn't like brakes; it wants to go fast. In about half of all lethal prostate tumors, PTEN is knocked out.

As you might expect, when this happens–think of a bunch of rowdy high school kids having a wild party when someone's parents go out of town–cancer cells behave more aggressively. "The loss of PTEN leads to uncontrolled cancer cell growth and the prevention of cancer cell death," says De Marzo. Normally, in the cycle of life of all cells, new cells are born and others die; this keeps the population in check. In cancer, many cells that should die stop dying. "PTEN is one of the few genes whose loss has been consistently associated with aggressive prostate cancer."

PTEN loss is a powerful predictor of which prostate tumors are likely to recur or metastasize. In the past, it has been expensive and cumbersome for scientists to try to measure this. Thanks to a novel antibody that was tested and validated extensively by De Marzo's laboratory, this may soon change. The new test, called a PTEN IHC test, is less expensive, faster, and much easier for pathologists to interpret.

Let's take a moment here to give you yet another alphabet soup–sounding name, knowing full well that you've probably had it up to here with such abbreviations. This one's worth remembering: IHC. It stands for "immunohistochemistry," and it's a type of test that involves using antibodies to "stain" cells in a highly specific way. With IHC tests, certain antibodies–think of tiny heat-seeking missiles targeting a plane–attach themselves to key markers on cells. Have you ever used a highlighter to mark important passages in a textbook? It's the same idea; molecules are "lit up," showing things pathologists couldn't see before.

De Marzo's IHC test does this for PTEN, and it will be available for widespread routine use soon. In studies led by pathologist Tamara Lotan, a colleague of De Marzo's at Johns Hopkins, scientists discovered a strong correlation between the loss of PTEN and the signs of *aggressive prostate cancer*. In other research, Lotan, De Marzo, and their colleagues found that PTEN loss correlated with *faster recurrences* after radical prostatectomy.

Lotan, along with De Marzo and Hopkins pathologist Jonathan Epstein, has found that the PTEN test can help identify an important subtype of noninvasive tumor called *intraductal carcinoma of the prostate*. Intraductal cancers spread in ducts within the prostate and don't venture outside the gland, but they keep bad company: they are linked to highly aggressive and often deadly invasive prostate cancers. Intraductal cancers are often difficult for pathologists to diagnose under the microscope, but Lotan has shown that these tumors have almost always lost PTEN, and this finding may help pathologists "better recognize these tumors and identify men who are at risk for developing metastases and lethal prostate cancer."

Also using the new assay, De Marzo and his colleagues have established a timetable of what happens in many prostate cancers on the genetic level–key molecular changes that can pinpoint precisely how prostate cancer develops and progresses to become a lethal disease. "We showed that PTEN loss happens after the fusion of two genes, TMPRSS2 and ERG," says De Marzo. (This fusion occurs in about half of all prostate cancers in Caucasian men, but is not as common in men of African ancestry.)

The Hopkins scientists hope the test for PTEN loss will become an important part of the diagnostic arsenal. Say a needle biopsy shows that a man apparently has low-risk cancer. Does he need treatment right away? When PTEN loss is present in low-grade prostate cancer, it strongly indicates that higher-grade cancer is lurking nearby. Men whose prostate biopsies show loss of PTEN are "significantly more likely to harbor tumors at radical prostatectomy that are higher-grade than those without a loss of PTEN," says De Marzo.

Other Genetic Tests

Prostate cancer lags behind breast cancer in the widespread use of genetic tests—and more importantly, in treatment that's based on those findings. For example, a test called Oncotype DX, for women with lymph node–negative, estrogen receptor–positive breast cancer, can help tell which women can safely avoid chemotherapy. "If you could take a test and know that you have cancer that is not going to be aggressive, wouldn't you want to do it?"

"We aren't quite there yet," De Marzo says, but he believes such tests are coming.

Making Sense of the Gleason Score

Under a microscope, prostate cancer is a mess. Imagine some work of modern art, a painting with countless shades of gray—some nearly white, some nearly black, most subtle variations of shades in the middle. This is prostate cancer—a hodgepodge, a mixed-up batch of cells that range from almost normal looking to are so poorly differentiated and obviously diseased that they could never be considered normal.

The concept here is known as heterogeneity, and it's one of the most frustrating aspects in determining how serious a man's prostate cancer is. A pathologist looks at cores of tissue taken in a needle biopsy, in which cells from one part of the prostate may look one way and those from another part may look completely different. So vexing is this, in fact, that for years, pathologists felt that it was impossible to classify, or grade, prostate cancer cells at all.

Then Donald F. Gleason did what nobody else was able to do: he made sense out of these cells. For years, Gleason, the reference pathologist for the Veterans Administration Cooperative Urological Research Group, studied thousands of prostate cancer biopsies. Gradually, he was able to identify five specific patterns of cancer cell architecture that could be seen under a low-powered microscope (see fig. 5.2). Basically, Gleason said you can't make sense of every

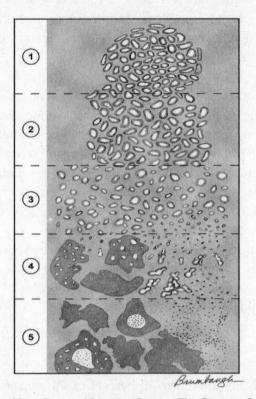

FIGURE 5.2 The Many Faces of Prostate Cancer: The Gleason Scoring System

This is prostate cancer—a hodgepodge, a mixed-up batch of cells that range from the almost normal looking (pattern 1) to so poorly differentiated and obviously diseased that they could never be considered normal (pattern 5). The Gleason system of evaluating prostate cancer is based on these five specific patterns of cancer-cell architecture. Pathologists add the number of the most common pattern to the number of the second most common pattern and use this score—such as 3 + 3 = 6, or 3 + 4 = 7—to assess the aggressiveness of prostate cancer. Recently, these scores have been reclassified into grade groups 1 to 5. Image courtesy Jonathan Epstein.

single cancerous cell, but there seem to be some identifiable patterns here. He labeled each cancer pattern 1 through 5. Which pattern was the most common? Which pattern was the second most common? Gleason figured out that if he added those two types together, this score, now known worldwide as the Gleason score, would be a pretty accurate way to determine how aggressive the cancer cells are.

Gleason's original system had more than twenty-five different possible combinations. That has recently been simplified into a new system, called "grade groups," by pathologist Jonathan Epstein at Johns Hopkins. The World Health Organization (WHO) has accepted Epstein's new system, and your hospital may already be using it. Here's what you need to know:

- **Grade Group I:** Gleason score 3 + 3 = 6. Low-grade cancer. Gleason 6 is as good as it gets. Epstein describes cancer in Grade Group 1 as having "an indolent nature, and no metastatic potential." Many men in this category can safely choose active surveillance.
- **Grade Group 2:** Gleason score 3 + 4 = 7. Intermediate grade. Some men in this category may also be candidates for active surveillance, or for radiation therapy instead of surgery, depending on their age, extent of cancer, and general health.
- **Grade Group 3:** Gleason score 4 + 3 = 7. The score is the same, but there is a difference—more pattern 4 than 3—and this cancer needs to be treated with surgery or radiation.
- **Grade Group 4:** Gleason score 8.
- **Grade Group 5:** Gleason scores 9–10.

Gleason scores 8–10 tumors are high-grade. Fortunately, these are seen only in about 8 to 10 percent of all biopsies. In the past, Gleason scores 8–10 were combined, but Epstein separated them because they have significantly different prognoses.

What does all this mean? In an ideal world—one where men start getting screened for prostate cancer in their forties—prostate cancer is caught early. Let's say a fifty-eight-year-old man who otherwise is in very good health is diagnosed with Gleason 6 disease. "If he has surgery, and we look at his prostate and there's nothing but Gleason 6 cancer, we know that man is effectively cured," says Angelo De Marzo. One recent Johns Hopkins study conducted by Epstein and colleagues showed that out of 14,000 men who had surgery and were found to have Gleason 6 cancer confined to the prostate, "zero of those 14,000 men had lymph node metastases. *Virtually no one at Hopkins has ever died of prostate cancer if he had Gleason 3 + 3 cancer that was confined to the gland,*" which means there was "no extraprostatic extension, or seminal vesicle invasion *on the pathology of the removed prostate*." (The seminal vesicles are near to the prostate, and sometimes when prostate cancer expands, it reaches them.)

In fact, some doctors have been questioning whether Gleason 3 + 3 disease should even be called cancer. Not so fast, says De Marzo, for one very important reason: "The malignant potential seems like it's not there, but there are lots of reasons to keep calling it cancer, and the biggest one is that if men have Gleason 6 on their biopsy, and you take out their prostate, between 20 and 40 percent of them will actually turn out to have a higher-grade tumor found in the radical prostatectomy specimen. The biopsy missed it."

Another important reason is uncertainty: Does the cancer change over time? Say a man has Gleason 6 cancer on a biopsy, and a year later, Gleason 7 is found. You might think, "Well, that Gleason 7 was there all the time, and it was just missed." But are you sure? Nobody knows the answer to this question for certain. "There are some suggestions that cancer grade can progress," says De Marzo. "Theoretically, it can happen. We just don't know what fraction of the high-grade cancers started out as low-grade."

It's like those drawings you may have seen of the "Evolution of Man," where there's an ape, then a Neanderthal-type knuckle-dragger, then a basic human. Does high-grade cancer spring forth as a Gleason 9? Or did it start out as something that's easier to treat?

In the future, De Marzo believes, we will be able to make much better-informed decisions. Some blood tests using molecular tools can help determine whether cancer shows aggressive potential; De Marzo anticipates that urine tests will prove even more helpful. "The prostate is directly connected to the urinary system. I think urine will eventually beat blood as a test in a few years." One such test, discovered by William Isaacs at Johns Hopkins, is called PCA3. The basic PSA test is prostate-specific, but not cancer-specific. PCA3 is much more cancer-specific. Although it is not meant to replace the PSA test, it can be used as another test to help determine if a repeat biopsy is needed. If the PCA3 score is low, the odds of a positive biopsy are lower.

Molecular-based tests won't replace the Gleason grading system, De Marzo notes. But these tests, combined with better imaging, will add to it—eventually, doctors hope, reducing unnecessary biopsies, making biopsies smarter by targeting where to stick the needle, highlighting aggressive cancer that needs to be treated, and helping give peace of mind to men who truly have indolent cancer that may not ever need to be treated.

Nationally, "there's a big variability in the expertise of the pathologist reading prostate biopsies," says De Marzo. "It can be very difficult. But it's not good to have a situation where not all patients get their biopsy read by a true expert." Molecular tests will help make sure that "everyone gets the same answer. You can't argue with the future of molecular testing. It will help level the playing field."

Grade Group	Gleason Score
1	3 + 3
2	3 + 4
3	4 + 3
4	4 + 4
5	9 or 10

The Gleason score ranks the amount of *differentiation* seen in the cancer cells (see fig. 5.2). Basically, the pathologist determines how clear-cut the cells' structures and edges are. The architecture of normal, well-differentiated cells involves distinct, clearly defined borders and clear centers. "They're like little round doughnuts," says Epstein. When cancer becomes poorly differentiated, the cells seem to melt together into malignant clumps. These cancers are the most aggressive. They run rampant, sweeping through nearby tissue and launching missiles into distant sites in the body, no longer respecting boundaries—their own or those of other cells. Well-differentiated cancers, in contrast, tend to progress very slowly.

Cancers with a high grade are more likely to be margin-positive (to have cancer that has penetrated the prostate wall to a point where it can't all be removed in surgery; more on this in chapter 7), and more likely to have spread to the seminal vesicles. With a high grade, there's also a greater likelihood of cancer spreading to the lymph nodes.

How Prostate Cancer Spreads

First, of course, it grows inside the prostate. (Most—about 72 percent of cancers—begin in the peripheral zone, 20 percent start in the transition zone, and 8 percent start in the central zone. For more on the prostate's zones, see chapter 1.) It reaches and then penetrates the prostate wall, also called the capsule. Then it starts to creep along the wall of the prostate, heading north toward the seminal vesicles. As the tumor penetrates the capsule of the prostate, it rarely extends more than one or two millimeters beyond it. That's the reason that men with capsular penetration can still be cured by surgery. In advanced cases, the tumor ultimately extends into the bladder, the urethra, and the pelvic side walls; however, it hardly ever reaches directly into the rectum. Biologically, for whatever reason—certain growth factors, perhaps, or supporting structures—prostate cancer cells seem to need the particular environment that spawned them. However, once the tumor has matured enough to live on its own beyond the prostate—that is, once it can grow around the seminal vesicles—it is more likely to have spread to distant sites. That's why the finding of cancer cells around the seminal vesicles is so important. It is a sign that this cancer can survive outside the environment of the prostate. When doctors speak of distant metastases of prostate cancer, they generally mean it has hitched a ride via the bloodstream or lymph system to the lymph nodes (channels that run throughout the body), the bones—the spine, ribs, or pelvic bones—or the lungs.

Note: Prostate cancers don't always spread in an orderly fashion, like a marching band in a parade, from point A to point B to point C—from the prostate to the seminal vesicles to the lymph nodes and beyond. Sometimes, especially when there is high-grade disease, even though the cancer is still confined within the prostate, a few cells can invade blood vessels or the lymph system. If the cells have become sophisticated enough to survive on their own, outside the main tumor, they can spread the cancer to a distant site. This is why, even though a cancer may be confined within the prostate with no obvious cells outside the organ, distant metastases can still develop.

What About Perineural Invasion?

As cancers grow, they compress normal tissue, looking for elbow room—spaces with less resistance, where they can spread. It just so happens that nerves are usually surrounded by some empty space. For cancer, this is the real estate equivalent of a nice suburban lot with a big backyard. Thus, it's not uncommon to find prostate cancer in the spaces around the nerves; this is called perineural invasion. Because the nerves are most common close to the surface of the prostate, the finding of perineural invasion on a biopsy suggests that the cancer is close to the edge of the prostate and may well have penetrated the capsule. However—this is important to keep in mind—*cancer that has penetrated the capsule can still be cured*. This makes perineural invasion a paradoxical finding, because although men with perineural invasion are more likely to have capsular penetration, they may still be cured with local treatment (surgery or external-beam radiation therapy) alone.

It was previously thought that nerve-sparing surgery should not be performed on the same side as the perineural invasion. However, this has turned out not to be an issue because of a fine distinction: the tumor is surrounding the *nerves to the prostate*, not the nerves responsible for erections. New York University urologist Stacy Loeb studied men with perineural invasion who underwent a radical prostatectomy at Hopkins, and her findings show good news. Although these men had more aggressive cancer, the presence of perineural invasion by itself was not a predictor that their cancer would come back, and the nerve-sparing procedure had no effect on their risk of developing rising PSA after surgery. However, another study from Johns Hopkins on men who received radiation showed that men with perineural invasion on their biopsy had a higher chance of PSA failure (an increase in PSA levels following treatment, indicating that the cancer may have returned) and prostate cancer–related death. Similar results have been confirmed by other groups. For this reason, at Hopkins, men with perineural invasion on their prostate cancer biopsies who choose radiation therapy typically receive treatments that include the addition of hormones and increased radiation dosages to the prostate.

Rare Forms of Prostate Cancer

Almost all—95 percent—cancers of the prostate are of a type called adenocarcinoma. These are cancers that form in the tiny glands within the prostate (see fig. 1.2). But there are some rare exceptions. One of these is small-cell carcinoma. This form of cancer develops in different cells, called neuroendocrine cells, in the prostate. Small-cell carcinoma of the prostate is very similar to small-cell carcinoma of the lung. It grows rapidly and is very difficult to cure. The main treatment is chemotherapy (discussed in chapter 12). It is rare for small-cell carcinoma to be diagnosed initially; usually, it's found in patients who were diagnosed with "regular" prostate cancer (adenocarcinoma) that was not controlled by surgery, radiation, or chemotherapy. In these men, cancer typically comes back as a large pelvic mass or as metastases to such organs as the liver. The tip-off to this diagnosis is that small-cell carcinoma does not make PSA. Thus, if a man has a large, local cancer and a low PSA level, he should be evaluated for small-cell carcinoma.

Another rare form of prostate cancer is transitional-cell carcinoma. (Note: This is different from cancer that is found in the prostate's transition zone.) This cancer arises from the prostatic ducts and the prostatic urethra, the stretch of urethra that runs through the prostate. It is the same kind of cancer often seen in men with bladder cancer—which means that if this diagnosis is made, a man should be checked for bladder cancer as well—and the treatment is often directed at removing both the prostate and bladder.

BIOPSY: WHY YOU SHOULD GET A SECOND OPINION

You're a pathologist staring at cancer cells under a microscope—just a few tiny cores of tissue—and a man's life may depend on what you have to say about it. You make the call: your word is a huge part of the treatment decision making. So think, think—what about those funny-looking cells over there? Is it cancer?

A prostate biopsy can be a pathologist's worst nightmare. "Of all biopsies, prostate biopsies are probably the hardest," explains Johns Hopkins pathologist Jonathan Epstein, who is world-renowned for his expertise in judging prostate cells. "You're dealing with such a limited amount of tissue, and cancers tend to creep around the benign gland" rather than forming a solid mass. Imagine a Tootsie Roll wrapped in paper. The cancer is like the paper, a veneer over an expanse of healthy tissue. And the veneer is often maddeningly ambiguous. So not only can the hollow-core biopsy needle overshoot and miss the cancer, but the cancer cells it does get don't always match the pictures in the textbooks.

One result of this is the biopsy being labeled atypical—a diagnosis that appears in about 5 percent of biopsies at most institutions, says Epstein. "Basically, what that means is that a pathologist will see something that he thinks could be cancer but is not comfortable calling cancer." For many patients, the next step is having a repeat biopsy—and the value of this is often questionable, he says. "The problem is, in about 20 percent of cases, the biopsy can miss cancer—so even if it's negative, it doesn't mean the patient *doesn't* have cancer; in fact, the cancer can be extensive. We've seen some missed entirely. They were called totally benign, yet they were cancer." So the first step, before you brace yourself for a repeat biopsy, should be to get a second opinion on the "atypical" diagnosis. (This is easier than it sounds and can be done by mail; your doctor simply sends your pathology slides to another pathologist to see if the diagnosis is the same.)

Another problem Epstein has found is that many pathologists seem just as likely to overdiagnose cancer. "There are many mimickers of prostate cancer under the microscope, and people not as familiar with prostate biopsies can diagnose cancer when it's not." About 1.5 percent—six to eight men—of the patients who come to the Brady Urological Institute each year with a diagnosis of prostate cancer have been misdiagnosed. "We switch the diagnosis. We say, 'This is not cancer; this is benign.'"

Perhaps the best option in the case of tricky diagnoses, says Epstein, is to have the slides sent to an expert. "About 70 to 80 percent of the time, it can be resolved as being definitively benign or definitely cancer." Even biopsies that seem straightforward deserve another look. "We recommend getting a second opinion before anybody undergoes any form of treatment," says Epstein. "It's just as important as getting a second opinion for surgery or radiation. You could have the best surgeon in the world, but if you don't have the right pathology, you could have the wrong thing done for you."

On this point, Epstein is blunt: "We have done numerous studies showing the reproducibility of Gleason scores" at academic medical centers and in the general pathology community, looking at the Gleason score based on a biopsy and then comparing it to the actual specimen removed during surgery. Although the "before" and "after" Gleason scores are usually in excellent agreement at academic medical centers, "by and large, the Gleason grading that's performed in the community is disappointing. All across the map, it doesn't correlate with what you see in a radical prostatectomy. People are having decisions made—surgery or radiation, or watchful waiting—based in part on a Gleason grade when it's not accurate."

In conjunction with the Association of Directors of Anatomic and Surgical Pathology, Epstein has developed a series of frequently asked questions (FAQs) to help patients understand their pathology reports, which you can find at www.adasp.org/FAQs.

Finally, sarcoma of the prostate is very rare. These tumors arise from the stroma, the smooth muscle and connective tissue within the prostate, and they can be very large at the time of diagnosis. Treatment, as with "regular" prostate cancer, is based on the extent of the tumor. Rarely, other types of cancer, such as gastrointestinal stromal tumors, involve the prostate. Because these tumor types are so uncommon, men who have them should be referred to a center that specializes in treating the rarest forms of cancer.

The Diagnosis Is Cancer: What Next?

Do you need further tests? That depends. At this point, you and your doctor have much of the information you need to determine the extent of your cancer and to decide on a course of treatment. The Gleason score tells you the kind of cancer cells you have. The next step is to estimate the extent—how far these cells may have spread. This is called determining the *clinical stage* of the cancer (or staging the cancer). Is cancer confined to the prostate? Or has it spread, and if it has, how far?

The Stages of Prostate Cancer

The staging of prostate cancer used to be based on the Whitmore-Jewett staging system, which had four basic categories, ranging from cancer too small to be felt to cancer that had metastasized to the lymph nodes and bone. However, it became clear that more refinements were needed for localized cancer categories, and for this reason, the International Union Against Cancer and the American Joint Committee on Cancer have promoted the use of the TNM Classification of Malignant Tumors system. (This system is used in many forms of cancer.) "T" represents the local extent of the tumor, "N" indicates the presence of metastases to the lymph nodes, and "M" indicates distant metastases. The T stage is divided into eight categories *depending on whether the cancer can be felt (an area of firmness is often referred to as a nodule) during a rectal examination*—and if so, how extensive it is. If your prostate feels normal on examination, you have T1 disease; the T2 category describes cancer that can be felt in half of one lobe, one entire lobe, or both lobes. Note: Many men, and

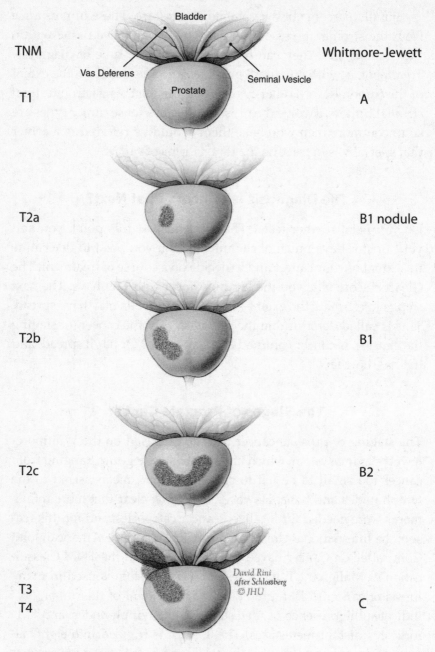

FIGURE 5.3   The Stages of Prostate Cancer

This illustration, using both the TNM and the Whitmore-Jewett staging systems, shows prostate cancer in all its stages, ranging from cancer that's too small to be felt to cancer that has spread to the seminal vesicles.

even some doctors, confuse bilateral biopsies with bilateral palpable disease. If your cancer is present on biopsy in both lobes of the prostate but nothing can be felt on examination, you have T1 disease.

TABLE 5.1

TNM STAGING SYSTEM

Stage	Description
T1a	Not palpable in a rectal exam; found incidentally, when benign tissue is removed by a TUR; 5 percent or less of the removed tissue is cancerous
T1b	Not palpable; found incidentally, but greater than 5 percent of the tissue removed by the TUR is cancerous
T1c	Not palpable; identified by needle biopsy because of elevated PSA level
T2a	Palpable; involves less than half of one lobe of the prostate
T2b	Palpable; involves more than half of one lobe but not both lobes
T2c	Palpable; involves both lobes
T3, T4	Palpable; penetrates the wall of the prostate and/or involves the seminal vesicles
N+	Has spread to the lymph nodes
M+	Has spread to bone

Where Do I Stand?

Is the cancer so small that it may not need to be treated? Is it bigger than that but still localized within the prostate and curable? Or has it spread to a distant site? By themselves, the various tests you've had aren't enough to paint the whole picture. For example, the rectal exam is not able to pick up microscopic cancer that has spread to the prostate wall and beyond. Because of this, *the rectal exam tends to underestimate the stage of cancer.* Studies have found that a significant number of cancers initially staged as T2b end up being classified as higher because the cancer has invaded the seminal vesicles or lymph nodes. One reason for this is that the rectal exam is subjective; it depends on the experience and perceptiveness of the doctor performing it. Another is that the rectal exam can give information *only* about the prostate gland itself—and not even all of it, at that. And it certainly can't tell anything about the nearby pelvic lymph nodes or bones. Also, if a man has had other surgery on the prostate—a TUR, for instance, for BPH—this can cause the prostate to feel different on a rectal exam.

What About PSA?

This section is very important. Please read this and keep it in mind as you are talking with your doctor about your treatment options and potential for cure.

We know a high PSA level can signal the presence of cancer. As always, though, PSA is tricky. As a tumor gets bigger, the PSA level generally goes up. However, as the tumor grows, it can eventually be overrun by more malignant, poorly differentiated cancer cells that have a higher Gleason score. These poorly differentiated cells are different from normal prostate cells: they make less PSA. In fact, these cancer cells elevate PSA less per gram of tissue than well-differentiated cancer cells do—which means that as cancers grow, the PSA level doesn't always go up in a directly corresponding way. That's why the PSA level can be normal even when cancer has spread to the seminal vesicles or pelvic lymph nodes, or it can be higher than expected in men with cancer that's confined to the prostate. PSA levels do not accurately estimate the growth of cancer. Thus, the true meaning of a PSA level can't be interpreted without knowing the Gleason score. As you will see in the Han tables (Table 5.2), for any given PSA level, your chance of curability depends on your Gleason score or Gleason Grade group.

In the past, before surgery we tried to estimate the chance of cure by predicting the extent of cancer that we would find during the radical prostatectomy—the *estimated* pathologic stage—using the Partin tables. However, once we had the actual data on curability, we learned that the Partin tables *underestimated* the chance of cure. For example, if a man has prostate cancer that is non-palpable (T1c), Gleason 3 + 4 (Grade Group 2), and a PSA between 4 and 6, the Partin tables would predict that the risk of tumor outside the prostate was 30 percent. But when patients like this were followed for ten years, *91 percent were cured*. Why? Because when prostate cancer extends outside the prostate, it rarely travels more than two or three millimeters away from the capsule, or wall of the prostate, and *this amount of tissue is normally removed with surgery*. For this reason, we no longer use the Partin tables to estimate curability. However, you will often encounter radiation oncologists who will try to discourage you from having surgery based on this flawed reasoning. If this happens, please show them this section of the book.

The Han Tables

Once we had long-term data on PSA levels in men who underwent surgery, Johns Hopkins urologist Misop Han developed these tables (see Table 5.2) based on more than two thousand consecutive men who underwent radical prostatectomy between 1982 and 1999 and estimated the likelihood that a man's PSA level will be undetectable ten years after surgery. Because men in recent years have better results (because of earlier diagnosis and important surgical refinements), these tables have been corrected to reflect the improvement in survival that comes from diagnosing cancer earlier.

THE HAN TABLES

Using PSA, Gleason score, and clinical stage, these tables predict the likelihood that a man will have an undetectable PSA level ten years after surgery and therefore give a very clear picture of the probability of cure. The numbers in parentheses indicate that only 5 percent of the patients fall on either side of those limits.

How to Use These Tables

Find your clinical stage, biopsy Gleason score (GG; from the left column) and your PSA level (from the top row) obtained before surgery. The intersection of the two is your probability of having an undetectable PSA level (less than 0.2 ng/ml) ten years after surgery. In the parentheses next to each percentage is the 95 percent confidence interval. A broader range means that this percentage is less certain than a narrower range.

TABLE 5.2

PERCENTAGE OF MEN WITH UNDETECTABLE PSA LEVELS AT 10 YEARS FOLLOWING RADICAL RETROPUBIC PROSTATECTOMY FOR STAGE T1C DISEASE

T1c Cancer	PSA 0–4	PSA 4.1–10	PSA 10.1–20	PSA >20
Biopsy Gleason score 5 (GG1)	99 (95–100)	97 (91–99)	94 (80–98)	87 (59–96)
Biopsy Gleason score 6 (GG1)	97 (91–99)	95 (83–98)	90 (69–97)	81 (47–94)
Biopsy Gleason score 3 + 4 (GG2)	95 (83–98)	91 (72–97)	84 (54–95)	73 (33–91)
Biopsy Gleason score 4 + 3 (GG3)	89 (67–97)	83 (53–95)	74 (36–92)	62 (18–88)
Biopsy Gleason score 8–10 (GG4-5)	79 (40–94)	71 (30–91)	61 (18–87)	50 (06–84)

PERCENTAGE OF MEN WITH UNDETECTABLE PSA LEVELS AT 10 YEARS FOLLOWING RADICAL RETROPUBIC PROSTATECTOMY FOR STAGE T2A DISEASE

T2a Cancer	PSA 0–4	PSA 4.1–10	PSA 10.1–20	PSA >20
Biopsy Gleason score 5 (GG1)	98 (94–100)	96 (88–99)	92 (74–98)	83 (50–95)
Biopsy Gleason score 6 (GG1)	97 (89–99)	93 (79–98)	87 (61–96)	75 (37–92)
Biopsy Gleason score 3 + 4 (GG2)	93 (78–98)	88 (64–96)	79 (44–93)	65 (22–89)
Biopsy Gleason score 4 + 3 (GG3)	86 (58–96)	78 (43–93)	67 (26–89)	53 (10–84)
Biopsy Gleason score 8–10 (GG4-5)	72 (30–92)	63 (20–88)	63 (20–88)	39 (03–78)

PERCENTAGE OF MEN WITH UNDETECTABLE PSA LEVELS AT 10 YEARS FOLLOWING RADICAL RETROPUBIC PROSTATECTOMY FOR STAGE T2B/C DISEASE

T2B/C Cancer	PSA 0–4	PSA 4.1–10	PSA 10.1–20	PSA > 20
Biopsy Gleason score 5 (GG1)	98 (92–99)	95 (83–99)	89 (66–97)	77 (38–93)
Biopsy Gleason score 6 (GG1)	95 (85–99)	91 (72–97)	83 (51–95)	68 (25–90)
Biopsy Gleason score 3 + 4 (GG2)	90 (71–97)	84 (54–95)	73 (33–91)	57 (13–85)
Biopsy Gleason score 4 + 3 (GG3)	81 (48–94)	72 (32–91)	59 (15–86)	43 (04–80)
Biopsy Gleason score 8–10 (GG4–5)	65 (19–89)	54 (11–84)	41 (04–78)	28 (01–72)

Several other sets of data are also available to predict outcomes after treatment, including the Kattan nomograms, CAPRA score, and D'Amico risk categories. The goal behind all these is to combine multiple factors together to estimate what will happen in the future. One final note: Men who develop an elevation of PSA still benefit from the huge effect that eradicating the primary tumor has on prolonging their survival (see page 180).

What Do I Do with All This Information?

First of all, know that although these figures are as accurate as we can make them, *they are just statistics*. There are no absolutes; every man's situation is different. Thus, factors beyond cold, hard numbers can be terribly important in determining the best course of action. For many men with low-risk cancer, active surveillance is a good choice (for a discussion of this, see chapter 7). What if you're in a situation where a cure is unlikely but possible? For a man in good health who otherwise could expect to live for at least ten to fifteen more years, *the side effects of radical prostatectomy are low enough that it's worth it to attempt a cure.* For older men or men with other health problems (because radical prostatectomy, a major operation, does take a certain physical toll) who are more likely to have severe side effects from surgery and less likely to receive the same benefit, radiation is probably a better choice.

So take this information as your starting point. Consider carefully your overall health and potential longevity. Then you and your doctor can decide whether it's reasonable to select curative forms of therapy or simply to adopt a policy of active surveillance, in which the tumor is treated only after there is evidence of progression.

And finally, *whatever your finding, don't get discouraged.* Even cancer in the highest stages can be controlled and kept at bay indefinitely, sometimes for many years. *There is always hope.* Even men with cancer in their lymph nodes can live for many years clinically disease-free (without any symptoms). There is much more about this in later chapters.

Factors That May Affect Your Outlook

Age

Age is one of the most important considerations in making a decision about treatment, and it's also one of the hardest. For most of us, on the scale of unpleasant things to do, estimating how many more years we have left to live would rank right up there with having a root canal. But now is the time for you to make an honest appraisal of your general health. If you appear to have localized cancer but you've got some other significant medical problems, then it may be necessary only to keep an eye on the tumor, a treatment that's called active surveillance. You might also opt for one of the less strenuous forms of treatment. On the other hand, if your family has a history of longevity (if your parents lived into their eighties or nineties), your blood pressure is low, you don't have diabetes, you don't smoke, and you have no history of heart disease, then you may live long enough to *need* to be cured, and your cancer may be aggressive enough that it requires aggressive therapy. The National Comprehensive Cancer Network (NCCN) guidelines recommend the use of the Social Security Administration tables for estimating life expectancy, which you can find at www.ssa.gov/OACT/STATS/table4c6.html. These guidelines recommend adjusting the values, based on a man's health. A man who's in the top quartile (twenty-fifth percentile) of health should add 50 percent, and a man in the lowest quartile should subtract 50 percent. Similar tables that are specific to African American men are also available at https://www.cdc.gov/nchs/data/nvsr/nvsr65/nvsr65_08.pdf. Again, nobody—especially not the government—knows for sure how long anyone will live; these are just estimates based on data from many people.

We used to believe that prostate cancer was an "old man's disease"—rather doddering, slow to progress, and more harmless than cancer in younger men. We don't believe that anymore. Research has shown that in older men, prostate cancer is often more aggressive than it is in younger men, and it's often diagnosed at a later stage. A recent study reported the striking observation that men *diagnosed* with prostate cancer at age seventy-five or older account for 53 percent of prostate cancer deaths, despite making up only 26 percent of the population and having a higher risk of death from other causes.

Why is this? Simply because the cancer has been there longer, and because men who are diagnosed at a later age may not have undergone regular screening. As prostate tumors grow, they become more heterogeneous and poorly differentiated. They accumulate more mutations and become more aggressive. Prostate cancer generally is a slow grower. In its early stages, it can take months or even years for a tumor to double in size. Before a tumor ever gets big enough for a doctor to feel—about 1 cubic centimeter in volume—it has to double at least thirty times. But after this, it takes only about ten more doublings for prostate cancer to become fatal—when it reaches 1 kilogram in volume. Each time the tumor doubles, there are more mutations. The cancer begins to grow faster; it becomes more aggressive, and the cells learn how to live outside the comfortable environment of the prostate. *So in healthy older men, it may be wise to undertake aggressive therapy if it is likely that they will be living for many more years.*

Being of African Descent

As we have discussed, African American men are not only more likely to develop prostate cancer but also more likely to die from it. In fact, black men from any country are more prone to prostate cancer than any other men. And even though we don't understand exactly why this is, the main thing that we do understand very clearly is that *black men with prostate cancer may have a more aggressive cancer and should talk to the doctor about how to manage it best.*

Stage T1c Cancer

Of all the categories of prostate cancer, this is probably the one that's hardest to make precise predictions about, because it contains a broad spectrum of tumors—from the tiniest, which need no treatment, to some that are quite extensive. We studied nearly 1,200 men with stage T1c disease who underwent a radical prostatectomy at Johns Hopkins between 1988 and 2000. We found two major determining factors in these men: a PSA level greater than 10 ng/ml or a biopsy Gleason score of 7 or higher. In men *without* either of these risk factors, the odds of having an undetectable PSA level at ten years were 96 percent. For men who had either of these risk factors, ten years after surgery, 73 percent had an undetectable PSA level. In this study, about one-third of the men had high-risk T1c disease. Beyond this, there are two distinct subcategories of stage T1c disease.

Low-Volume T1c Cancer

In chapter 3, we discussed how a Caucasian man in the United States has a 1 in 8 chance of being diagnosed with prostate cancer during his lifetime. But there is also another very important statistic. If a man with no signs of prostate cancer is hit by a car and undergoes an autopsy, there is a 50 percent chance that a few cancer cells will be found in his prostate. These cancers are considered incidental and not likely to progress to the point where they would ever have been diagnosed—unless this man had a prostate biopsy. And that explains the problem with low-volume cancer. Maybe men who are diagnosed with it just got an autopsy before their time.

The advantage of any screening program for cancer is that it's designed to detect cancer early. The disadvantage is that some cancers may be found at such an early stage that they don't need to be treated. This can be the case in men with T1c cancer: a number of these men have low-volume cancers. Do you? And does this mean you're one of those lucky men whose cancer won't ever grow enough to cause trouble? Your PSA density or free PSA and the findings reported by the pathologist on the needle biopsy can help here. If the pathologic findings suggest that you may have a small tumor, your PSA density should not be more than 10 to 15 percent of the weight of your prostate. If it's higher, this suggests that something more than benign disease is responsible for your elevated PSA level, and that the needle biopsy just didn't find it. Similarly, if the PSA is coming from BPH, your free PSA should be high—above 15 percent. If it's less than 15 percent, then it is likely that cancer, not benign disease, is causing your PSA to rise—in which case, the cancer is probably more significant than it seems. Finally, the amount of cancer present on the biopsy is important. If fewer than three of the biopsy samples were positive for cancer, and no more than 50 percent of each biopsy core contains cancer tissue, that suggests a low-volume cancer.

If you have been diagnosed with a small cancer that is not life-threatening, you may be a candidate for watchful waiting, or active surveillance. Active surveillance, which we'll discuss more thoroughly in the next chapter, means monitoring the situation and not making a decision about treatment until it's more clear that your cancer poses a significant threat. Here are some factors that can help predict which cancer is significant and which is not. *Note: These factors apply only if the cancer is not palpable and if the biopsies have included at least six cores.*

Stage T1c Cancer Is Significant If...
It's found in three or more needle cores; or
It's present in greater than half of any one needle core; or
The Gleason score is 7 or higher (Grade Group 2 or greater); or
The PSA density is greater than 0.1 to 0.15; or
The free PSA is less than 15 percent.

Stage T1c Cancer May Not Be Significant If...
It's found in only one or two needle cores; and
It makes up less than half of each needle core; and
The Gleason score is 6 or lower (Grade Group 1); and
The PSA density is less than 0.1 to 0.15; and
The free PSA is greater than 15 percent.

The key word here is *predictive*. (Remember, any clinical stage is a prediction. The only certainty is pathologic stage.) This prediction is the best we have, based on all we know, and it's only about 75 percent accurate. This means that about 75 percent of the men who are predicted to have low-volume cancer actually are found to have it when they undergo radical prostatectomy.

What about the remaining 25 percent? The news is good: although there's more cancer, it is almost always confined to the prostate and curable. However, 25 percent is a large number of men with significant prostate cancer.

If your health is otherwise good, you expect to live at least ten years, and you decide to select active surveillance, you will need to watch this cancer like the proverbial hawk. For starters, if you did not have twelve samples taken during your biopsy, you should have a repeat biopsy to make sure there isn't more cancer than the original biopsy suggested. Even for men who had an adequate biopsy, other tests can be helpful to confirm that the staging is correct. Marker tests and MRI (discussed on page 161) can provide additional information beyond PSA, stage, and grade for men with newly diagnosed prostate cancer to help you and your doctor make the best treatment decisions. For more on this, see chapter 7.

Very High PSA

You have T1c disease, but your PSA level is through the roof. Is it still possible that you may have curable disease? There is an unusual form of prostate cancer in which men with curable disease can have very high PSAs—as high as 300 ng/ml, for example. How can this be? The cancer is in the transition zone—the site where BPH develops. This ring of tissue surrounds the urethra, and if cancer is here, it may be trapped in the center of the prostate by a thick band of smooth muscle. In this location, tumors can grow to be quite large without escaping the prostate. This is the site, too, of the low-grade Gleason tumors, as discussed above, that probably wouldn't be diagnosed if it weren't for a TUR procedure. For reasons we don't understand, tumors here are usually well differentiated, and *men with transition zone cancer can usually be cured.* How do you know if you have it? First, cancers in the transition zone are hardly ever felt during a rectal exam, because they're smack in the middle of the prostate. Second, they're hard to diagnose, and a typical patient will have undergone two or three negative biopsies before the cancer is found. And finally, the tumors are usually lower than Gleason 7 (Grade Group 2). If these criteria apply to you, you may well have curable cancer.

Transrectal Ultrasound and Staging

Most studies have found transrectal ultrasound to be a rather mediocre predictor of the presence of cancer that has penetrated the prostate's wall, or capsule, and to be downright poor in finding cancer that has reached the seminal vesicles. Most lesions that show up on ultrasound are not cancer, and most cancers are not seen on ultrasound. In two studies, only 30 percent of tumors that had spread to the seminal vesicles could be found by ultrasound. One investigation of thirty men undergoing radical prostatectomy found ultrasound's sensitivity in spotting cancer that had worked its way beyond the prostate's capsule was a lowly 5 percent. Another study, comparing ultrasound and pathological staging in 121 men, found ultrasound's overall accuracy in staging was only 66 percent—better, but still not reliable enough. And a multicenter study of 230 men found that ultrasound correctly staged 66 percent of locally advanced cancer and only 46 percent of cancers confined to the prostate.

Ultrasound's main difficulty is its inability to "see" microscopic cancer spread. So, to sum up: ultrasound's primary purpose is to guide the biopsy procedure, and no definitive decisions about a man's course of treatment should be made on the basis of ultrasound alone. Moreover, ultrasound readings shouldn't be the cause of a man's exclusion from surgery that potentially could cure his disease.

Imaging Tests for Staging Prostate Cancer

Thank goodness we have such powerful tools as the PSA blood test and the Gleason score to help us understand what we're dealing with in each man with prostate cancer. The one thing we don't have in our diagnostic workshop is the ability to see the exact extent and location of cancer within the prostate. Such imaging would make life so much simpler! For example, we wouldn't have to guess where to put the needle during the biopsy; we'd already know. And we would have a much better idea whether a man truly had a small amount of cancer in his prostate.

Who needs imaging? The NCCN recommends a CT scan of the pelvis or MRI in men diagnosed with clinical stage T3 or T4 cancer, or in men with T1–T2 disease, if their likelihood of lymph node involvement is more than 10 percent. To make this determination, go to http://urology.jhu.edu/prostate/partin_tables.php .

MRI Scan

Magnetic resonance imaging (MRI) is painless and noninvasive; it gives a three-dimensional scan of the body, producing images that are like slices of anatomy. It creates better pictures than CT scans (see below), but it's expensive and slow; the average scan takes about forty-five minutes.

The appeal of MRI is that it produces beautiful images of the prostate that can help at multiple steps in the process. MRI can be used to detect suspicious areas, graded from 1 (lowest) to 5 (highest), using a scoring system called PI-RADS. These lesions can then be used to target the biopsy.

MRI can be used for staging in men with prostate cancer, including whether the tumor extends beyond the prostate or involves the lymph nodes. MRI also shows the bones in the pelvic region. However, MRI cannot accurately predict the local extent of a tumor and patients need to be careful in placing too much confidence in the findings. The NCCN guidelines do not recommend it for that purpose.

Although being inside an MRI machine has been described as "like being a sardine in a can," fewer than 5 percent of patients actually become claustrophobic. To help prevent this, some hospitals play soothing music while patients are being imaged. Although it's easier said than done, it really helps to relax, close your eyes, and, if you can, try to go to sleep. The newest generations of MRI machines are moving away from the torpedo-tube design and are more open.

CT Scan

Getting a computed tomography (CT) scan basically means having a circular series of X-rays taken by a machine that goes around the body. A computer then puts the pictures together, generating images that, as in MRI, are like slices of anatomy. The CT tube in which a patient lies is bigger than that of an MRI machine, so claustrophobia is not such a problem, and this technology is faster than MRI. However, the pictures aren't terribly good. (One way doctors can enhance CT images is to give patients an intravenous dye; however, this can cause an allergic reaction in some people.)

When it comes to imaging the prostate, CT has turned out to be something of a dud. It can't visualize cancer in the prostate, and it's not very good at showing cancer that has spread beyond the prostate. This is mainly because CT looks for sizable masses. It can't spot tiny invasions, and sadly, this is how most prostate cancers spread to new territories. (For example, the overwhelming majority of metastases to the lymph nodes start out on a microscopic level.)

In detecting localized spread of prostate cancer (beyond the prostate wall or into the seminal vesicles), CT has been found to have a sensitivity of 50 percent at best. It also has an unfortunate false-positive rate in diagnosing prostate cancer in the seminal vesicles. We do not recommend routine CT scans for men who appear to have localized disease. In men with advanced disease, where we are concerned that cancer may have spread to the lymph nodes, MRI is the preferred means of imaging.

Bone Scan (Radionuclide Scintigraphy)

In a bone scan, doctors inject into the bloodstream a radioactive tracer, a chemical that's attracted, like a magnet, specifically to bone. (This substance is harmless and soon passes out of the body.) Then, using a device called a gamma camera, doctors take pictures of the bones. Normal bone absorbs the radioactive tracer at a lower level. But in areas of new growth—of bone regeneration, as in a healing fracture or cancer—the tracer accumulates; more is absorbed, and this surplus shows up as a "hot spot" on the image.

Bone scans are not perfect. Many men feel that if their bone scan is negative, they're home free. Unfortunately, that's not always true. Microscopic prostatic cancer cells, as we've discussed earlier in this chapter, can sneak out of the prostate and move into bone. But these cells are called micrometastases for a reason—they're tiny. It could take five, ten, or even fifteen years for them even to show up on a bone scan. Thus, a negative bone scan doesn't mean you don't have micrometastases, so it's not very sensitive. Worse, it's not terribly specific. Any form of bone disease will show up as a hot spot mimicking cancer: a new or old fracture, infection, arthritis—anything that's got to do with the bone in question. For example, one man with newly diagnosed prostate cancer went through a terrible scare because a hot spot suggested the cancer had spread to his skull. It turned out to be an old football injury. The man's prostate was removed, and his PSA remains undetectable. But he and his family experienced needless stress at an already stressful time. Thus, routine bone scans are not useful for all men with localized prostate cancer. In patients with PSA levels lower than 10 ng/ml, Gleason scores of 7 or lower (Grade Group 2), and clinically localized disease, bone scans are typically not performed unless a man is experiencing bone pain. This is because his likelihood of metastases is extremely low, and most of the lesions the scan is likely to pick up aren't cancer anyway.

Who needs a bone scan? The NCCN recommends a bone scan for patients with T1 and PSA greater than 20, T2 and PSA greater than 10, Gleason score of 8 or greater, and T3/T4 or symptoms. For these men at higher risk of advanced disease, a bone scan can be very helpful. If it demonstrates that cancer has spread to bone, the treatment at this point is clear—hormonal therapy and possibly also chemotherapy, depending on the extent of disease. If the bone scan is inconclusive, more tests will be necessary to find out what form of bone disease is present. Plain X-rays can rule out the presence of benign conditions, such as an old fracture, arthritis, or Paget's disease (in which there is an overgrowth of bone). If these X-rays are clear, it is possible there is a small bit of underlying cancer—in which case, the next step is usually an MRI scan of bone. If the answer is still not clear, rarely, some men undergo biopsies of bone to exclude metastases.

Optional Imaging Tests for Staging Prostate Cancer

PET Scan

Positron emission tomography (PET), a noninvasive imaging technique, can show precisely where areas of cancer are hiding within the body. It has the unique ability to show specific biochemical processes, such as tumor glucose metabolism, within the body. It uses radioisotopes that release positrons (positively charged particles) as they decay. The release of these radioactive substances can be measured with a radiation detector and then fused to standard CT images, taken along with the PET scan.

Tumors, like normal cells, use glucose; in fact, some types of cancer use a lot of it, and this can be highlighted with a radioactive sugar. Most prostate cancers, however, break down glucose at a relatively low rate, so we use alternative radiotracers to look for prostate cancer. In the United States, three radiotracers are available for prostate cancer imaging. The first is $Na^{18}F$, a substance used by bone as it tries to repair itself when metastases have invaded it. Note: This test cannot detect prostate cancer in areas other than bone—in the prostate itself, for example, or the lymph nodes. The other two are ^{11}C-choline and ^{18}F-fluciclovine (also known as Axumin or ^{18}F-FACBC). Unlike $Na^{18}F$, both of these can detect prostate cancer in all areas of the body. ^{11}C-choline is taken up by rapidly dividing prostate cancer cells, where it becomes trapped. ^{18}F-fluciclovine is a synthetic amino acid that is transported into prostate cancer cells.

These radiotracers offer the greatest clinical value in helping detect tiny sites of prostate cancer in men with a rising PSA after radiation or surgery. However, neither ^{11}C-choline nor ^{18}F-fluciclovine is specific to prostate cancer cells; both agents can accumulate in inflammation, for example. Scientists are actively looking for compounds that are more specific for prostate cancer; these include molecules targeting the androgen receptor (^{18}F-FDHT) and prostate-specific membrane antigen (PSMA), found on the surface of prostate cells. The results of PSMA-targeted PET, developed by Martin Pomper at Johns Hopkins, are particularly encouraging, and an imaging agent targeting this protein will likely be approved for use in the near future (see chapter 10).

Chest X-ray

Although the presence or absence of cancer in a man's lungs can help doctors in staging prostate cancer, metastases to the lungs are very rare in men with localized prostate cancer. A chest X-ray, then, is optional, but definitely not necessary. The greatest value of this test is in detecting heart and lung disease rather than the spread of prostate cancer. Chest X-rays are often performed in men having surgery as part of routine preoperative testing.

Lymphadenectomy

Just as the best way to stage cancer is to look at it after the fact (after it's been removed during surgery), the best way to check the lymph nodes in the pelvis for cancer is to go in there and get them—to remove them surgically and let a pathologist examine them. If a large, suspicious-looking lymph node is seen on an imaging study, it is possible to do a needle biopsy (similar to a needle biopsy on the prostate) without surgery. However, when prostate cancer metastasizes to the lymph nodes, the nodes rarely become enlarged. Thus, if it's essential to know the status of the lymph nodes, surgical removal is necessary. However, this could all change once PSMA PET scans (see page 325) are approved.

The lymph nodes can be tested during a prostatectomy operation, with the patient remaining under anesthesia during a rapid pathological examination (see chapter 8). However, this technique, called frozen section analysis, often misses small amounts of tumor. So again, if it's absolutely essential to know whether cancer is in a man's lymph nodes, the best approach is surgical removal with permanent sections to examine the pathological specimen (this takes two days). This can be performed laparoscopically or through a small, three-inch open incision. Recovery from both procedures is similar. This procedure is not commonly performed nowadays, since current thinking is that even men with extensive local disease may still benefit from surgical removal of the prostate, in addition to radiation, hormonal therapy, or other forms of treatment.

To Sum Up

Take a deep breath. You've had a lot to deal with, and there's a tremendous amount of information to digest. You are not alone. For most men, the diagnosis of prostate cancer is unexpected—like a sudden punch in the stomach. As with any other unexpected calamity in your life, you've got to face it square-on and collect all the facts. At your fingertips are three facts you will probably come to know as well as your Social Security number—your PSA level, Gleason score, and clinical stage. With just these three facts, almost immediately you have a good idea of where you stand. The cancer either appears to be clinically localized to the prostate—the most common scenario in the United States today because of improved diagnostic testing—or the cancer has spread locally but does not appear to be present at distant sites; or rarely, less than 10 percent of the time, the cancer has been caught later, and it has spread either to the lymph nodes or bone. Once you have reached the point of knowing where you stand, your next move is to examine the options for treatment and find the one that you feel is best for you.

Another thing: *Many common statistics are based on men who were diagnosed with cancer at least a decade ago.* If you have just been diagnosed with prostate cancer, there is no question that you're better off—chances are, you've been diagnosed a lot sooner and at a much more curable stage. The long-term success stories of you and other men newly diagnosed haven't been written yet. With the explosion of new treatment strategies for advanced disease, our ability to control cancer is only getting better and better. There is more hope now than ever. Do not let yourself get discouraged.

Now on to chapter 6, where, based on what you now know, we'll examine your options.

6

WHAT ARE MY OPTIONS?

This chapter was written with expert opinion from Edward M. Schaeffer, M.D., Ph.D.

THE SHORT STORY:
The Highly Abridged Version of This Chapter

What's the best treatment for prostate cancer? This is a trick question. There is no single best treatment, because prostate cancer isn't a one-size-fits-all disease. It's different in every man. A better question: What's the best treatment for your prostate cancer? The two most important factors to consider are the aggressiveness of the cancer (clinical stage, PSA, and Gleason grade grouping) and your life expectancy (based on your age and general health).

Thirty-five years ago, most men were diagnosed with prostate cancer at an older age and with more advanced disease, and many of them died within a few years. Today, thankfully, the tables have turned. Now most American men are diagnosed with localized prostate cancer that is curable. It is possible today to prevent a man from dying a painful death of prostate cancer fifteen or twenty years in the future. The goal is to achieve this and leave the patient with an excellent quality of life—cured of cancer, continent, potent, and as if nothing had ever happened.

In this chapter, we will review how we assess the aggressiveness of a cancer and a man's life expectancy to determine which treatment is best for him. If you have localized prostate cancer, active surveillance, surgery, and radiation therapy are proven options. If you have been diagnosed with more advanced disease, take heart: there are many new treatment approaches to extend the duration and quality of your life, and promising new drugs are showing great results in clinical trials.

The best thing you can do now is educate yourself—not just about prostate cancer, but about the doctors who treat it. You're building a bridge here, and you can go only so far by yourself. Ultimately, you are going to have to find a physician you trust, to help you find your way through this very complicated disease.

I Have Cancer...How Do I Begin to Think About My Options?

Prostate cancer is a complicated disease—so complicated, in fact, that it's unique in every man. Your brother-in-law had prostate cancer? Your neighbor, too? And now you—three men with three distinct cancers. There is so much variability here. Because the disease is completely different from man to man, you may find the treatment that's best for your neighbor is not the one that's best for you. You can't go by anybody else's experience with prostate cancer, because you've each got your own custom-made case. And yet, you're all part of the same club, a group nobody wants to join—the reluctant brotherhood of men with prostate cancer.

What's the best treatment? This is a trick question. There is no single best treatment because, again, prostate cancer isn't a one-size-fits-all disease. There are many factors—not only the clinical stage of your particular cancer, but your own age and general health—involved in choosing the treatment that's right for you. Your personal preferences are paramount here: Some men, for example, would rather take action—even if their cancer is incidental—than drive themselves crazy with worry, living from one PSA test or biopsy to the next in active surveillance. To other men, the idea of surgery is so disturbing that they would rather take their chances with diet, meditation, and other lifestyle changes than go under the knife. For some men—such as an eighty-one-year-old man with diabetes and congestive heart failure—any form of aggressive treatment, with side effects and recovery time, would not only be unhelpful but could produce complications that would make the "golden years" needlessly unpleasant. For others—a seventy-six-year-old man who swims two miles a day, has two teenage children, and whose parents who died in their nineties—not going after this disease aggressively would be uncharacteristic and unthinkable. Only you know how you really feel about this.

Thirty-five years ago, most men were diagnosed with prostate cancer at an older age and with more advanced disease, and many of them died within a few years. Today, thankfully, the tables have been turned. Now most American men are diagnosed with localized prostate cancer that is curable. The use of PSA testing has given us a five- to ten-year lead time in diagnosis. It is possible today to prevent a man from dying a painful death from prostate cancer fifteen or twenty years in the future. Now the goal is to achieve this *and* leave the patient with an excellent quality of life—cured of cancer, continent, potent, as if nothing had ever happened, and as if the diagnosis and treatment of cancer were just a rough patch on the road. If you have localized disease (this includes locally advanced disease), you have three main treatment options: active surveillance, surgery, or radiation therapy. As you work through your decision, ask yourself questions like these: What's more important? Knowing that you're cured of cancer but realizing there's a trade-off—in other words, you might have some side effects from treatment? Or would it be better for you to get the treatment with the fewest side effects, hoping that you may die of something else before cancer catches up?

The first step in understanding what will be the "best" treatment for you is to assess your overall health.
If you have localized disease, the big, blunt question you need to ask yourself is this: *How long am I probably going to live?* Nobody wants

to think about this question, but there it is. In men over sixty-five who don't have heart disease or another form of cancer, life expectancy can vary tremendously, from two years to thirty-seven years. The factors that can shorten your life expectancy, in order of importance, are hypertension, smoking, diabetes, consuming more than four drinks of alcohol a day, and not exercising. On the other hand, if your family has a history of longevity (if your parents lived into their eighties or nineties), your blood pressure is low, you don't have diabetes, and your HDL (the good kind of cholesterol) is high, you don't smoke, and you have no history of heart disease, then you may live long enough to *need* to be cured, and your cancer may be aggressive enough that it requires aggressive therapy.

The National Comprehensive Cancer Network (NCCN) guidelines recommend the Social Security Administration tables for estimating life expectancy (www.ssa.gov/OACT/STATS/table4c6 .html). These guidelines recommend adding 50 percent for patients in the top twenty-fifth percentile of health and subtracting 50 percent for those in the lowest twenty-fifth percentile. Similar tables that are specific to African American men are also available at https://www.cdc.gov/nchs/data/nvsr/nvsr65/nvsr65_08.pdf.

And next, how old are you? This is different from the question about your life expectancy. If you are in your fifties or younger, even if the odds of a cure don't appear to be in your favor, *you will tolerate surgery better than an older man will, and you should probably consider it.* If you are older, the situation gets a bit more complicated. Men over seventy who undergo radical prostatectomy are more likely to have problems with impotence and incontinence. (Note: Both of these can be treated, and the rates of complications vary significantly depending on the expertise of the surgeon who performs the operation.) Men over seventy are also *more likely to have more cancer* than younger men. For example, in men with stage T2 cancer (the kind of cancer that can be felt on rectal examination), the tumor is more often organ-confined in men in their fifties than in men in their seventies. Why? Because in the older men, the cancer has been there longer and has had a chance to grow and possibly to become more malignant. Johns Hopkins urologist H. Ballentine Carter studied five hundred men with stage T1c disease who underwent radical prostatectomy. He found that older men were more likely to have Gleason 7 (Grade Groups 2 and 3) tumors than men in their fifties, and that age was a statistically significant factor in the prediction of curability.

Let's consider the case of one sixty-five-year-old man: He's in otherwise good health, he has a tumor that needs to be treated, and he can reasonably expect to live at least twenty to twenty-five more years. His cancer is curable now. If he does nothing about it, he may miss his golden opportunity for a cure. Although we have markers that can help us estimate whether cancer has the potential to be aggressive, we don't know if or when it will make that leap beyond the prostate. Even in its earliest stages, prostate cancer doesn't always spread in logical, easy-to-predict steps.

At the other end of the spectrum is a man in his eighties. Even if his cancer is organ-confined and curable, will he live long enough for aggressive treatment to be worthwhile? Older men are less resilient; aggressive treatment—particularly surgery—is much harder on them. Is it worth risking incontinence, a result of surgery, or rectal bleeding, a result of radiation, in an eighty-five-year-old man? If his disease progresses to the point where he has difficulty with urination, there are many ways to treat such symptoms, ranging from a TUR (to relieve urinary obstruction) to hormonal therapy. For older men, *the number of years of life*—the long-term survival—is not nearly as important as the *life in those years*—the quality of life.

Early hormonal therapy: Just say no. You may feel, desperately, that your older father who has localized disease, no symptoms, and no spread of his cancer still needs *something* done, and there are many urologists who will suggest it's time to start hormonal therapy. *Don't do that!* As we'll discuss in chapter 12, there are many adverse side effects associated with hormonal therapy, like new-onset diabetes, cognitive impairment, and an increased risk of death from cardiovascular disease. Indeed, in a study of 65,000 older men diagnosed with localized prostate cancer, those who received early hormonal therapy did not live as long as those who started it later. Another study of older men found that there was *no benefit* to early hormonal therapy, even in men who had a high Gleason score.

How Aggressive Is My Disease?

Most prostate cancer grows relatively slowly. When it's localized (confined within the prostate), it can take years for a tumor to double in size. And here is the confounding thing: cancer can stay in the prostate indefinitely. It takes a long time and many steps involving subtle genetic changes before a normal cell, which is designed to live and die, becomes a cancer cell—before some switch is activated that makes the cell think it's immortal—and before such cells start dividing endlessly. (As we've discussed earlier, in high-risk men, some of these steps are shortened.)

We are now working on molecular and genetic tools that can help us "see inside" a cancer cell to help us understand its potential for aggressiveness. We're getting better at predicting, but for now, we still can't "mind-read" localized prostate cancer.

What determines aggressiveness? Several factors, including the cancer's Gleason group, your PSA level and the physical exam. Imaging scans that check for metastatic spread of the cancer also come into play here, but are typically needed only for men with higher grade or higher stage disease (more on this later). When we put all these pieces together, we come up with a "risk grouping" or "risk stratification" for your cancer.

There are many different published risk groupings, but I believe the most widely accepted and applicable are the guidelines from the National Comprehensive Cancer Network (NCCN), which include five main categories for men with localized or locally advanced disease (see Table 6.1). These guidelines can be found at www.nccn.org. Let's look at the risk groups.

TABLE 6.1

PROSTATE CANCER RISK GROUPS—AS DEFINED BY THE NCCN

Risk Group	Clinical stage (on digital rectal examination)	PSA	Biopsy findings
Very low (All criteria must be met)	T1c (non-palpable)	< 10 ng/ml, AND PSA density < 0.15	Gleason score ≤ 6, AND ≤ 2 cores with cancer, AND < 50% involvement of any core with cancer
Low (All criteria must be met)	T1c (non-palpable), OR T2a (palpable on less than half of one side of the prostate)	< 10 ng/ml	Gleason score ≤ 6
Intermediate (Any single criterion)	T2b (palpable on more than one-half of one side of the prostate, OR T2c (palpable on both sides)	10–20 ng/ml	Gleason score 7 (either 3 + 4 = 7 or 4 + 3 = 7)
High (Any single criterion)	T3a (palpable lesion extends outside the prostate)	> 20 ng/ml	Gleason score 8-10
Very high#	T3b (palpable lesion invades seminal vesicles), OR T4 (tumor is fixed or invades adjacent structures other than seminal vesicles)	> 20 ng/ml	Primary Gleason pattern 5 (Gleason score 5 +3, 5 + 4, or 5 + 5), OR > 4 biopsy cores with Gleason score 8–10 cancer

* Cancers are assigned to the highest risk group for which they meet one criterion (clinical stage, PSA, or biopsy findings).
# Very high-risk prostate cancer is defined either by the clinical stage, or by having two or more high-risk features, or by having primary Gleason pattern 5 disease.

Very Low-Risk Prostate Cancer

Men in this group have *all* the following: a normal rectal exam; a PSA lower than 10; Gleason 3 + 3 = 6 (Grade Group 1) cancer; fewer than three biopsy cores positive for prostate cancer, with less than

50 percent cancer in each core; and a PSA density of less than 0.15 ng/ml/gm. (PSA density is a number that correlates the size of the prostate with a man's PSA number. For more on how PSA density is determined, see page 105). This is a very long list! However, it's important to note that for a man to have very low-risk prostate cancer, he needs to meet all these strict criteria.

If you have very low-risk prostate cancer, what treatment should you consider? You've got a lot of options, and much of the decision-making depends on your age and overall health. For men with very low-risk prostate cancer and a life expectancy less than twenty years, active surveillance (AS) is a very good option. Important note: AS is not a "one-way street." If you and your doctor begin AS and something changes—either in your cancer, or in your personal preferences—you can initiate treatment. AS is not a recommended long-term strategy for men who can expect to live longer than twenty years. We'll discuss this in further detail in chapter 7, but statistically speaking, in most men with more than twenty years' life expectancy, the cancer will change and require intervention. For these men, AS is probably better viewed as a means of delaying treatment for several years.

Men with very low-risk prostate cancer do not need any radiographic imaging to determine if their cancer has spread or metastasized. It's not necessary. Low-volume, low-grade prostate cancer is not capable of metastasizing. We think over time, low-grade, low-volume prostate cancer can grow locally within the prostate—but even so, Gleason 6 prostate cancer does not have the genetic capability to metastasize to other parts of the body. Men who are strongly considering AS may want to consider obtaining a multiparametric MRI (mpMRI) to help confirm that surveillance is a good option. Your doctor may also recommend genetic tests to evaluate the degree of aggressiveness of your cancer. The true utility of these tests in AS is the focus of much research. For men who are unsure if AS is a good option, I find that these tests (presently offered by GenomeDx, Myriad Genetics, and Genomic Health) can be helpful pieces to the puzzle of choosing the right treatment.

IF YOU HAVE STAGE T1A/B DISEASE

If you have not had a transurethral resection (TUR) of the prostate, you can skip this section. About 5 percent of men who undergo surgery for the treatment of an enlarged prostate turn out to have some cancer found in the tissue that's removed. These men can be subclassified into stage T1a, if 5 percent or less of the tissue is involved with cancer, and T1b, if more than 5 percent is involved or if the Grade Group is 2 or higher.

In a study performed at Hopkins in 1976, we determined that when 5 percent or less of the tissue was cancerous and lower than Gleason 7, only 17 percent of the men went on to develop more advanced cancer within seven years; this is now the classification for stage T1a disease. But when more than 5 percent of the removed tissue was cancerous, 68 percent of these men went on to develop cancer progression within seven years; this now is the classification of stage T1b disease. It is felt that the amount of cancer in almost all these patients is significant enough to warrant therapy.

Further analysis has shown that when men with stage T1a disease undergo radical prostatectomy, about 25 percent of them turn out to have a significant amount of cancer in the prostate—the kind of cancer that's found in men with palpable tumors. So some men with stage T1a cancer require treatment, and some don't. How to tell the difference? Our old friend PSA comes back to help us again. As it turns out, the level of PSA three months after the TUR can be helpful in identifying men at highest risk of cancer progression. If the PSA level is greater than 10, all these men are likely to have significant cancer remaining, and all should have definitive therapy before it's too late. If the PSA is less than 1.0 ng/ml, virtually all the men with stage T1a disease have an insignificant amount of cancer and can probably be followed safely with an active surveillance protocol involving careful follow-up—with rectal examinations, PSA tests every six months to one year, and mpMRIs.

What about the patients in the middle, with PSA levels between 1 and 10—the range for about half the men with T1 disease? These men are similar to the low-risk category of men discussed below. If they are young and healthy, they should consider definitive treatment.

Low-Risk Prostate Cancer

Men in this group have either no palpable cancer or an abnormality found only in one half of one side of the prostate; Gleason 6 (Grade Group 1) cancer; and a PSA lower than 10.

If you have low-risk prostate cancer and your life expectancy is more than ten years, you should consider curative treatment with either radiation or surgery. Although active surveillance is a possibility for men with low-risk prostate cancer, the likelihood that the cancer will progress is higher than for men with very low-risk disease. The criteria for low-risk cancer do not specify the *amount* of cancer detected on biopsy. Therefore, a man with a clinical stage of T2a or lower, PSA lower than 10 ng/ml, and Gleason score 6 cancer technically meets low-risk criteria—even if cancer is detected in 100 percent of the tissue cores (usually twelve) taken during his biopsy! So be very careful in looking at these criteria. Also, men who have cancer found in multiple biopsy cores have a greater risk of progression than do men with only one or two cores positive. However, active surveillance and watchful waiting are excellent ways to manage this type of cancer in a man whose life expectancy is less than 10 years.

Intermediate-Risk Prostate Cancer

Men in this group have Gleason 3 + 4 = 7 (Grade Group 2) *or* Gleason 4 + 3 = 7 (Grade Group 3) disease *or* a PSA between 10 and 20 ng/ml *or* an abnormality felt during the rectal exam that is confined within the prostate but involves more than half of one lobe.

It's important to note that men are characterized with intermediate-risk prostate cancer if they have *only one of the above criteria*. (This differs from very low-risk and low-risk disease, where men must meet *all* the criteria outlined.) Another important thing to understand about intermediate-risk disease is that there's a broad spectrum of disease aggressiveness here. All intermediate-risk prostate cancer is not alike. For example, a man with Gleason 3 + 4 = 7 cancer in 10 percent of one biopsy core has a far different disease than a man with Gleason 4 + 3 = 7 cancer in twelve of twelve cores.

If you have intermediate-risk prostate cancer, you really need to know how extensive your cancer is. It is essential that you choose the treatment that offers the best chance of cure now; a wrong choice here could present problems down the road. Men with intermediate risk (particularly Gleason Grade Group 3) disease will likely need additional tests to help determine the cancer's stage, or extent. These may include a bone scan and CT or MRI scan. In general, men who have both an abnormal rectal exam and a PSA of 10 or above should get both a bone scan and CT scan.

Treatment Options

Most men with intermediate-risk prostate cancer should consider curative treatment with either surgery or radiation. Note: Many men with intermediate-risk prostate cancer who are interested in radiation will also need a short course of androgen deprivation therapy (ADT, discussed further in chapter 9) to bring testosterone down to very low levels. *This is only temporary*—four to six months—and although nobody likes it, ADT has been shown to make a huge difference in prognosis. ADT improves the ability of radiation to kill high-volume, high-grade prostate cancer, and it is far better to take it for a few months now and cure your cancer than to end up taking it for many years down the road if the cancer becomes metastatic.

Surgery is also a very good option (see page 206). Talk to your surgeon about the lymph node dissection (removal) that you will need to undergo; intermediate-risk disease does have the capacity to spread to the lymph nodes and beyond, and it's important to undergo a thorough staging workup before surgery and lymph node dissection during the radical prostatectomy. One key advantage for surgery in men with intermediate risk prostate cancer is the ability to avoid ADT; another is that removing the tumor and the lymph nodes improves survival and can delay any return of PSA for many years.

High-Risk Prostate Cancer

Men in this group have: either Gleason score 8 (Grade Group 4) or Gleason score 4 + 5 (Grade Group V) cancer; *or* PSA greater than

20 ng/ml; *or* a rectal exam that shows firmness extending beyond the prostate.

If you have high-risk prostate cancer and your life expectancy is more than five years, you should seek active treatment, which may mean surgery and/or radiation. If you choose radical prostatectomy, your surgeon will need to perform an extended lymph node dissection (removal). This is important from a prognostic perspective: *some men who have cancer in the lymph nodes are cured when the lymph nodes are removed.* Talk to your surgeon about the extent of the lymph node dissection. For some men with high-risk prostate cancer, surgery may not be enough; about one out of every three or four of them may also need radiation to their pelvis and pelvic lymph nodes. Note: Having radiation after surgery is not necessarily a failure of surgical treatment; instead, postoperative radiation is sometimes administered when very aggressive features are seen on the final pathology report, with the goal of eradicating the cancer.

If you are considering radiation as your main form of treatment, there are several options to consider. One is external-beam radiation *and* two to three years of ADT. An alternative radiation-based treatment strategy is external-beam radiation plus brachytherapy seeds, with or without ADT. Work from an emerging trial suggests that the combination of both types of radiation without ADT may be a more effective way to control aggressive cancers. One concern here is that the combination of external-beam radiation and brachytherapy seeds delivers a lot of radiation to the prostate; this raises the risk of side effects, including urinary problems.

You may be asking yourself, "Why are my treatment options so complicated?" The answer lies in the aggressiveness of this type of cancer. I often explain to patients that attacking the cancer on more than one front (called multimodal treatment) can be life-saving when the disease is more aggressive. Not all men with high-risk cancer need multimodal treatment. However, if you are in this category, it is very important to talk to a surgeon and a radiation oncologist, or to go to a prostate cancer Center of Excellence, because managing high-risk disease is not always straightforward.

Very High-Risk Prostate Cancer

Men in this group have multiple high-risk prostate cancer features: more than four biopsy cores with Gleason 8–10 cancer (Grade Group 4 or 5); *or* Gleason score of 5 + 4 (as opposed to 4 + 5); *or* a rectal exam that shows firmness extending beyond the prostate into the seminal vesicles, pelvic sidewall, or bladder. If you have very high-risk prostate cancer, you need comprehensive treatment (outlined on page 177), ideally at a cancer Center of Excellence. You also may wish to participate in a clinical trial.

In men with very high-risk disease, primary treatment with surgery or radiation may not always cure the cancer. Many men who have this type of extensive cancer will eventually develop a rising PSA following treatment. (Important note: In recent years, we have stepped up treatment of intermediate, high-, and very high-risk cancer, and hope that by going after it aggressively up front, we will change these statistics.)

You may wonder, "If my PSA comes back, did I go through all this treatment for nothing?" I believe in appropriate men that primary treatment of these tumors is highly beneficial. Important scientific evidence suggests that metastatic prostate cancer develops mostly from the prostate and pelvic lymph nodes (see below). Thus, controlling the disease at its source could minimize the risk of metastasis; we are still trying to answer this question.

Men with Regionally Advanced or Metastatic Prostate Cancer

If you have regionally advanced or metastatic prostate cancer, take heart: there has never been a time of more hope. This is one of the most exciting and expanding areas of prostate cancer treatment, which we will discuss in chapter 13. Briefly, new hormonal and radiation therapies are helping us control this disease for years, sometimes even for decades. Important new avenues of treatment are showing exciting results, putting some men with widely metastatic disease into what appears to be complete remission. Finally, scientists are cracking the code of the immune system, figuring out how to reactivate it after cancer has put it to sleep with "checkpoints," or brakes. New immunotherapy drugs are showing great success in several forms of cancer, including prostate cancer. These drugs don't work for everyone, but exciting new drugs that target different checkpoints are being tested as we speak. Scientists are also focusing on specific inherited genes, and already a few gene-targeting drugs—which have shown success against other forms of cancer—are showing promise against prostate cancer. New "nanotechnology" that targets individual prostate cancer cells is killing prostate cancer in European and Australian studies, soon to start here. Finally, all the research that has been under way for a decade or more is achieving critical mass and extending survival longer than ever before.

EVEN IF YOU HAVE HIGH-RISK CANCER, ELIMINATING THE MAIN TUMOR MAKES A BIG DIFFERENCE

What if you have been diagnosed with a tumor that may be difficult to cure? Maybe you've looked up your PSA, Gleason score, and clinical stage on the Han tables (Table 5.2, page 152) and it looks like your chance of having an undetectable PSA ten years after surgery is not great. Maybe you are worried that you are going to die. Don't despair. I want you to know that things are not as bad as you may be imagining. And let me make a promise to you: I do not lie.

Here are some facts that don't show up on tables but are real and very important:

First, PSA is very sensitive in detecting residual cancer cells after treatment. So yes, you may have some cancer cells left in there—but that fact, by itself, is not going to kill you, or even make you feel sick. It can take many years before those cells ever show up on a scan or cause symptoms.

Next, even if your initial treatment did not completely cure you, it still can have a powerful effect in prolonging your life! When I began my training, we were taught to perform big operations for little cancers and little operations for big cancers: in other words, to operate only on patients who we thought were curable. But for years, we have seen a phenomenon, and now there is scientific evidence to back up what we have observed: *eliminating the primary tumor can prolong survival, even if it doesn't cure the patient.* Yes, there may still be cancer, but it has taken such a huge hit that it may never recover. Or, if it does start to come back, it still may take many years before it gathers enough numbers to cause a problem.

With that in mind, let's examine the concept of eliminating the cancer with surgery or radiation therapy in men where the chance of cure is not high. In other words, what about treatment in men with high-grade disease?

If you look at Table 5.2, you will see that if you have a Gleason score of 8, the ten-year probability of an undetectable PSA following surgery is pretty low. Yet, in the famous Scandinavian trial discussed on page 182, *the greatest survival benefit following surgery was in young men with Gleason 8 disease.*

Years ago, the established first step in radical prostatectomies was to remove the lymph nodes and send them off to the pathologist for frozen sections. If cancer was detected in the lymph nodes, the prostate was not removed and the incision was closed. Why? Because we assumed that the cancer had already spread and the patient could not be cured. We don't do that anymore, because we now know that if you remove the prostate in these men, they are going to live longer than they would if we left it in place.

But what about men treated with radiation? We now know that in men with locally advanced disease, radiation to the prostate combined with ADT prolongs life more than ADT alone. Why?

There is a growing body of evidence in other cancers—metastatic ovarian cancer, gastrointestinal cancers, and kidney cancer—that treating the primary tumor and giving systemic therapy improves survival. First, removing the primary tumor reduces the cancer's ability to continuously metastasize. Second, we now know that when tumor cells escape the prostate, they often recirculate back into the prostate—revisiting the mother ship, in effect—in a process called "self-seeding." This helps accelerate tumor progression. And finally, we have known for more than one hundred years that tumor cells will selectively colonize organs with "favorable soil." A scientist at Cornell named Rosandra Kaplan was the first to show that the first thing that happens at the metastatic site is not the arrival of tumor cells, but of bone marrow-derived cells that "prepare the soil" by altering the microenvironment. It has been proposed the growth-promoting factors and immunosuppressive cytokines produced by the prostate may be involved in this process. For all these reasons, men with advanced disease may benefit from eradication of their local tumor. Indeed, there are now clinical trials in men with low-volume metastatic disease to determine whether radiation to the primary tumor will improve their outcome. We suggest you strongly consider treating the primary tumor. Our goal with this book is to help you fight your disease and win.

Does Treating Localized Prostate Cancer Save Lives?

The best study that addresses this question began in 1989 in Sweden. The Scandinavian Prostate Cancer Group, made up of physicians from Sweden, Finland, and Iceland, embarked on a courageous trial, published in the *New England Journal of Medicine*, that has changed the way prostate cancer is perceived worldwide. In the study, nearly seven hundred men with localized, mostly intermediate-risk prostate cancer were randomly assigned either to watchful waiting or to radical prostatectomy. Because this study began before PSA testing, most of the men had more aggressive cancers than we diagnose today. For this reason, the effect of treatment was more dramatic than it would be if the study were repeated in a group of men who had been screened. What happened to these men provided the first concrete evidence of something American doctors had believed anecdotally for years—that *treating localized disease reduces deaths from prostate cancer.* Ten years after the study began, half of deaths in the watchful waiting group were from prostate cancer. Because radical prostatectomy reduced the likelihood of dying of prostate cancer by 40 percent, there was a statistically significant reduction in *death from all causes* in the group that underwent surgery. After fifteen years of follow-up of men who were younger than sixty-five when they entered the study (and those most likely to benefit from treatment), men who underwent surgery experienced an across-the-board, 50-percent relative reduction in death from all causes, death from prostate cancer, and the development of metastatic spread to bone. In an article accompanying the updated fifteen-year report, the Scandinavian researchers looked at the side effects in all of the men, and by four years they found that the quality of life in both groups was the same—largely because the progression in the watchful waiting patients required them to receive additional treatments and hormones.

The PIVOT Study

Another attempt to shed light on prostate cancer treatment was the national PIVOT (Prostate Cancer Intervention Versus Observation Trial) study, led by a Minnesota internist and a Seattle urologist and funded by the Department of Veterans Affairs and the National Cancer Institute. In this study, carried out in the PSA era, men were randomly assigned either to radical prostatectomy or watchful waiting. Although the study was originally designed to recruit two thousand healthy men with at least a ten-year life expectancy, it actually recruited only 731 men. By ten years, 40 percent of these men were dead from other causes, and at fifteen years, 60 percent. Although there was no reduction in deaths from prostate cancer in men with low-risk disease at ten years (something we have known for thirty years), there was a *60 percent decrease in metastases and a 40 percent reduction in cancer deaths in men with PSA greater than 10.* Despite these positive findings, the authors proclaimed that surgery didn't save lives. The *New York Times* summarized the findings this way: "A new study shows that prostate cancer surgery, which often leaves men impotent or incontinent, does not appear to save the lives of men with early stage disease, who account for most of the cases, and many of these men would do just as well to choose no treatment at all."

How could the findings from the Scandinavian study be so positive and this one not? Ruth Etzioni, an outstanding epidemiologist from the Fred Hutchinson Cancer Research Center, analyzed the two studies side by side. She concluded that "the absolute results were different because there were fewer deaths from prostate cancer in PIVOT—but the relative benefit was similar." She went on to say that the PIVOT trial "should not be interpreted as evidence that surgery is not efficacious in reducing prostate cancer mortality."

So what did the authors of the PIVOT trial actually do? They said they were going to randomize healthy men who were candidates for surgery to watchful waiting; but instead, they randomized old, sick men who weren't good candidates for surgery to radical prostatectomy. What should the authors have concluded? The a man with a life expectancy of ten years or less who has low-volume disease does not need surgery. This study provides no useful information for a healthy man in his forties, fifties, and early sixties. Unfortunately, many men and their general doctors still do not understand this.

The gold standard for knowing whether any form of treatment for localized prostate cancer works is determining if it reduces deaths. The problem is that it takes a long time to get that answer, and ten years is not long enough. There is a famous study from Sweden where more than two hundred men with early, low-risk prostate cancer were *observed without treatment* for three decades. At ten years, only 10 percent of the men had died from prostate cancer but after twenty years, more than 50 percent had succumbed to the disease.

The Prostate Testing for Cancer and Treatment (ProtecT) Trial

This study from the United Kingdom is the latest randomized trial to evaluate the best treatment for localized prostate cancer. It randomized 1,643 men who had been diagnosed based on PSA screening to active monitoring, prostatectomy, or radiation. About 80 percent had low-risk cancers. This study showed several important things. First, at ten years, there was no difference in prostate cancer-specific deaths among the three initial treatments. However, they also showed that 44 percent of men in active surveillance went on to require treatment with surgery or radiation, and that rates of metastases were three times higher in the active monitoring group compared to the active treatment groups. Thus, from this study, it is clear that surgery and radiation were equally effective in reducing the risk of metastases *at ten years*. This is a very powerful study, and because it was just recently reported, we have a lot more to learn from it.

What are its limitations? First, the monitoring of untreated patients used in this study was much different and much less intensive than the measures we use in our AS programs, which are designed to detect progression of disease and treat it as soon as possible. For this reason, the rates of progression and metastatic disease in the ProtecT participants were higher than we would expect in this country. The second limitation of ProtecT is the experience of the surgeons in the study. When ProtecT began, urologists in the United Kingdom were not as experienced as surgeons in the United States at performing radical prostatectomy. Today, with added experience, their outcomes are much improved. The study's third limitation is that most men treated with radiation also were treated with ADT at the same time. Thus, in these men, there could have been more side effects. In summary, ProtecT is a very important study. It supports the findings from the Scandinavian trial that active treatment of prostate cancer reduces metastatic disease. It also supports the role of AS for some men, but underscores the need for careful selection of these men for surveillance.

What Do All These Studies Tell Us?

Prostate cancer can be a lethal disease in some men, while in other men, it can move very slowly, with no obvious progression over the course of many years. There is no one-size-fits-all answer here. With that in mind, it's time to take what we've talked about, look at all the treatment options, and decide which one is best for you.

Which treatment is better? We know for certain (see the discussion of the Scandinavian study on page 182) that radical prostatectomy saves lives.

It cures cancer, and for years, the results of radical prostatectomy have been the gold standard against which all other forms of treatment are compared. Radiation cures cancer, too. Most physicians agree that, for men with prostate cancer in its early stages, it would be difficult to show a definite difference in cure rates between radical prostatectomy and external-beam radiation. The results with both treatments are good.

For many men, a big advantage of radical prostatectomy is simply knowing that the prostate—and the cancer inside it—has been completely eliminated. It's out of there. Also, after a radical prostatectomy, the PSA levels are undetectable, which provides peace of mind; after radiation therapy, the PSA levels do not always decrease to the undetectable range, because some normal prostate tissue survives. The disadvantages are the side effects—namely the risks of impotence and incontinence. And although most patients recover quickly with little pain following radical prostatectomy, it is major surgery even when done with the laparoscopic, robotic procedure, and the body must be strong enough to handle it. (For a detailed discussion of radical prostatectomy, see chapter 8.) In men under sixty-five who undergo treatment by a surgeon who is an expert, the side effects of surgery and radiation therapy are similar, with the exception that rectal problems are rare following surgery. In men over seventy, surgery carries a higher risk of incontinence and impotence. Note: The side effects of surgery are highly variable, depending on the skill and experience of the surgeon.

Radiation therapy's great advantage is that it isn't surgery. For this reason, it has been the preferred option for men who are older or who have other medical problems. In the past, there was also concern that the long-term effectiveness of radiation was unproven, as most men who received it were old enough to die of other causes. More recently, however, there have been short-term studies reporting that radiation can be effective in younger men. Radiation has side effects of its own—impotence and injury to the rectum (see chapter 9). To some degree, the chances of side effects with external-beam radiation are less operator-dependent than with surgery or seed implantation, although your best bet is to receive treatment at a center where experienced radiation oncologists treat many men with prostate cancer.

So What Do I Do?

First, educate yourself. Learn everything important there is to know about your own cancer—your clinical stage, PSA level, and Gleason score. These will help you understand your cancer risk group. Then begin to explore your options. We've done our best to cover them all in this chapter, and specific forms of treatment are covered in greater detail in the next chapters. Get a second opinion, and a third if you need it, and talk to other patients. If you can't get some names from your doctor, call a prostate cancer support group (see Where to Get Help, page 503) or another organization that specializes in prostate cancer. Be your own advocate, and take heart: there is much you can do to make sure you get the best treatment possible.

What if you don't like any of the options? Maybe you're worried about the complications of surgery and of radiation therapy. Maybe you're also questioning whether your cancer really needs to be treated, because right now you feel terrific. And what about all the health stories in the newspaper and on TV? Every day, there's another new breakthrough in cancer treatment. Maybe some new form of treatment will come along. What if you bite the bullet, undergo treatment for prostate cancer, and open up the newspaper the next morning only to see the headline "Cure for Prostate Cancer Discovered—No Side Effects!"

Or maybe, like some men, you think you can achieve a time-out by putting your prostate on "hold" by taking hormones. The problem there is, as we'll discuss later in this book, some prostate cancer cells respond to hormonal therapy. But others don't—and unfortunately, it is the cells that don't that eventually could kill you. So if you take hormones, your PSA level will plummet—even though, as we'll discuss later on, this is not the same as making the cancer go away completely—and the tumor may shrink clinically. But the cells that can eventually prove fatal *aren't affected at all.* So taking hormones doesn't cure you, and it doesn't really put the problem on hold. It doesn't stop the clock in the cells that are immune to it. Even worse, it causes significant side effects.

But what about the miracle cure that could come along any day now? Well, there's the "test of time" issue. *Even if a new form of treatment were developed today, it would take fifteen to twenty years before we knew whether it really worked.* That's the problem with prostate cancer. Localized disease progresses very slowly; this is why we can't tell if a treatment is working right away.

So, as nice as it would be for a new form of treatment that cures cancer without side effects to come along tomorrow, the truth is that there is no way to know whether that treatment will actually cure prostate cancer. The answer to that question, every time it's asked, takes many years to determine.

How can you think calmly when you're riding a roller coaster? Most men who find out they have prostate cancer feel physically great. They have no symptoms. They're taking some doctor's word for it—not only that there's a cancer growing inside them, but that the cancer could kill them if they do nothing. Or, unfortunately, some men are being told the opposite. They're given false assurances that the cancer will grow slowly and it's okay if they don't do anything but watch its progress, or that they can change its course by starting hormonal therapy years before they may ever actually need it.

Throughout this book, we've emphasized that your best hope of surviving prostate cancer is to educate yourself, to learn all you can about a disease that's deceptively simple—which is actually so complicated that many doctors don't understand it.

Now we're at the crossroads. *Educating yourself is just half the battle—the half you can control. The other half involves a leap of faith. You must find a doctor you can believe in, and then you must be able to accept that doctor's advice.* We talk about finding a good surgeon in chapter 8, but this is more than that—your doctor must be adept and knowledgeable but must also inspire your trust. Ultimately, in matters of illness, this is something everybody must do. Even we doctors (keeping in mind the old adage "The doctor who treats himself has a fool for a patient") must put our trust in the hands of another physician when we get sick. This is because—as educated as you may be, or as much as you've learned about this disease, or as accustomed as you are to taking charge of your life—you can't be objective, and somebody needs to be. Make sure this somebody is the best you can find, and then be prepared to follow the plan this doctor believes is best.

7

ACTIVE SURVEILLANCE

This chapter was written with expert opinion from Jeffrey J. Tosoian, M.D., Stacy Loeb, M.D., and Edward M. Schaeffer, M.D., Ph.D.

THE SHORT STORY:
The Highly Abridged Version of This Chapter

What Is Active Surveillance?

Active surveillance (AS) could be summed up by something Ronald Reagan once said: "Trust, but verify." It is not for everyone, but if you have low-risk, slow-growing, low-volume prostate cancer, it might be right for you. The key word here is *active*—not "do nothing." AS involves careful monitoring to make sure your cancer is what all evidence suggests it is: indolent. That's the *trust* part: an evidence-based belief that you have the kind of cancer that just sits there, causes no harm, and never grows. Indolent cancer is like the pet rock of cancers; it doesn't do much, and it doesn't need to be treated now—or maybe ever. But here's the *verify* part: regular testing is essential to detect any changes in the cancer, and to treat it promptly with the aim of curing it. AS has the immediate advantage of allowing men to avoid unpleasant treatment and its side effects, often for many years. If you're interested in AS, this chapter will cover what you need to know—whether you're an ideal candidate, what to expect for follow-up, and the risks and benefits of choosing AS over immediate treatment. Then it's up to you to answer the most important question: If you're eligible, is AS right for you?

Do I Really *Not* Need Treatment?

When I tell a man he doesn't need immediate treatment for his newly diagnosed cancer and that we plan to just watch it, he doesn't always welcome this news. Doesn't cancer kill people? Isn't this risky? The answer is, many prostate cancers need to be treated. Yours does not look like it's one of them. Let's look at a couple of statistics: Today, 1 in 8 men will be diagnosed with prostate cancer during his lifetime. However, if a man over age fifty who has never been diagnosed with prostate cancer is killed in an automobile accident and undergoes an autopsy, there is a more than 50 percent chance that the pathologist will find small amounts of cancer—indolent cancer—in his prostate. This is cancer that would never have caused trouble and may never even have been detected.

So the question here, as we mentioned in chapter 5, is, have you just had an autopsy before your time? That's why it is important to pause and make certain that the cancer is not significant (see very low risk prostate cancer on page 173)—and, if you choose AS, to make sure your tumor remains small and does not begin to grow and become aggressive over time. An estimated 40 percent of all newly diagnosed prostate cancers don't need immediate treatment.

Why Should I Consider AS?

AS could be summed up by something Ronald Reagan once said: "Trust, but verify." It is not for everyone, but if you have low-risk, slow-growing, low-volume prostate cancer, it might be right for you. The key word here is *active*—not "do nothing." AS involves careful monitoring to make sure your cancer is what all evidence suggests that it is: indolent. That's the *trust* part: an evidence-based belief that you have the kind of cancer that just sits there, causes no harm, and never grows. Indolent cancer is like the pet rock of cancers; it doesn't do much, and it doesn't need to be treated now—or maybe ever. But here's the *verify* part: regular testing is essential to detect any changes in the cancer, and to treat it promptly with the aim of curing it. AS has the immediate advantage of allowing men to avoid unpleasant treatment and its side effects, often for many years.

And yet, the idea of living with cancer and choosing not to treat it right away can be difficult to comprehend. Why would anyone choose to live with prostate cancer but not treat it? Why do experts consider active surveillance the best option for some men with prostate cancer? Years of treating and researching prostate cancer have shown us that many tumors are not the fast-growing, aggressive cancers that can be lethal. In fact, prostate cancer is generally considered a slow-growing cancer. Furthermore, because prostate cancer is most often diagnosed in older age, men with less aggressive cancers are more likely to die *with* their prostate cancer rather than *of* it. So if a cancer appears to be slow-growing, there are good reasons to think about not treating it immediately.

Important point: Cancer doesn't always stay indolent; in fact, maybe it was never truly indolent. Maybe it's the proverbial wolf in sheep's clothing: maybe, from the initial biopsy and test results it appears to be low-risk and low-volume, but actually more cancer is there and the biopsy needle just missed it. So be aware that if you choose AS, you may not stay on it forever if your cancer undergoes a "grade reclassification"—that is, if you have another biopsy and it suggests that more cancer is present, or that the cancer is not as slothlike in personality as it first appeared. If this happens at some point, you may need to have surgery or radiation.

There is good evidence to support AS. True, we don't have a crystal ball that will accurately predict which cancers will eventually prove more aggressive, but we do have your PSA level, Gleason score, and a number of other tests to help provide an educated prediction of how your cancer will behave. Furthermore, with the type of active monitoring described in this chapter, we now believe that the vast majority of men who choose active surveillance have a similarly low risk of dying from their cancer compared to those treated immediately. (One notable exception: A recent study, the ProtecT Trial described in Chapter 6, followed a more passive approach to monitoring, *without* standard biopsies during follow-up. Those men did have a higher risk of progression and metastatic disease—but they weren't closely monitored!) Remember, active surveillance involves *close monitoring with the expectation to initiate curative treatment* if the cancer later appears to be more aggressive. For many men, it makes sense to hold off on immediate treatment and preserve excellent quality of life.

Who Is the Ideal Candidate for AS?

How dangerous is your cancer? Figuring this out involves a process called *risk stratification*. Prostate cancer risk groups traditionally have been defined based on three factors: the clinical stage of the cancer, the PSA level, and the appearance of the cancer cells under the microscope (this is "pathologic grade," discussed in chapter 5).

Low-, intermediate-, and high-risk groups were established in research led by Anthony D'Amico, a professor of radiation oncology and prostate cancer specialist at the Brigham and Women's Hospital. The D'Amico Risk Groups were based on the likelihood of cancer recurrence after treatment with either radical prostatectomy or radiation therapy. These classifications also help predict the risk of metastatic disease and of death from prostate cancer, and were adopted by the National Comprehensive Cancer Network (NCCN) to help guide treatment selection. The NCCN also recognizes two additional categories: "very low-risk" and "very high-risk" prostate cancers. The NCCN risk groups are used by clinicians and researchers around the world and provide an excellent basis for the discussion of active surveillance (see Table 7.1).

TABLE 7.1

WHO IS A CANDIDATE FOR ACTIVE SURVEILLANCE (AS)?

Risk Group	Clinical stage (on digital rectal examination)	PSA	Biopsy findings	Does NCCN recommend considering AS?**	Do we recommend considering AS?**
Very low (All criteria must be met)	T1c (non-palpable)	<10 ng/ml, AND PSA density <0.15	Gleason score ≤ 6, AND ≤ 2 cores with cancer, AND < 50% involvement of any core with cancer	Yes	Yes
Low (All criteria must be met)	T1c (non-palpable), OR T2a (palpable on less than half of one side of the prostate)	<10 ng/ml	Gleason score ≤ 6	Yes	Yes, in cases of low-volume cancer (see text)
Intermediate (Any single criterion)	T2b (palpable on more than one-half of one side of the prostate, OR T2c (palpable on both sides)	10–20 ng/ml	Gleason score 7 (either 3 + 4 = 7 or 4 + 3 = 7)	Maybe considered for Gleason score 3 + 4 = 7 if < 50% of biopsy cores are positive and no other intermediate risk factors are met	No
High (Any single criterion)	T3a (palpable lesion extends outside the prostate)	> 20 ng/ml	Gleason score 8-10	No	No
Very high#	T3b (palpable lesion invades seminal vesicles), OR T4 (tumor is fixed or invades adjacent structures other than seminal vesicles)	> 20 ng/ml	Primary Gleason pattern 5 (Gleason score 5 + 3, 5 + 4, or 5 + 5), OR > 4 biopsy cores with Gleason score 8–10 cancer	No	No

* Cancers are assigned to the highest risk group for which they meet one criterion (clinical stage or PSA or biopsy findings).

** These recommendations assume the patient has a life expectancy of ten years or more. Patients with very low-, low-, or intermediate-risk cancers and a life expectancy less than ten years are recommended by the NCCN to undergo observation with monitoring for symptoms, in which case palliative treatment is pursued (watchful waiting).

Very high-risk prostate cancer is defined by either (1) the clinical stage or (2) men with multiple (two or more) high risk features or (3) primary Gleason pattern 5 disease.

Men with Very Low-Risk Prostate Cancer

In 1994, genitourinary pathologist Jonathan Epstein of Johns Hopkins introduced clinical criteria for "insignificant" prostate cancer. Additional research has confirmed that cancers meeting the "Epstein criteria" are *extremely unlikely to spread beyond the prostate.* The NCCN definition of very low-risk prostate cancer is based on Epstein's findings. To be considered very low-risk, a cancer must have clinical stage T1c (tumor is not palpable on exam nor visible by imaging), PSA lower than 10 ng/ml, PSA density lower than 0.15 ng/ml/g, Gleason score of 6 or lower (Grade Group 1), no more than two biopsy cores positive for cancer, and no more than 50 percent of any biopsy core involved with cancer (see Table 7.1).

There is universal agreement that some men with very low-risk cancer are excellent candidates for active surveillance. In fact, AS is the NCCN's primary recommendation for men with very low-risk cancer and a life expectancy of ten to twenty years. For very low-risk cancer in young, healthy men with a life expectancy of at least twenty years, AS is considered one of three recommended options, along with radiation therapy and radical prostatectomy.

How can we be confident that AS is safe for very low-risk men? Thankfully, today we have more than twenty years' experience in managing very low-risk cancers with AS. In 1995, urologists at Johns Hopkins University and the Sunnybrook Health Sciences Centre in Toronto initiated AS programs for selected men with small, low-grade prostate cancers. Initial reports from these institutions were promising, and other institutions began their own AS programs. The end result is a combined experience of more than ten thousand men managed with AS at several institutions around the world (more on this later in this chapter).

Who Else Is Eligible for AS?

Men with low-risk prostate cancer can also consider AS depending on their overall health.

Beyond the *very low-risk* population, there is no consensus as to exactly who else should be offered AS. The American Society of Clinical Oncology recommends active surveillance as an option for most men with *low-risk* cancer. Low-risk disease is defined by the following criteria: clinical stage T1–T2a (tumor is nonpalpable or palpable but involves no more than one-half of one side of the prostate), PSA lower than 10 ng/ml, and Gleason score of 6 or lower (Grade Group 1).

Low-risk and very low-risk are different. (Note: Together, very low-risk and low-risk groups are considered "favorable-risk.") As we will discuss further in this chapter, research has confirmed that AS is a reasonable approach for most men with low-risk disease. But this comes with a very important caveat: The criteria for low-risk cancer do not specify the *amount* of cancer detected on biopsy. Therefore, a man with a clinical stage of T2a or lower, PSA lower than 10 ng/ml, and Gleason score 6 cancer technically meets low-risk criteria—even if cancer is detected in 100 percent of the tissue cores (usually twelve) taken during his biopsy! So be very careful in looking at these criteria. Also, men who have cancer found in multiple biopsy cores have a greater risk of progression than do men with only one or two cores positive.

Men with Favorable Intermediate-Risk Prostate Cancer

More recently, some guidelines have even suggested active surveillance as an option for certain men with "favorable" intermediate-risk cancers. The NCCN defines intermediate-risk disease as clinical stage T2b or T2c (tumor involves more than half of one side of the prostate, or both sides), PSA between 10 and 20 ng/ml, or Gleason score 7 (Grade Group 2 or 3). Note: There are two kinds of Gleason score 7 cancers, which is why they fall into two different Grade Groups. When there is more Gleason grade 3 (less aggressive) than grade 4 (more aggressive) cancer, that is Gleason score 3 + 4 = 7 (Grade Group 2). When there is more of grade 4 than grade 3, that is Gleason score 4 + 3 = 7 (Grade Group 3). The higher grade indicates a more aggressive cancer, and more aggressive cancers need to be treated.

Is AS safe for some men with Gleason score 7 cancers? *We do not recommend AS for men with Gleason score 7 cancers who have a life expectancy of at least ten years.* These cancers have a significantly higher potential to spread and be aggressive than does Gleason score 6 disease—and remember, what pathologists see in biopsy needle samples is often different from what they see when they examine the whole prostate specimen after surgery. There could be more cancer in there, and it could be of a higher grade. We just don't know. Some studies indicate that men with intermediate-risk cancers benefit the most from immediate treatment. The AS experience in men with Gleason score 7 cancers is limited, but recent reports from AS programs in Toronto and Sweden confirm what one would expect— these men did not do as well on AS as did men with very low- and low-risk. We will summarize these findings later in this chapter.

What Happens During AS?

Most AS programs require a repeat "confirmatory" biopsy performed within a year to fifteen months of your initial biopsy. As its name suggests, this is done to confirm that the cancer is, in fact, as slow-growing as it first seemed and to help rule out the presence of hidden, higher-grade cancer. From there, AS commonly proceeds with PSA tests every three to six months and a rectal exam every six to twelve months (see Table 7.2). If there is any cause for concern—a significant rise in PSA, for example, or any change detected in the exam, you'll need a repeat biopsy. If there are no worrisome changes, you will still need to get biopsies from time to time—but it is unclear just how often these need to be performed. For years, at Johns Hopkins, we erred on the side of caution and recommended yearly biopsy to men on AS. Other programs have intervals of up to five years between biopsies. Of course, having more frequent biopsies minimizes your risk that a higher-grade cancer will go undetected; but the trade-off is that biopsies are uncomfortable, and each biopsy slightly raises your risk of having a complication such as bleeding or infection. The good news is that advances in technology are giving us new tests that can help decrease the need for frequent biopsies.

Are There Tests to Confirm I Have a Low-Volume Cancer?

Yes. Multiparametric MRI (mpMRI, discussed in chapter 5) can provide a "high-resolution map" of the prostate. Data from Johns

TABLE 7.2

EXPECTED MONITORING DURING ACTIVE SURVEILLANCE*

Assessment	PSA measurement	Clinical examination	Repeat "confirmatory" biopsy	Subsequent biopsies	Imaging studies
Common recommendations	Every 3–6 months	Every 3–12 months	Yes	Every 1–5 years AND in the presence of changes in PSA, prostate exam, or other tests	Research indicates MRI may be useful in some settings

* This table summarizes the recommendations of several institutions but does not account for specific institutions' monitoring approaches. For further detail regarding institution-specific recommendations and a discussion of the positives and negatives of more intensive versus less intensive monitoring, see: Tosoian JJ, Carter HB, Lepor A, Loeb S. "Active surveillance for prostate cancer: current evidence and contemporary state of practice." *Nat Rev Urol*, 2016; 13: 205–15.

Hopkins suggest that if a man is eligible for AS and has a negative MRI (one that shows nothing suspicious that could be cancer), there is a very good chance that he is indeed a good candidate for AS. However, mpMRI is not perfect; it is estimated to miss about 15 percent of cancers with Gleason scores of 7 or greater (Grade Groups 2–5). Further, it is unclear whether repeat mpMRI remains useful after a man has been on AS for some time. This is why mpMRI is only one part of the monitoring plan—and why we have backups to our backup tests, to give us the most comprehensive picture possible. New tests such as the Prostate Health Index (PHI, a blood test discussed in chapter 4) can also help predict whether you are at a higher risk of needing treatment to cure the cancer.

Will My Cancer Change in the Future?

Well, if we could know this for sure, there would be no need to monitor some cancers at all. But take heart: precision medicine has entered the prostate cancer arena, and several new genetic tests can help predict how aggressive a specific cancer will be. One advantage of these molecular tests is that they can predict cancer's aggressiveness long before any changes can be seen under the microscope. Note: These tests have not been extensively researched in the setting of AS, so we're still figuring out exactly how to interpret them and which one may be best. Edward Schaeffer, who, in addition to being a urologist, has a Ph.D. in molecular biology, tells me that these tests offer similar information—they all look at the molecular underpinnings of the cancer. Since these tests will need to be interpreted by your urologist, he recommends working with your urologist to determine which (if any) could be most helpful for you.

How Do I Know If AS Is No Longer Safe?

Although you have a low-grade cancer today, it may not remain that way forever. Even a "safe" cancer can change over time, and as this happens, its DNA becomes less stable; the cancer can develop new mutations and become more aggressive. It is possible for a tumor to change from a low-grade, indolent-appearing cancer into high-grade, aggressive cancer. This is why active surveillance is so *active*: we are looking for this, hoping not to find it, but ready to take action if we do. If your cancer turns out to be more aggressive, you will need treatment with surgery or radiation

Triggers for Intervention

What changes, exactly, are we talking about? When should a man move from AS to treatment? In the past, some AS programs recommended treatment based on substantial rises in PSA over time (termed high "PSA velocity" or short "PSA doubling-time"). Unfortunately, changes in PSA levels are not accurate in predicting tumor aggressiveness in this setting. Today, most programs recommend treatment only if the pathologist finds changes in the tissue obtained at biopsy. If, on a repeat biopsy, your Gleason Grade Group changes—if your Gleason score changes from 6 to 7, for instance—your cancer should be treated.

In men with *very low-risk* disease, it also makes sense to consider treatment if the disease no longer meets the strict entry criteria for AS—for example, if the *amount* of cancer found in a biopsy increases above two needle cores, or cancer is found in more than half of the tissue in any single core. For men with *low-risk disease*, because there is no clear threshold for what defines "too much" cancer, deciding on treatment based on the amount of cancer detected in the biopsy cores is less straightforward. At Johns Hopkins, men who have more than three cores of cancer almost always undergo treatment. In the *favorable intermediate-risk* group, an increase in the amount of Gleason 4 disease should trigger a discussion about treating the cancer.

Other findings: Changes found in the rectal exam or in PSA levels should warrant a biopsy that may not have otherwise been planned. Changes in MRI or PHI can also signal that the disease is becoming more aggressive and prompt further investigation.

How Do Men Do on AS?

If you're considering AS, the tables at the end of this chapter can help give you a sense of what to expect. However, it is important to realize that two decades is probably not enough time to provide definitive conclusions; although the largest AS programs began in 1995, the majority of patients enrolled more recently and have only been followed for five or six years. We don't have definitive "forever" results yet; those will take many more years to determine.

Will I End Up Needing Treatment?

Maybe; results vary. Treatment is most often pursued after higher-grade cancer is detected, and the likelihood of detecting a change in the cancer grade depends on how intensively one is being monitored—"the more you look, the more you find." At Johns Hopkins, where most men in AS have undergone yearly biopsies, the rates of treatment tend to be higher. On the other hand, in the Sunnybrook program—where biopsies are scheduled every three to four years—the rate of treatment is lower. As you may imagine, there's a notable tradeoff. Less intensive monitoring means fewer men getting treatment. It also raises the odds of a dangerous cancer going undetected during follow-up, and places men at a somewhat higher risk of having cancer spreading beyond the prostate or even becoming fatal.

Of the five published AS programs with adequate follow-up (see Table 7.3), four of them reported the proportion of men who needed treatment five years after beginning AS. This ranged from 24 percent in the Sunnybrook program to 40 percent at the University of California, San Francisco. Three programs reported the treatment rate ten years after diagnosis: 37 percent at Sunnybrook, 50 percent at Johns Hopkins, and 53 percent in Göteborg. These findings suggest that within five years, about one-third of men on AS will need surgery or radiation, and within ten years, half will undergo treatment.

TABLE 7.3

REPORTED 10- AND 15-YEAR AS OUTCOMES BY RISK GROUP*

	Treatment		Metastatic disease		Death from prostate cancer	
	10-yr	15-yr	10-yr	15-yr	10-yr	15-yr
Johns Hopkins						
Favorable risk	50%	57%	0.6%	0.6%	0.1%	0.1%
Sunnybrook						
Favorable risk	36%	42%	4%	5%	2%	3%
Intermediate risk	39%	52%	9%	18%	3%	11%

* Reliable research of outcomes is dependent on several factors including, but not limited to the amount of follow-up accrued at the time of publication, the number of patients in the cohort, the variation of patient risk within each group, and the type of analysis performed to estimate these probabilities. For simplicity, these factors are not represented in the table. Furthermore, the table does not include an exhaustive list of all AS programs, but of two large programs that have prospectively enrolled men on AS since 1995. As such, the table includes a limited perspective of the AS experience and should not be interpreted as a reliable representation of expected outcomes.

1 Data obtained from: Tosoian JJ, Mamawala M, Epstein JI, Landis P, Wolf S, Trock BJ, Carter HB. "Intermediate and Longer-Term Outcomes From a Prospective Active-Surveillance Program for Favorable-Risk Prostate Cancer." *J Clin Oncol*, 2015 Aug 31;JCO.2015.62.5764.

2 Data obtained from: Musunuru HB, Yamamoto T, Klotz L, Ghanem G, Mamedov A, Sethukavalan P, Jethava V, Jain S, Zhang L, Vesprini D, Loblaw A. "Active Surveillance for Intermediate Risk Prostate Cancer: Survival Outcomes in the Sunnybrook Experience." *J Urol*, 2016 Dec;196(6): 1651–8.

Risk of Metastatic Disease and Death from Cancer

Good news here: The risk of metastasis or death from prostate cancer appears to be exceedingly low in men who are carefully selected and monitored on active surveillance. Of nearly 1,300 men enrolled in the Johns Hopkins program, 71 percent had very low-risk cancer and 29 percent had low-risk cancer. Since the program began in 1995, only two men have died of prostate cancer, and five men have developed metastatic disease. The likelihood of developing metastatic disease within fifteen years of enrolling in AS was 0.6 percent, and the risk of dying of cancer was only 0.1 percent.

By comparison, the Sunnybrook program has reported a 5.7 percent likelihood of cancer death at fifteen years from diagnosis. The reasons for this discrepancy appear to be patient selection—23 percent of the men in the Sunnybrook program were considered intermediate-risk—and, as discussed above, less intensive monitoring. Research from the Sunnybrook experience has helped to clarify the risk of AS in men who do not meet very low- or low-risk criteria. Sunnybrook investigators recently compared outcomes between the intermediate-risk and favorable risk (very low-risk and low-risk) groups. They reported that the risk of metastatic disease fifteen years after diagnosis was 18 percent in the intermediate-risk population, as compared to 5 percent in the favorable-risk population. The corresponding risks of death from prostate cancer were 11 percent versus 3 percent, respectively. These numbers help illustrate why we do not recommend AS in healthy men with intermediate-risk cancer.

Is AS the Same as Watchful Waiting?

Not at all. *Watchful waiting* is the traditional "wait and see" approach. There is no intention to cure the cancer, nor to provide any treatment unless symptoms develop; thus, no specific follow-up tests are required. This is primarily used in older men and men with other health problems who are diagnosed with a prostate cancer that is unlikely to cause harm during their lifetime. Watchful waiting does not mean your doctor has written you off; it means you undergo treatment for specific symptoms if and when you need it.

If you have no symptoms, you simply live your life and return to the doctor if any symptoms develop. Note: Although it is very tempting to want to do *something*, and there are many urologists who used to recommend giving hormonal therapy (androgen deprivation therapy, or ADT) at this stage, *don't do it!* Many serious side effects are associated with ADT (see chapter 12), including a higher risk of developing diabetes, cardiovascular disease, and even cognitive impairment. In a study of 65,000 older men diagnosed with localized prostate cancer, the men who received early hormonal therapy were more likely to die. Another study of older men found that there was no benefit to early hormonal therapy (before symptoms of metastasis), even in men who had a high Gleason score.

Who Should Consider Watchful Waiting?

A good rule of thumb is that if you are not healthy enough to undergo treatment, observation is the best approach. You may already sense that you fall in this category; if not, it may be time for a frank discussion with your primary care doctor to discuss your overall health.

Is AS Right for You?

Although programs vary in intensity of monitoring, if you undergo AS, you can expect to get follow-up PSA tests, rectal exams, and biopsies, maybe for many years. If you are a young man, say, age fifty, and you could reasonably expect to live another forty years, this could mean that you will get your prostate stuck with needles many, many more times in your life. Biopsies have their own risks (discussed in chapter 5). You may not want to subject yourself to this.

You will also have to live your life knowing you have cancer. Can you handle this? Some men can't. Thinking about the cancer in there makes them anxious. To them, it's like a time bomb—when actually, it may not be a time bomb at all, but more of a clock just happily ticking away, not causing harm—and they end up having surgery or radiation just for the peace of mind. But there are risks of side effects with treatment, as well (discussed in the next chapters). Weigh them carefully.

On the other hand, if you can live with it—trusting that the follow-up monitoring will detect any change and that if you need to get treatment, you won't miss that window of treatment when the cancer is still confined to the prostate—then active surveillance may be a good option for you.

Only you can answer this question. Take some time to consider how each approach to management would affect the aspects of life you value most, and discuss the tradeoffs with your doctor and those closest to you. Remember, the "right" answer is the one that is best for *you*.

How About Combining AS with Drugs? Will That Make It More Effective?

Several studies have looked at whether taking certain drugs could slow the progression of prostate cancer or put it on hold indefinitely. For instance, could 5-alpha reductase inhibitors such as finasteride (Proscar) or dutasteride (Avodart) be helpful in AS? As we discussed in chapter 3, these drugs block the conversion of testosterone to dihydrotestosterone (DHT). Unfortunately, because there is not much 5-alpha reductase in prostate cancer, these drugs don't help stop prostate cancer. What they're much better at, and what they were originally intended for, is treating a different kind of growth in the prostate associated with benign enlargement. That particular kind of prostate tissue is chock-full of 5-alpha reductase and does respond well to drugs designed to inhibit BPH.

If that were the only problem—that these drugs don't really work on prostate cancer—this would be concerning enough, but there's more. These drugs are not without side effects, such as erectile dysfunction and breast swelling. But the major problem is that they give men a false sense of security, because they lower their levels of PSA by 50 percent. Start taking one of them, and your PSA is cut in half. Whew! What a relief! That's pretty dramatic; isn't this a good sign? No, it's a cause of false optimism, because the decrease is only in the PSA made by benign disease—not by cancer. In a small study carried out by a pharmaceutical company, when men on active surveillance were treated with dutasteride, it reduced the risk of cancer progression from 24 percent to 19 percent at eighteen months; however, by three years, progression in the two groups was the same. Because active surveillance involves follow-up for many years, this finding is insignificant. In a Johns Hopkins study, urologist Ashley Ross, looking at the patients in the Johns Hopkins active surveillance program, was unable to demonstrate any improvement in men who were taking finasteride.

Let's take this a step further, because there are advocates who do. Some doctors advise men on AS not only to take the 5-alpha reductase inhibitors, but to do it in combination with LHRH agonists and an antiandrogen (these forms of hormonal therapy are discussed in detail in chapter 12). The idea here is that these men can "buy some time" until a new cure comes along that has few or no side effects. This is a false promise. What these individuals fail to tell patients is that these drugs will do nothing to slow down the growth of prostate cancer cells that are not controlled by hormones (these are called hormone-insensitive cells; see chapter 12), and in prostate cancer, these are the ones that can ultimately kill you.

It gets worse. To someone who has seen curable young, healthy men miss their chance to be cured, it's sickening. These advocates also deceive patients about the side effects of these ineffective drugs. No problem, they say—the side effects can be reversed if you take additional medications. Got impotence? Take sildenafil (Viagra). Still more disturbing, advocates of this regimen reject the concept that early ADT increases cardiovascular risk (see chapter 12). Beware of anyone who tells you Viagra will restore your love life if you are on hormonal therapy, and that there is no need for you to be concerned about worsening of cardiovascular disease. In chapter 12, we quote guidelines developed by the American Heart Association, the American Cancer Society, and the American Urological Association advising men who are going on hormonal therapy to recognize the potential for worsening of diabetes and increased risk of cardiovascular death.

So we've seen things that don't work. Is there anything that you can do, if you're on AS that might slow down the cancer? Yes. Read the recommendations in chapter 3 on lifestyle and dietary changes that are known to decrease the risk of prostate cancer. Remember, at autopsy, 50 percent of men are found to have a bit of prostate cancer, but only 1 in 8 men actually develops the disease. What's the difference? We believe it relates to factors that encourage the cancer cells to grow and to progress. That's also the same mechanism responsible for progression in men who are undergoing active surveillance. Although there is no reliable study that proves this, it makes sense. Don't go overboard by going on a severe diet and taking every pill you can find in a health-food store that promises "prostate health." Just follow the sensible recommendations in chapter 3, remain vigilant by scheduling follow-up visits with your doctor to make sure the cancer has not changed, and don't take drugs that will simply mask the progression of cancer and fail to treat the real problem.

8

RADICAL PROSTATECTOMY

This chapter was written with expert opinion from Edward M. Schaeffer, M.D., Ph.D.

THE SHORT STORY:
The Highly Abridged Version of This Chapter

Never underestimate prostate cancer. It is a formidable adversary that springs up in several places—on average, three to seven separate areas inside the prostate—at once. Although with MRI imaging we can do a better job of pinpointing cancer's location, we can't always see the clear outline of where a prostate tumor begins and ends. Thus, to cure the disease, we can't just treat the spots of cancer that we can see; we must eliminate the entire prostate.

If cancer is confined to the prostate, there is no better way to cure it than with radical prostatectomy. The goal of all other forms of treatment for prostate cancer is to be as good as this "gold standard." Today, radical prostatectomy cures the vast majority of men with cancer confined to the prostate—even if cancer has penetrated the wall, or capsule, of the prostate. If the operation is performed by an experienced surgeon, preserving potency is common, and serious incontinence is very rare.

But radical prostatectomy is not for everybody. It is intended for the otherwise healthy man who can reasonably expect to live for at least another ten to fifteen years. In other words, it is for the man who is going to live long enough to need to be cured. It is not ideal for a man already burdened by significant health problems.

The radical prostatectomy used to be an operation of last resort; there were so many side effects—excessive blood loss, incontinence, and impotence—that many men said they would rather have the disease than the cure. That changed in the early 1980s, with the development of the anatomical approach now known as the Walsh procedure—the preservation of anatomic structures that previously had been unknown to surgeons, including the urinary sphincter and the nerve bundles that are responsible for erection. These advances permitted thousands of men to have an excellent cancer operation, while preserving and accelerating recovery of urinary control and sexual function.

THE LAPAROSCOPIC/ROBOTIC PROCEDURE

Laparoscopy is basically surgery through tiny holes, or ports, instead of a larger incision. It begins when a fiber-optic camera, about the size of a pen, is threaded into the body through a port; this camera guides the surgeon throughout the procedure. Then surgical instruments are inserted through other small ports.

Robotic-assisted approaches have advanced traditional laparoscopy in two significant ways. First, the robotic camera actually has two "eyes," and this is a good thing; it allows the surgeon to see the inside of the body in three dimensions. It gives us depth perception. Traditional laparoscopy uses a single lens or eye, which only allows the surgeon to see in two dimensions. Second, the robotic surgical system includes extremely precise, tiny instruments that are "wristed." They move like a hand. So in the robotic procedure, we have extremely magnified, 3-D vision of the pelvis and prostate along with microscopic wristed instrumentation. The robotic surgical system is a powerful tool in the prostate surgeon's arsenal; however, like all powerful tools, it is only as good as the hand holding it. The robotic system needs a skilled operator to use it safely and to maximal advantage. One key advantage the robotic-assisted laparoscopic approach offers is a near bloodless field. "It allows surgeons to see the prostate and its adjacent anatomy as well as Dr. Walsh with his open procedure," says Edward Schaeffer, M.D., Ph.D., Chairman of Urology at Northwestern University. He cautions: "It is important to remember that the fancy robot is not a surrogate for a good surgeon! A skilled prostate surgeon must know the anatomy cold and understand all the subtleties of the disease and the operation."

In radical prostatectomy, as with all surgical procedures, the outcome is operator-dependent—which is why, whichever procedure you select, it is essential that you have an experienced surgeon. This is just as important, maybe even more so, with the laparoscopic/robotic techniques. Remember, *the operation is not performed by the machine, but by the surgeon who tells the machine what to do.*

We also discuss in detail the complications that can occur in the days and months after the operation. For a detailed discussion of cancer control outcomes with all forms of treatment for localized disease—surgery, radiation, and cryo/thermal ablation, see chapter 10.

Radical Prostatectomy–The Gold Standard

Never underestimate prostate cancer; it is a formidable adversary. In its own way, prostate cancer is much like the Hydra, the many-headed, hard-to-kill monster of Greek myth. It's what scientists call multifocal, which means it springs up in several places at once inside the prostate. A cancerous prostate has, on average, three to seven separate tumors growing inside it, in both lobes. Thus, to cure the disease, we can't just take out a few of these spots of cancer; we must eliminate the entire prostate.

If cancer is confined to the prostate, there is no better way to cure it than with radical prostatectomy. The goal of all other forms of treatment for prostate cancer is to be as good as this gold standard. Having said that, we must add right away that radical prostatectomy is not for everybody. It is intended for *healthy men with curable disease*, who are expected to live for at least another fifteen years. In other words, it is for the man who is not only curable but who's going to live long enough to need to be cured.

What if you're somewhere in the middle of these two ends of the spectrum? What if you're a young, active man, but the statistics say there's only a fifty-fifty chance your cancer can be cured? *If surgery is the best way to cure you, then you should do it.* This often refers to men with high-risk disease (a PSA level greater than 20 ng/ml, or clinical stage T3a disease, or a Gleason score between 8 and 10). *Men in this situation should realize that if they are going to be treated with radiation, they will also receive hormonal therapy, with all of its side effects* (see chapter 12) *for two to three months before and for up to three years after treatment.* Many men do not want to do this, and would rather have surgery and get it over with. Is this a good idea for you? In a recent review of radical prostatectomies performed on high-risk patients, we found that men who had only *one* of these three high-risk features (that is, *either* a PSA greater than 20 *or* clinical stage T3a disease *or* Gleason 8 to 10 disease) did very well. At ten years after surgery, PSA levels were undetectable in 68 percent, bone scans were negative in 84 percent, only 8 percent died of prostate cancer, and 71 percent never received hormonal therapy. It's worth making this point again: Hormonal therapy is something no man should begin lightly. It has significant side effects, and if it can be delayed for years or avoided altogether, it should be.

What if you're a man in his early seventies, in excellent health, with curable disease and a family history of longevity? Is surgery right for you? It may well be. Why? Because as men live longer, the prostate cancers that develop in them tend to be more aggressive.

As we discussed in chapter 7, older men often have more advanced disease, because it has been there longer. However, older men are more prone to side effects after surgery than younger men are, and it is very important to consider the quality of the years ahead. How would you feel if you never regained full control over urination? Also, what if you had complications and were not cured? On the other hand, if an older man selects a less effective form of treatment, has a long life, and the cancer comes back, he may end up asking himself "what if"—what if he had gone for surgery the first time around? This can be a tough decision.

Many men of any age hate what this decision entails—being forced to look in the mirror, the necessary assessment of their own health aside from prostate cancer. You may find it helpful to look back at the section in chapter 6 on the Scandinavian study. Although this study clearly demonstrated that surgery increased survival, the main beneficiaries were men who were younger than sixty-five at the time of surgery. For men over age sixty-five, there was no improvement in cancer-specific survival—mainly because many men died of other causes before they died of prostate cancer. On the flip side, men today in the United States are healthier than ever. And here's yet another statistic, an important one to consider: very healthy men who are seventy live an average of eighteen additional years. Talk to your doctor, talk to your family, and really think about the best way to manage your cancer.

Today, radical prostatectomy provides excellent cancer control and cure for men, even if cancer has penetrated the wall, or capsule, of the prostate. Serious bleeding is very rare, and if the operation is performed by an experienced surgeon, the preservation of potency is common, and few suffer from serious incontinence.

Evolution of an Operation

Surgery to remove the prostate as a treatment for cancer was first performed in 1904 at Johns Hopkins by Hugh Hampton Young, the pioneering first director of the Brady Urological Institute. Young's procedure, called the radical perineal prostatectomy, was a success. Six and a half years later, when the patient died of other causes, an autopsy showed that his prostate cancer had been cured.

In the late 1940s, another approach called the radical retropubic prostatectomy was developed, and like Young's operation (which is still used today, although not as often as the retropubic approach), it proved extremely effective in stopping prostate cancer in its tracks.

The early radical perineal and retropubic operations had a definite downside—two devastating side effects, incontinence and impotence. Every man who had a radical prostatectomy was impotent, and as many as 25 percent had severe problems with urinary control. Worse was the extreme, often life-threatening bleeding that went along with the retropubic approach. It's no exaggeration to say that the operation used to be performed in a sea of blood. In that era, many men believed that the side effects from surgery were almost worse than having the disease, and surgeons did not want to operate because of the life-threatening blood loss.

The harshness of the procedure and its aftereffects were the catalysts for change, inspiring the anatomical discoveries that have drastically reduced these side effects. As a result of these discoveries, *when radical prostatectomy is performed by an experienced surgeon,* younger men should remain potent, and few should have serious problems with urinary control. Today, radical prostatectomy is the most certain way to cure men with cancer that's confined to the prostate.

Crafting a Kinder, Gentler, Better Operation

How did radical prostatectomy change? My role in this operation began in the 1970s. Like many urologic surgeons, I was appalled by the blood loss in these men. With the goal of finding surgical methods to lessen the bleeding—so we could actually see what we were doing instead of blindly feeling our way—I studied the anatomy of the venous drainage surrounding the prostate and developed some new techniques, which did two things. First, *with less bleeding, the operation became safer.* And with what we call a bloodless field, critical structures—which previously had been unrecognized and damaged simply because there was too much blood in the way to see them— could be looked for and saved. More precise dissection and reconstruction reduced the likelihood of significant urinary incontinence to 2 percent, and even these men are not incontinent all the time.

Breakthrough in Understanding Potency

But what about impotence? It had always been assumed that impotence was caused by damage to the nerves that controlled erections, but nobody knew exactly where those nerves were located. However, because all men were impotent following surgery, everyone believed the nerves must run *through* the prostate and that it would be impossible to preserve them. Impotence was assumed to be the price of curing the cancer.

It didn't make sense to me that the nerves from one organ would run through another organ. Around this time, something unbelievable happened. In 1977, one of my patients returned for a follow-up visit three months after surgery and reported that he was totally potent. To me, this news was staggering. How could this man be potent if the nerves that control potency were inside the prostate that I had removed? Furthermore, if this could happen to one man, then why *only* this one? Why weren't *all* men potent after radical prostatectomy?

The key had to be these elusive nerves. If we could just figure out where they were—and then find a way to save them but still cure prostate cancer—then men would no longer be faced with an either-or situation. They could be cured of cancer *and* remain potent.

Fast-forward to 1981. I was at Leiden University in the Netherlands, where my friend Pieter Donker had just retired as chairman of urology. He specialized in neurourology, the treatment of neurological conditions that affected bladder function, and I visited him at his laboratory. He was using a dissecting microscope to trace the nerves supplying the bladder in a stillborn male infant. In adult cadavers, he explained, the abdominal contents compress the pelvic organs into a thick pancake of tissue and formaldehyde dissolves the fat between tissue planes—making it impossible to study these microscopic structures. For this reason, no one had previously dissected the nerves to the bladder. I asked Donker if he knew the location of the branches of the nerves that controlled erections. He said that he had never looked. We got to work. Four hours later, we were jubilant. We could see clearly that the nerves were outside the capsule of the prostate—and that, indeed, it was possible to completely remove the prostate and preserve sexual function!

Over the next year, we worked together on this project long-distance, and then we met again. In the infant cadaver, the location of these nerves had become clear. But how could we apply these findings in stillborn infants to the complicated recesses of the pelvis in adult men? It was like having a schematic drawing and trying to identify a burned-out transistor in your television set. During this year, I had noticed something important: there was a cluster of arteries and veins that traveled along the edge of the prostate in the exact location where these nerves were found in the infant cadaver. Perhaps these blood vessels acted as they do elsewhere in the body— maybe they provided a scaffold for these microscopic nerves. And maybe we could use these bundles as landmarks. Donker agreed.

In March 1982, I tested this theory while performing an operation called a radical cystectomy, removal of the prostate and bladder, in a sixty-seven-year-old man. I had never seen or heard of a patient who had been potent after this operation. But ten days after surgery, this man stated that he awoke in the morning with a normal erection. And then on April 26, 1982, I performed the first purposeful nerve-sparing radical prostatectomy on a fifty-two-year-old professor. This man regained his sexual function within a year and has remained complication-free—and cancer-free—ever since.

Better understanding of the anatomical terrain also led to several important observations. Now that we've learned exactly where the scalpel can and cannot go, depending on the extent of a man's cancer, it has become possible either to save these nerves deliberately or to remove more tissue by cutting these bundles away—in surgical terms, to create wider margins of excision—than we previously had believed possible. It used to be that surgeons never excised these nerves because they were adherent to the rectum; instead, surgeons just cut the nerves and unknowingly left them in place. However, with these anatomical techniques, we now have a better chance of removing all the cancer. Many people call this a nerve-sparing operation, but a more accurate description is that it's an anatomic radical prostatectomy, because there are actually two things going on here: one is preserving the nerves; the other is creating wider margins—by excising the nerves when necessary, removing as much tissue as possible around the cancer—making this a better cancer operation.

At the same time these discoveries were taking place, an anatomist provided an entirely new insight into the location of the sphincter responsible for urinary control. Previously, we believed that the pelvic floor muscles opened and closed like sliding doors. But it turns out that the sphincter is a tubular structure embedded in the veins that had once bled so much during surgery. This observation explained why the anatomic approach improved the results of urinary continence: in controlling the venous bleeders and making the bloodless field, we did a better job of preserving this sphincter.

WILL I BE FERTILE AFTER SURGERY?

For most couples, there is good news after a radical prostatectomy: they can safely discontinue birth control measures. That's because the vas deferens (see chapter 1), which carries sperm, is completely divided, and there is no way a woman can become pregnant during intercourse. But what happens to the sperm that continue to be produced by the testes? They are absorbed by the epididymis (this is what happens after a standard vasectomy as well).

However, many men who undergo radical prostatectomy today may not have completed family planning, says Northwestern University urologist Robert Brannigan. If you're not ready to close this door forever, the safest and simplest thing to do is store sperm before surgery (via a process called cryopreservation). There is also a plan B available for men who have already undergone radical prostatectomy and then decide they want to have children. Basically, it involves a simple outpatient procedure called "sperm aspiration," in which a tiny needle is used to harvest sperm from the testis or epididymis. Whether the sperm was cryopreserved before prostate surgery or aspirated afterward, it is most commonly used in a process called in vitro fertilization (IVF) with intracytoplasmic sperm injection (ICSI). "The sperm are injected directly into eggs that have been harvested from the patient's partner. After a period of incubation, one or two fertilized eggs (embryos) are then transferred into the female partner's uterus." But the best bet, if there's even a remote chance that you may want more children after surgery, is to plan ahead and store your sperm.

If you undergo a radical prostatectomy, you need to understand that there are three important goals: removing all of the tumor, preserving urinary control, and preserving sexual function. Sexual function is number three, because if it is lost, there are many ways to restore it. *Men who are impotent following radical prostatectomy have normal sensation, normal sex drive, and can achieve a normal orgasm.* The one element they may be lacking is the ability to have an erection sufficient for intercourse, and that can be restored by drugs such as sildenafil (Viagra), tadalafil (Cialis), and vardenafil (Levitra), or by other means. (For more on erectile dysfunction, see chapter 11.)

Are You in Good Hands?

The complications from a radical prostatectomy ought to be minimal, but they can be devastating. A bad surgeon can ruin your life. This is why it is essential that you find the best surgeon you can. Get this done right.

FOR BEST RESULTS, FIND A HOSPITAL WHERE THEY DO A LOT OF RADICAL PROSTATECTOMIES

When it comes to finding a hospital for radical prostatectomy, a Johns Hopkins study has found a simple rule for potential patients to keep in mind: experience counts, especially if you want the best chance of being cured.

"Radical prostatectomy is a complex, notoriously difficult surgical procedure," says epidemiologist Bruce J. Trock. The study confirms what many in the medical community have known for years: the best results—fewest side effects and greatest control of cancer—are found at academic medical centers where the urologists specialize in this complicated operation.

The study, headed by Robert Wood Johnson scholar and Hopkins urology fellow Lars Ellison, compares the recurrence of prostate cancer at a hospital to the number of prostatectomies performed at that hospital. What does hospital volume have to do with the results of surgery? A lot, explains Trock, who also took part in the study—particularly when the procedure is a hard one for surgeons to master. This study was published in the *Journal of Urology*.

Ellison and his colleagues evaluated more than twelve thousand men aged sixty-five or older from hospitals in Arizona, California, Connecticut, Iowa, Utah, and Washington State who underwent radical prostatectomy between 1990 and 1994 and who were followed through 1999. The researchers determined hospital volume based on the number of prostatectomies performed in men aged sixty-five or older from 1990 to 1994—low (1–33), medium (34–61), high (62–107), or very high (108 or more). Then they looked for evidence of prostate cancer recurrence in these men—the start of hormonal therapy or radiation therapy more than six months after radical prostatectomy.

They found that the low-volume hospitals had more patients with low-grade disease and local tumor stage, both of which indicate a better prognosis. This suggests that hospitals with less experience prefer to operate on the men most likely to do better, explains Trock. Even so, low- and medium-volume institutions had significantly higher rates of treatment for cancer recurrence—25 percent and 11 percent higher, respectively—than did very high-volume institutions. The higher recurrence rates at lower-volume institutions could be because the surgeons' experience—and also their techniques—vary widely. Ellison and colleagues found as much as a 25 percent difference in cancer control between low- and very high-volume hospitals. "The anatomy of the prostate and biology of a tumor can vary tremendously among patients," concludes Trock. "Surgeons at high-volume institutions encounter the full range of this diversity and are prepared to deal with it."

In another study involving surgeons at a number of large institutions, investigators found that the *total* number of open radical prostatectomies a surgeon performed—not in a week or year, but over a cumulative period—made a difference in cancer control. Patients who underwent surgery by a urologist who had performed more than 250 radical prostatectomies had the best chance of being cured.

Doctor A is a nice, personable young doctor whose empathy for your condition appealed to you immediately. That's great. Now, what else do you know about him? He's got a terrific bedside manner, but is he a board-certified urologist? What training has he had? Does he know—and use—the nerve-sparing techniques, the anatomical approach to radical prostatectomy? How many of these operations does he do a year? What success has he had in preserving potency and continence? (If he can't or won't give you his rate of success as compared to reports from other surgeons or to results published in medical journals, this may be a red flag, and perhaps you should look elsewhere.) You should be able to get a good idea of his success rate in numbers or percentages. And if he hasn't done very many of these operations—ideally, hundreds—you might want to find a more experienced surgeon. Look at it this way: Do you want to be one of the patients he's learning on? Do you want to be part of someone's learning curve?

When you're looking for a surgeon, you don't necessarily want some brand-name academician or a specialist in *other areas* of urologic surgery. You want to find a doctor who performs *this particular operation*. Often. Preferably, a doctor who does this operation several days a week. Even better, a surgeon who has dedicated his or her life to doing this one operation.

Doctor B is another nice doctor, a respected, fatherly man who's been operating in your town for as long as anybody can remember. Just looking at him inspires confidence. Swell. But does he also keep up with the latest research? Does he continue his education regularly, brushing up on old surgical skills as well as mastering new techniques?

Doctor C is Mr. Technology. His hospital is widely advertising the new multimillion-dollar robot it just acquired (and now must pay for). This robot, Doctor C promises, will do everything: reduce blood loss, get you back to work earlier, and give you a much better likelihood of retaining continence and potency. The robot, however sophisticated, is not performing the surgery; it's just a tool in the hands of Doctor C.

There's no getting around it: radical prostatectomy is a tricky operation, one of the most difficult in medicine. A good surgeon can handle unexpected or excessive bleeding without panicking, but also—thinking of your long-term quality of life—won't damage the microscopic nerves necessary for erection. An experienced surgeon knows how to preserve these nerves *and when it's safe to do so*. You don't want someone whose knee-jerk reaction to the biopsy is to cut, cut, cut. For example, if the biopsy is positive on the right side and your surgeon says, "We'll take out the nerves on the right side and on the left, too, for good measure—I'm interested in getting out all the cancer," you should find another surgeon. For one thing, the biopsy being positive on the right side doesn't mean the nerves on the right side are involved in the cancer. For another, it's unlikely that such a surgeon will actually remove the nerves on either side.

A more probable scenario is that he'll cut the nerves and leave most of them in place. Excising these nerves widely is as difficult as preserving them, because they're adherent to the rectum, and it takes great skill to cut them out completely.

Then there's the surgeon who says, "We don't care about side effects; I'm just there to get out all the cancer. We can always put in an artificial sphincter [for control of incontinence] and give you shots or a penile prosthesis [for impotence]." Again, probably not the right surgeon for you. Your ideal surgeon should get out all the cancer *and* make every effort to minimize side effects.

Remember, you don't want a surgeon who's "pretty good" at removing the prostate, you want a surgeon who "lives, eats, and sleeps" prostate cancer and radical prostatectomy. And you can't assume that every urologist does this well. There are no second chances here; this is a one-shot operation. *You are looking for the one surgeon who will perform the one radical prostatectomy you will ever receive in your life, the one operation that will cure your cancer.* You want a surgeon who isn't going to leave some cancer behind and who knows how to minimize trauma to your body during surgery so you don't wind up incontinent, impotent, or both. (Note: Unexpected trouble can crop up in any operation; nobody can help that. But the unexpected is less likely to happen with an experienced surgeon.) So ask questions, such as:

- How many of these operations are performed at your hospital per year? (You want the answer to be sixty-two or more.) How many have you personally performed in your professional career? (More than three hundred is a good answer.)
- What percentage of your patients have positive margins? (Stated another way, how often is cancer left behind?)
- In patients like me whom you have operated on, at one to two years, what percentage have to wear a pad, and how many have recovered erections sufficient for intercourse? How do you collect data on your patients? Do you know their long-term outcome? (If the answer is something like, "Only if they let me know," find someone who keeps better tabs on his or her patients. Urologists who don't know their own results may not realize that their

technique should be better. And if the urologist can produce statistics but you don't like those results, get another opinion.)

Ask to talk to the urologist's patients. Find out how they're treated—how hard is it to get the doctor when you have a question or need help? If they've had postsurgical complications, how did the doctor treat them?

Finding the right physician may mean that you must travel to a major medical center in another city. This may mean that you'll be away from home for four days. But after that, even though you will be wearing a catheter for a week or two (see below), the recovery from this operation is usually speedy, and follow-up communications can usually be carried out over the telephone (for example, if you have your follow-up PSA tests done in your hometown, you can have the results sent to your surgeon and discuss them—or any complications or troubling issues, such as incontinence or impotence—over the phone).

HOW TO FIND THE RIGHT SURGEON: A CHECKLIST

- **Look for a high-volume center.** If a hospital does a lot of radical prostatectomies, and does them well, then everyone is going to be better at helping you. The nurses know how to take care of recovering radical prostatectomy patients, and there is a wing or set of beds just for these men—and not also appendectomy or hysterectomy patients, whose post-op needs are very different. Edward Schaeffer, Chairman of Urology at Northwestern University, refers patients to two websites. One is the National Cancer Institute's website (www.cancer.gov/research/nci-role/cancer-centers/find), which designates "cutting-edge cancer treatments to patients in communities across the U.S." The other is a website showing National Comprehensive Cancer Network (NCCN)–designated cancer centers: www.nccn.org/patients/about/member_institutions/qualities.aspx.
- **Look for a place where different specialties work together.** Top centers have multidisciplinary teams—experts from different specialties including urology, radiation oncology, medical oncology, and pathology—working together on prostate cancer. Some men are perfect candidates for surgery; others might do better with

radiation, and if you are one of those, you need at least to speak with a radiation oncologist before you decide on surgery. Other men need to talk to a medical oncologist as well. Prostate cancer is a complicated thing, and there is no "one size fits all" answer for every patient. With the multidisciplinary approach, you get the opinion of a team of experts, not just one, and the benefit is a more thorough and thoughtful approach to your treatment.

- **Ask the surgeon about results.** I follow my patients for life, and that's what a good surgeon should do—so we know, twenty years after the fact, whether the PSA is still undetectable, whether there was any incontinence, whether erections returned on their own or with help from medications or other treatments, etc.
- **Ask more than one doctor to recommend the best prostate surgeon in your area.** (Note: Some doctors are in practice groups, and recommend the specialist in that group. This is why it's good to ask different doctors in different practices.)
- **Beware of the reviews or ads on the Internet.** "It is unclear to me who actually goes to these sites and makes the comments," says Schaeffer. Maybe it's the patients; maybe it's a buddy of the doctor putting in a rave review to get the number of five-star listings up. Or maybe it's a disgruntled colleague, or a competitor hoping to drive business away from that surgeon. Who knows? For the most part, says New York University urologist Stacy Loeb, "Online reviews are totally unreliable, so I am hesitant to tell men to rely on them. Speaking to other patients and local doctors is a much better idea." Loeb also recommends that you check with prostate cancer support groups in your area, and ask these men about their own experiences.
- **And finally, don't worry about offending the doctor with questions or by getting a second opinion.** You don't get to be a surgeon without being something of a tough cookie. People ask for second opinions all the time. Patients ask questions all the time. You are paying the doctor, not the other way around. (Note: That doesn't mean you should be rude or disrespectful; it just means you shouldn't feel intimidated or like you are being a bad guy simply for doing your homework.) If the situation were reversed, do you think your doctor would not make every effort to find the best possible surgeon? It's your prostate, it's your recovery, it's your life. You don't want to be one of those guys saying afterward, "My surgeon was not very good."

Questions You May Have Before Surgery

Why Do I Have to Wait Several Weeks for the Operation?

There should always be a delay of about six to eight weeks between the time a man's prostate cancer is diagnosed and the time he can undergo surgery. Many men are frustrated by this. They think, "I've got cancer, it's curable, and I want it out of there right now!" It's not that the hospital is overbooked; it's so you can have a better cancer operation.

Immediately after the needle biopsy, your body reacts—as it does to any injury—with inflammation and bleeding. That is not the ideal time for surgery. A biopsy is what doctors call an insult to the body—in this case, to the wall of the rectum, which is riddled with a dozen or more tiny holes and weakened. Think of how much easier it is to tear perforated paper than regular, intact paper. The body needs time to recover from this relatively minor insult so it will be ready for the really big one—major surgery. Even after two weeks, the punctures may have healed, but the prostate is now adherent to the rectum; it remains stuck to the rectum until the inflammation resolves. If surgery were attempted at this point, it would not be easy to release the rectum from the prostate—and the last thing the surgeon wants to do is make a hole in the rectum. In an attempt to protect the rectum, the surgeon may cut too close to the prostate, possibly leaving cancer cells behind. But after giving it a few more weeks, the inflammation heals, and the prostate is no longer sticky. The normal anatomy is restored, and it's easier for the surgeon to see the terrain.

We have studied hundreds of patients who underwent surgery and evaluated the delay between diagnosis and cure. With long follow-up, we found no significant difference in the ten-year cancer control rates of these men. Let these results reassure you that *there is no immediate urgency to perform surgery after you are diagnosed with prostate cancer,* especially if you have stage T1c disease and a biopsy Gleason score lower than 7. Take your time, and find the right doctor and hospital (see page 215).

Should I Stop Taking Aspirin, Herbal Remedies, and Vitamins?

Before surgery, when you give the doctor your medical history, be sure to mention if you've had any unusual problems with bleeding in the past (from dental work, for example). Aspirin and drugs such as ibuprofen (Advil, Motrin), and some herbal medications and supplements such as fish oil, can cause excessive bleeding; if you are taking aspirin or a similar drug regularly, make sure you stop *at least ten days before the operation.* But what if you have a stent for heart disease, a history of blood clots or irregular heartbeat, and are taking a blood thinner such as aspirin and clopidogrel (Plavix)? These are situations where it's important to consult with your cardiologist or hematologist. Often, surgery can still be performed, but it's best to talk with your entire health care team to understand the full risks and benefits.

Does It Matter If I've Had Previous Prostate Surgery for BPH?

This is how some men find out they have prostate cancer—when the prostate tissue removed in a TUR procedure or open prostatectomy (another procedure for BPH) is evaluated by a pathologist. Having had a prior BPH procedure makes the operation more difficult for surgeons to perform, but that doesn't mean it can't be done. It often is, and with great success. If you have had a recent TUR procedure, you may need to wait at least twelve weeks, until the inflammation from this operation has gone down, before having a prostatectomy.

Countdown to Surgery

One of the most important steps in recovering from a radical prostatectomy is the recovery of the gastrointestinal tract—mainly, the return of normal bowel movements. This return to normal happens much faster and with fewer complications if the bowels are empty when you undergo surgery. Thus, to help speed things along after surgery, you can work on improving your digestive tract *before* surgery. Be sure that your bowels are moving well for about two weeks before the operation; increase your daily intake of fiber, fruit,

ARE YOU IN SHAPE FOR SURGERY?

In any man, the prostate is not terribly accessible. It's way down there, deep in the pelvis. Reaching it is not only much more difficult in a man who is overweight; the extra fat can also interfere with performing a good cancer operation, preserving urinary control, and preserving potency.

Here, as an example of what can be done in just two months, is a diet plan developed by one of my patients, who was diagnosed with prostate cancer at age fifty-three. I agreed to operate on him under the condition that he lose at least 30 pounds.

Here's how he explains it: "I needed to lose the weight for my own health benefit, and a leaner patient would simplify the surgical procedure, improving my prognosis for success. I dropped from 224 pounds to 189 pounds between November 8 and January 8. I had surgery on January 15, stronger and leaner. Here's how I did it.

- Goal-setting and plotting expectations kept me motivated to lose weight continually.
- Actual weighing-in took place only twice a week, Monday and Thursday. There is too much weight shift due to water retention to recommend weighing in every day. I wanted to avoid setbacks. Every weigh-in should result in a legitimate loss.
- I didn't starve! It took only four days to get used to a daily diet, which roughly followed this pattern: Breakfast–Ultra SlimFast; tea or coffee. Lunch–salad (I was creative, using a variety of vegetables), cup of soup; Dinner–tossed salad, Lean Cuisine. These are delicious, come in many varieties, and provide a 'unit dose' of calories, about 230 to 290. I favor the spicier ones.
- I wrote down everything that I ate or drank, meal by meal, in a daily journal. Having to confront my sins in black and white kept me from committing them.
- Exercise played a key role. I worked out daily, varying the thirty- to forty-five-minute exercise between NordicTrack, treadmill, jogging, and briskly walking with my dog. This burned off one of the meals, so I netted out at two meals per day."

and liquids. If necessary, take a stool softener, or talk to your doctor about using a bulking laxative (such as Citrucel). Stick to clear liquids during the day before surgery. Then, on the night before surgery, take a laxative, and don't eat anything after midnight.

Anesthesia

Modern anesthesia is incredibly safe. For most men, general anesthesia is the preferred approach.

Surgical Approaches

Radical prostatectomy can be performed in four ways: open retropubic, laparoscopic, robot-assisted laparoscopic, and perineal. Because all these techniques use the same anatomy, we can use the same set of drawings to illustrate the basic steps in the procedure. Note: The order in which these steps are performed varies with each technique.

Anatomic Radical Retropubic Prostatectomy

How much information do you want? In this section, we're going to take you through the open radical retropubic prostatectomy step by step. But if you want to know even more or actually see these steps, you can find them on the Johns Hopkins Urology website: http://urology.jhu.edu/prostate/index.php. (The video is here—at the top of the page. Click on the arrows to advance to Radical Retropubic Prostatectomy—Detailed Description of the Surgical Technique.) Let's begin with a quick review of the territory. (It might help if, as you read this, you refer to figures 8.1–8.8.) The prostate (fig. 8.1) is located deep in the pelvis, surrounded by structures that are fragile and vulnerable to injury—the rectum, the bladder, the sphincter responsible for urinary control, some large blood vessels, and the bundles of nerves that are responsible for erection.

The operation begins with a 3-inch incision through the skin that extends from the pubic area halfway to the navel. Next, the muscles in the abdomen are separated along the midline and spread apart. They are not cut, which is one of the reasons men recover from this operation quickly, with little pain and with no long-term injury to their abdominal muscles.

The next step is the staging pelvic lymphadenectomy—dissection of the pelvic lymph nodes to make sure they're free of cancer (fig. 8.2). To do this, we remove a triangle of tissue on either side of the bladder; these triangles contain important lymph nodes. These lymph nodes are usually removed as part of the operation and sent along with the prostate to the pathologist, who then examines this entire "specimen," or bunch of removed tissue.

Today, a staging pelvic lymphadenectomy as a separate procedure (done several days ahead of time) is rarely performed. That's because there is emerging evidence that radical prostatectomy along with an extended lymph node dissection (removing cancerous

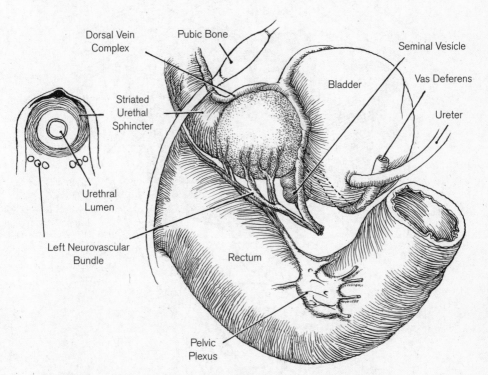

FIGURE 8.1   The Radical Retropubic Prostatectomy, Step by Step

You're looking at the prostate and surrounding terrain—the rectum and bladder; key nerves; veins; and the urethral sphincter, a tube-shaped structure that helps control urine. You can also see one of the two neurovascular bundles, the package of nerves critical for erection, which sit on either side of the prostate. Figures 8.1–8.8 by Leon Schlossberg, reprinted from Patrick C. Walsh, "Radical Prostatectomy: A Procedure in Evolution," Seminars in Oncology 21 (1994): 662–71. Used by permission, W. B. Saunders Company.

lymph nodes) may be beneficial in men with higher-grade and more advanced cancers. With lower-grade cancers (Gleason scores of 7 or lower) even when there is a tiny bit of cancer in a lymph node—without further treatment (such as hormonal therapy), up to 35 percent of men will have an undetectable PSA level, and 60 percent will have no sign of metastases on bone scans ten years later. Although

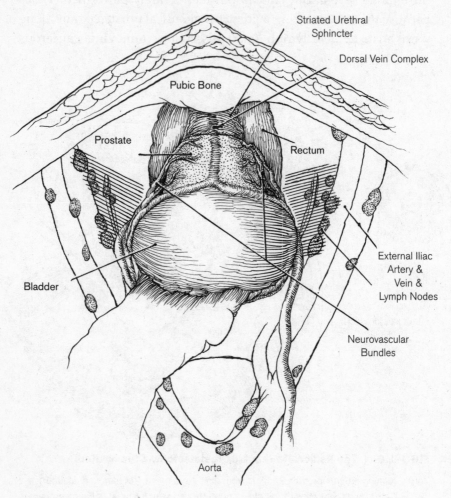

FIGURE 8.2   The Radical Retropubic Prostatectomy (Continued)

This is a schematic look at the prostate, bladder, and lymph nodes. It's the view the surgeon has after the abdominal incision has been made. Inside the shaded area are the lymph nodes removed during a staging lymphadenectomy.

some of these men may be cured, this does not mean the cancer won't eventually come back in other men. Because of the many emerging treatments for advanced prostate cancers (see chapters 12 and 13), men are living much longer, and we now think that "local control" of the prostate and lymph nodes can not only prevent problems with urinary tract obstruction and bleeding later, but also may delay cancer progression (see chapter 6).

Some surgeons do not perform lymph node dissection at all, because finding positive lymph nodes is—fortunately—so rare these days. That's understandable. However, one out of a hundred times, lymph nodes turn out to be positive in a patient in whom you would least expect it. Because we have found that these are also the exact patients who would benefit most from having these lymph nodes removed, we continue to do lymph node dissections in all patients. We are emboldened to do this because of the extremely low risk of complications associated with this, the ease with which a complete lymph node dissection can be performed in a short time, and the fact that more good can come from doing it than not.

Next, the major vein system that overlies the prostate and urethra (the dorsal vein complex) is divided and tied (see fig. 8.3). This is a crucial step; control of these veins makes a huge difference in the surgeon's ability to see what's happening, and it's particularly significant for what happens next—cutting through the urethra (see fig. 8.4). If the urethra is cut too close to the prostate, some cancer might be left behind. This is the most common location for a positive surgical margin—for the presence of cancer cells at the cut edge of the removed prostate specimen. Positive surgical margins are discussed later, but briefly, a positive margin can mean one of two things. It can mean that the tumor extends outside the prostate, to a point where the surgeon can't remove it all. But it often means simply that the boundaries of the prostate are indistinct, and the surgeon cut extremely closely along the edges of the prostate. This is the part of the operation where it's most difficult to see exactly where the prostate ends and the tissue outside it begins. If we err on the other side—if we cut too far away from the prostate—the urethral sphincter might be damaged, and such an injury can make a

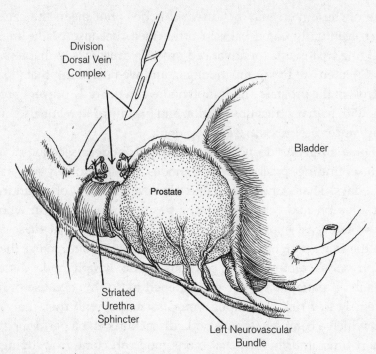

FIGURE 8.3   The Radical Retropubic Prostatectomy (Continued)

This is how the surgeon helps create the critical bloodless field—carefully cutting the dorsal vein complex, which travels over the urethra and prostate and carries a great deal of blood.

man incontinent. The surgical line here is literally not much more than a hairbreadth, and that's why, in this operation, the surgeon's experience counts.

Next, depending on the degree of cancer, the surgeon must make a decision that will affect the patient's potency—to leave intact the neurovascular bundles, the wafer-thin packets of nerves that sit on either side of the prostate, or to remove one or both along with the prostate (see fig. 8.5). These are the nerve bundles responsible for erection.

Remember the three goals of radical prostatectomy: removing the cancer, preserving urinary continence, and preserving sexual function, in that order. The primary goal here is not to preserve potency; it's to get rid of the cancer in a careful but thorough way. Fortunately, because most prostate cancers are now detected early in most men, it is usually possible to preserve the neurovascular

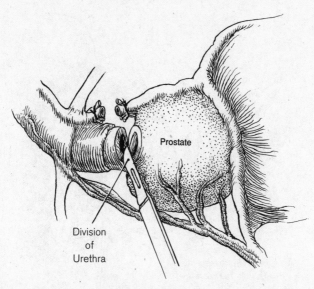

Division
of
Urethra

Prostate

FIGURE 8.4   The Radical Retropubic Prostatectomy (Continued)

The surgeon is now cutting the urethra, which runs through the prostate. This is another delicate procedure. Cutting the urethra too close to the prostate might mean some cancer is left behind, but cutting it too far from the prostate might mean damaging the urethral sphincter, which helps control urine flow. With great care, the prostate is separated from all the tissue and blood vessels that are connected to it.

bundles on both sides. These bundles are outside the capsule of the prostate; even when cancer penetrates the capsule, it travels only 1 or 2 millimeters—not much more than the width of a pencil point—away from it before turning northward, toward the seminal vesicles. Because the neurovascular bundles are, on average, about 5 millimeters from the prostate and because cancer—even when it penetrates the capsule—travels only 1 or 2 millimeters away from the prostate, we can usually preserve most of the neurovascular bundle on that side without creating a positive surgical margin. The neurovascular bundles are weblike structures, composed of microscopic nerves, arteries, veins, and connective tissue. At the time of surgery, the surgeon decides whether to preserve the entire web if it appears safe to do so; to preserve a portion of it (to be sure that there is enough tissue on the prostate to avoid a positive margin), or to widely excise the entire web (if there is extensive penetration of tumor outside the prostate). This is where the open operation performed by an experienced surgeon excels; using tactile feedback,

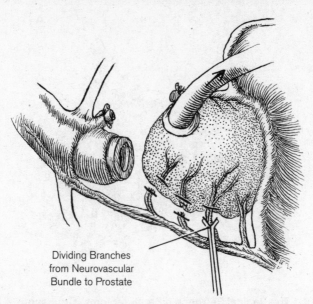

Dividing Branches
from Neurovascular
Bundle to Prostate

FIGURE 8.5   The Radical Retropubic Prostatectomy (Continued)

If it's possible—and today, for most men diagnosed with curable cancer, it usually is—the surgeon can preserve the neurovascular bundles on either side of the prostate. To do this, the surgeon gently separates each branch of these nerves and vessels from the prostate.

it is possible to sense resistance as instruments delicately separate structures. We can also palpate the capsule to determine whether it is hard (suggesting that tumor is penetrating the tissue), to assess the extent of tumor.

In sum, an experienced surgeon, during open radical retropubic prostatectomy, can maintain that delicate balance—knowing when these bundles should stay and when they must go; how to remove enough tissue to obtain a clear surgical margin, yet preserve the patient's sexual function.

It also helps to have good tools, including a fiber-optic headlight, which shines a powerful light directly into the surgical field, and magnifying glasses called loupes, like a jeweler uses. Using magnifying eyeglasses provides excellent three-dimensional magnification, much like the visualization associated with use of the laparoscope, or the robot (see page 234).

If it is necessary to remove one neurovascular bundle, it should go (see fig. 8.6). Remember, men (particularly young men) can remain

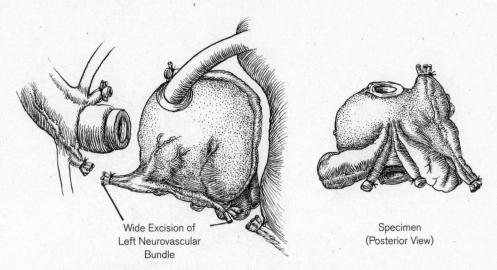

Wide Excision of
Left Neurovascular
Bundle

Specimen
(Posterior View)

FIGURE 8.6 **The Radical Retropubic Prostatectomy (Continued)**

If it is not possible to preserve these nerve bundles—if they have been reached by cancer—then the surgeon removes them along with the prostate. This is called wide excision. The surgeon cuts out as much tissue as possible surrounding the prostate in an aggressive attempt to get every last bit of cancer.

potent even if one bundle is removed and can still have normal sensation, sex drive, and orgasm even if both bundles are removed. There are plenty of men out there who haven't had prostate surgery who still have problems with erection. In other words, it may be a bullet you couldn't have dodged anyway. But again, there is help available, and you can still have a normal sex life (see chapter 11). Some surgeons will tell you that if they decide to remove one or both of the bundles, they will perform a nerve graft. Although this sounds attractive, this has been shown not to work. *If it is likely that you will need to have one neurovascular bundle removed, the best thing you can do to ensure your recovery of sexual function is to find a urologist who can do a good job of preserving the nerve bundle on the other side.*

There is no way for the surgeon to know for certain before the actual operation whether the bundles can be spared. The most common site of positive surgical margins is the apex of the prostate (where the sphincter meets the urethra), followed by the posterior (next to the rectum), and, last, the posterolateral area (near the neurovascular bundle).

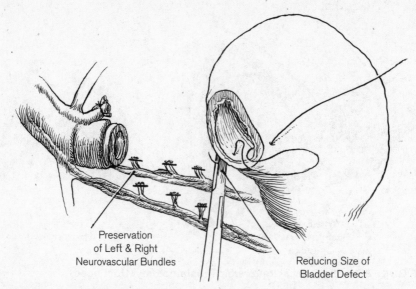

Preservation
of Left & Right
Neurovascular Bundles

Reducing Size of
Bladder Defect

FIGURE 8.7   The Radical Retropubic Prostatectomy (Continued)

This shows the situation after the prostate has been removed. Note how big the opening in the bladder is in comparison to the urethra. This must now be narrowed in size so the two can be connected.

Experienced surgeons don't make any decisions beforehand. We wait and assess the extent of a tumor during surgery. We can see it and observe how the prostate interacts with the tissues around it; we can also feel it. During surgery, if we feel cancer on the edge of the prostate—this can only be done during open surgery—the neurovascular bundle should be removed. It should also be removed if, at any point during its release (when we slowly peel it away from the rectum), it seems adherent or sticky. This is a red flag—it is often a sign that the cancer is beginning to escape the prostate. However, if no firmness is felt and the neurovascular bundle falls away from the prostate, it's safe to preserve it. As a final precaution, we double-check the bundles later in the operation. Once the prostate has been removed, the surgeon carefully examines the specimen, feeling every inch of it for hardness. If there is any suggestion that we need to go back and remove a bit more tissue, we can remove the bundle at that time. Unfortunately, with current laparoscopic and robotic techniques, many surgeons do not examine the prostate until the operation is completely finished and the patient is on his way to the recovery room.

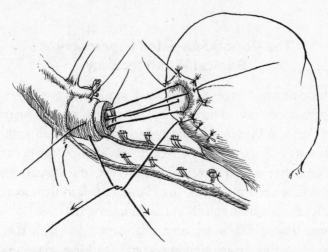

FIGURE 8.8   The Radical Retropubic Prostatectomy (Continued)

The operation's almost over now. Here the surgeon rebuilds the urinary tract, pulling the bladder down to bridge the space connecting the urethra and urethral sphincter.

If the surgeon decides to preserve the nerve bundles, the tiny branches that connect the nerves to the prostate are divided carefully. If, however, one or both bundles must be widely excised, the nerve bundles are cut near the urethra and beside the rectum.

Next, the surgeon goes to work on the prostate, making a cut to separate it at the bladder neck, which links the bladder to the prostate (see fig. 8.7). The seminal vesicles are removed, along with the vas deferens on each side (for the anatomy, see chapter 1). The goal here is to remove as much surrounding tissue as possible along with the prostate. Finally, the surgeon must carefully rebuild the urinary tract, hooking the bladder once again to the urethra and the urethral sphincter, which is responsible for urinary control. Note that the gap between the bladder and urethra—where the prostate used to be—is now filled by the bladder. Some men worry that the penis will be shortened—that the surgeon will pull it up to meet the bladder. This doesn't happen; instead, the bladder is mobile and can easily be pulled down to meet the urethra. The surgeon uses sutures, or stitches, to narrow the bladder neck so it matches the size of the urethra (see fig. 8.8). The Foley catheter is left in place after the operation to drain urine until the connection has healed and is watertight.

The Robotic-Assisted Laparoscopic Radical Prostatectomy

The robotic-assisted procedure is very similar to the laparoscopic radical prostatectomy—with one big exception: a robot (usually the da Vinci Surgical System), connected to special instruments, allows for some new refinements. The robotic-assisted procedure requires general anesthesia. In the robotic approach, the surgeon sits at a remote console controlling the instruments, but in the laparoscopic procedure, the surgeon stands at the operating table.

Again, this is major surgery, performed through tiny holes, or ports. First, the surgeon creates some working space inside the abdomen by pumping in carbon dioxide—like blowing air into a balloon. This "extra air" may fluctuate during the operation. Excessive levels of carbon dioxide can build up in the blood, and the inflation pressure sometimes needs to be adjusted; the anesthesia team monitors this closely. In the robotic procedure, the bottom of the operating room table is raised so the patient's feet are higher than his head. This causes the intestines to shift out of the way into

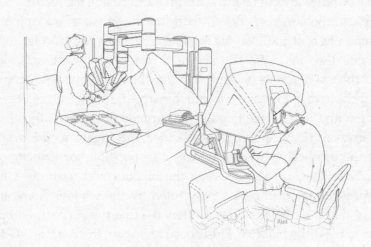

FIGURE 8.9   How Robotic Prostatectomy Works

Robotic-Assisted Laparoscopic Radical Prostatectomy: The surgeon, seated at the console (at right), controls the robotic arms that are connected to the patient. An assistant stands by the patient to exchange the robotic instruments and help the surgeon throughout the operation.

the upper abdomen, making still more room for the procedure to be performed. Next, pointed surgical instruments called trocars are introduced into the abdomen through small openings in the skin.

Then instruments, including a camera, are inserted into ports. Most robotic cases require five or six ports, each with a very small incision; the camera goes in the middle port, near the belly button. Next, the patient is positioned with his feet in the air. Gravity helps here; the bowels slide out of the way and give the surgeon a clear path to the prostate.

"In general terms, the steps are very similar to those of the open operation," says Edward Schaeffer, who trained at Johns Hopkins and is one of the world's foremost experts on the laparoscopic and robotic-assisted laparoscopic procedures. "I always adhere to the same surgical principles that Pat Walsh taught me when I learned the anatomic radical prostatectomy from him: meticulous technique, a bloodless field, and adherence to the anatomic and oncologic principles." The robotic procedure, like the open procedure, begins with a lymph node dissection. One major difference is where the surgeon starts the procedure: In an open radical prostatectomy, surgeons begin the operation at the apex of the prostate, closer to the feet, and work their way toward the bladder. With the robotic approach, surgeons begin at the bladder and work their way toward the feet; this difference in approach does not affect outcomes for patients. "Nerve preservation is approached in a very similar manner to the open procedure," Schaeffer continues, and no decision about whether to spare or remove the nerves is made until the time of the operation. "Although a surgeon can't feel the tissue during the robotic approach, the visualization of the prostate and neurovascular bundles is so outstanding that experienced surgeons can carefully observe how the prostate interacts with the tissues around it. Where there is adherence or stickiness of the nerve bundle to the prostate, this is an early warning sign of possible cancer coming close to the edge of the prostate or beginning to penetrate through its capsule. These visual cues give a skilled robotic surgeon the ability to make real-time adjustments during the operation." Once the prostate is freed from surrounding tissue, it can be removed and examined by the surgeon, just as in the open procedure, if there is any concern. The reconnection between the bladder and urethra is more precise with the robotic approach, Schaeffer notes. "This is where the tiny wristed instruments shine. We can carefully sew the bladder to the urethra, as with a precise sewing machine, ensuring a watertight connection. This significantly diminishes the formation of scar tissue at the bladder neck."

Which Procedure Is Better–Open or Robotic?

The better question, Edward Schaeffer says, is: Which procedure is right for me? "In the open approach we can feel the tissue, but the absolute magnification is less. In the robotic approach, the magnification is superior, but there is not haptic (touch) feedback. With the robotic technique, it is easier to achieve a bloodless field because the transected veins are compressed by the increased intra-abdominal pressure. My feeling is that each case is unique; each patient has different anatomy and a different extent of cancer, and each surgeon has a different degree of experience with each approach. I am lucky because I am a true Walsh disciple: I have been able to directly merge all the knowledge Pat Walsh taught me about the anatomic open approach with the precision and magnification of the robotic approach. Why is this so important? Because knowledge of the anatomy is more valuable than any surgical instrument or tool."

At Johns Hopkins, more than six hundred radical prostatectomies are performed annually, and the majority are now performed using the robotic approach. If the operation is performed at a large-volume center of excellence by an experienced surgeon, both are excellent options. Both open and robotic radical prostatectomy are associated with a steep learning curve, and the surgeon's experience matters. Let's look at a few specifics:

Recovery

Both procedures are similar. Patients are given a clear liquid diet on the night of surgery and encouraged to get up frequently and walk. The timing of discharge from the hospital—based on how the patient is doing and on his own preference, not on surgical approach—is usually one day and rarely more than two. There are not major differences in pain medicine requirements, and men in both groups receive the same instructions on returning to work and resuming physical activity. A urethral catheter is placed during surgery and kept in place for about a week, depending on how the patient is doing and the surgeon's discretion, rather than on the surgical approach used.

"One apparent difference between the two approaches is the skin incision," notes Schaeffer. Open surgery can be performed through a midline vertical or horizontal incision 3 inches in length, made just above the pubic bone. Robotic surgery involves five to six smaller incisions, ranging from 2/10 inch to 1/2 inch in diameter, around the level of the belly button. The relative cosmetic appeal of multiple smaller incisions higher on the abdomen versus a single larger incision lower on the abdomen is a matter of personal preference. While it is true that on average, the blood loss associated with the robotic approach is lower than that for open surgery, the need for blood transfusion is rare for either technique. *However, this will not be the case for surgeons with limited experience in performing the open procedure.*

Previous Surgery

"Technical factors can make one approach preferable for certain patients," Schaeffer continues. "Specifically, men who have undergone other major surgical procedures in the lower abdomen could be more suited for an open procedure or an *extraperitoneal* laparoscopic radical prostatectomy. This is because the robotic procedure is most commonly performed using a *transperitoneal* technique. Your intestines are enclosed in a sac called the peritoneum. During a transperitoneal technique, the surgeon cuts through this sac to get to the prostate; thus, any scarring from prior surgery may complicate things. In contrast, because the open technique is performed outside the peritoneal cavity, it steers clear of the whole area containing your intestines." If you have ever undergone major abdominal surgery, be sure to mention this to your surgeon; it could complicate the robotic approach.

The robotic procedure may be preferable for some men who have had laparoscopic surgery to repair a bilateral inguinal hernia, in which mesh was placed across the abdomen on both sides.

"Sometimes this mesh is placed right under where the incision needs to be made during open surgery. This can create scarring and complicate our access to the prostate." Because the robotic approach is transperitoneal, the surgeon is able to operate underneath the mesh and avoid going through it.

Being Overweight

Because the prostate lies deep in the pelvis, the operation is more difficult if a man is overweight, no matter which procedure we use. The best advice I can give an overweight man seeking radical prostatectomy is to lose weight through a healthy program of diet and exercise. Some surgeons believe that in overweight men, it is easier to perform the robotic procedure than open surgery. This may be true, Schaeffer says, "but for those who are severely overweight, robotic surgery is still extremely challenging and should be performed only by experienced surgeons. Furthermore, in men who are very overweight or morbidly obese, it can be very difficult for the anesthesiologist to ventilate the lungs because of the weight of the abdomen pressing on the diaphragm."

Cancer Control

The most important factor you should consider when choosing a surgical approach and surgeon is, will your cancer be cured? When prostate cancer is localized, complete surgical removal remains the best cure; but the key words here are *complete removal* of the tumor. So, it is important that you include a critical examination of surgical margin status in both procedures. At Johns Hopkins, the rate of positive surgical margins—having cancer cells present at the edges of the removed prostate—is less than 6 percent in men with organ-confined disease. When comparing margin rates between surgeons at Hopkins, Schaeffer noted that there was no difference in margin rates by approach. Rather, it was the experience of the surgeon that mattered most. Other institutions have reported positive margin rates with open surgery *up to 24 percent* for organ-confined disease. *This highlights the need for having an experienced surgeon perform the procedure.*

"A cautionary note is that 'expert' surgeons with the highest lifetime number of procedures comprise the minority of surgeons who are performing these operations and are often found at centers of excellence, including Northwestern University and Johns Hopkins," Schaeffer says. "You should realize that published margin rates for open or robotic prostatectomy from high-volume academic centers may not be generalizable to other settings."

The bottom line: The skill of your surgeon is everything. To paraphrase the MasterCard commercial: Cancer control? Priceless. I follow my patients for the rest of their lives. If they have any side effects or developments months, years, or even decades after the surgery, I know about it. When you talk to a surgeon, ask how the men who've had this procedure three, four, five years ago are doing. If the surgeon doesn't know, you might want to ask yourself why.

The Radical Perineal Approach

The radical perineal prostatectomy is rarely performed today. In this approach, the prostate is removed through a small incision in the perineum, the space between the scrotum and rectum. This is the original operation devised by Hugh Hampton Young, the Johns Hopkins surgeon who pioneered radical prostatectomy in 1904. Although this approach makes sense on paper, it has fallen out of favor, as the operating quarters are tight and cramped. To avoid bleeding, the prostate is removed with little surrounding tissue, making positive surgical margins (the presence of cancer cells on the removed edges of the tumor) more likely. This limits the surgeon's ability to make "real-time" adjustments during the operation if more cancer is detected. Also, a surgeon can't perform a lymph node dissection with this approach and preservation of the neurovascular bundles is extremely difficult and rarely successful. In sum, the limitations of this procedure outweigh its benefits.

After Surgery

Whether you had a robotic, open, or laparoscopic, procedure, a drain will be left in your abdomen until nothing flows through it;

this usually takes a day or two. Also, a Foley catheter, inserted into the penis and anchored by a tiny balloon in the bladder during surgery, will remain in place for one to two weeks. Note: To minimize your risk of getting a urinary tract infection, which often happens in men who have a catheter, you should begin taking an antibiotic such as ciprofloxacin (Cipro) or levofloxacin (Levaquin) the day before the catheter is scheduled to come out, and keep taking it for two to three days afterward. On the day the catheter is due to come out, be sure to drink extra fluids. Your doctor will want to make sure you are urinating with a strong stream. (Note: The time it takes to recover urinary control varies, and it is not likely that your urinary control will be perfect immediately. Your doctor just wants to make sure there is no urinary obstruction.)

The main reason for using the catheter is that it allows the newly connected bladder and urethra (this connection is called the anastomosis, if you hear your surgeon using this term) a chance to heal. *It is critical that the Foley catheter stay in place.* If it is inadvertently pulled out or removed too soon after surgery, this can be disastrous and may lead to permanent incontinence. Your catheter should be secured to your thigh, and you should examine its mooring often. The catheter may take some getting used to, but remember, it's only temporary, and its presence is helping your body heal. Depending on your surgeon's preference, the catheter will be left in place for one to two weeks.

Bleeding Around the Catheter

This looks scary, but it's pretty common, especially if you strain to have a bowel movement. Don't worry—it will stop. Also, don't worry if you see some blood in the urine. This usually has no significance and almost always resolves on its own—usually by the time the catheter is removed. Sometimes this bleeding happens spontaneously, and sometimes it's due to overexertion (walking too briskly, for example). If you see blood, flush it out by drinking a lot of fluids. This will dilute the blood so it won't clog the catheter, and it will also help stop the bleeding. If the bleeding around the catheter is persistent (lasting longer than a week), let your surgeon know. Sometimes old blood that has collected in the space where the prostate was removed drains through the urethra. If so, it's wise to delay removing the catheter until the bleeding has stopped.

Leakage Around the Catheter

Another scary phenomenon, but this, too, is usually nothing to worry about. Leakage can occur when you're up walking around or when you're having a bowel movement. It can usually be managed with the use of diapers or other absorbent materials. *Important:* If your catheter stops draining completely, lie down flat and drink a lot of water. If after one hour there is no urine coming through the catheter, it is possible that your catheter has become clogged or dislodged. Call your doctor right away.

Urinary Sediment

Another common, disconcerting problem, urinary sediment can manifest in several ways. You may see some old clots, which appear as dark particles, after you have had bloody urine. These usually go away on their own. Also, the pH balance of the urine (its acidity) changes throughout the day. After a meal, for example, urine often becomes alkaline. There are normal substances in the urine called phosphates. These can cause cloudy masses to appear in the urine if the urine has too little acid. (The urine also may appear cloudy if you have a urinary tract infection—see page 243.)

Bladder Spasms

These can be extremely painful and may feel similar to a cramp you get in your calf or foot. Fortunately, bladder spasms are not very common. The men most likely to have them are those who have been troubled by urinary symptoms before surgery (usually, men who have had BPH), who have developed a thickened bladder wall and a hair-trigger bladder that is easily irritated. In this case, the irritant is huge—the catheter—and the bladder is trying its best to push it out by contracting. The spasms may happen at random, or they may be provoked by an activity, such as having a bowel movement or going for a walk. If you have a bladder spasm, lie down until the contractions improve. If you have frequent spasms, you may be helped by medication. Nonsteroidal analgesics (such as ibuprofen) work quite well because they relax smooth muscle. For persistent spasms, tranquilizers such as diazepam (Valium) are usually able to control the problem.

Pain

You should receive pain medicine before you even wake up from the surgery. The key is to stay on top of the pain, says Schaeffer. "By being proactive about pain control, we use less pain medicine—particularly, narcotics—today than we did even five years ago." This is a good thing. Most patients receive an intravenous NSAID called ketorolac (Toradol). This, along with oral acetaminophen (Tylenol), is highly effective at managing postoperative pain. For men with additional discomfort or allergies to NSAIDs, oral narcotics can be used as supplementation.

You will walk a little bit the night of surgery. "Don't fret! Most men feel better once they are up on their feet." One or two days after surgery, you will be able to leave the hospital. Regardless of the surgical approach, most men report little pain, and it often comes from irritation of the abdominal muscles.

You can begin to eat the night of surgery, too. "I always tell my patients to take it slow and eat in small portions, because nausea from the anesthesia may persist," Schaeffer adds. When you leave the hospital, as soon as your doctor says it's okay, you can eat and drink whatever you wish—even alcohol, in moderation. The main thing is that you *avoid becoming constipated*. Remember, the prostate sits on top of the rectum; when it's removed, this part of the rectum is thin, fragile, and particularly vulnerable to injury for the first three months after surgery. *Therefore, it is critical that you* **do not** *have an enema or have your temperature taken rectally anytime soon. And it's absolutely essential that you have a bowel movement every day.* For many men, this is easier said than done; pain medications, inactivity, and slight dehydration (from not getting enough fluids before or after surgery) can all add up to constipation. To help keep things moving, you'll probably be given stool softeners or laxatives for several days. If you do become constipated, take mineral oil and milk of magnesia or polyethylene glycol 3350 (MiraLAX), but again, *do not use an enema*—you could perforate your rectum.

Caring for the Incision

You can take a shower as soon as you are discharged from the hospital. Your surgeon will either sew your incisions closed or use temporary skin clips (the surgical equivalent of staples, which are usually removed before you go home from the hospital). Some men develop an infection in the incision several days after they get home from the hospital. This usually manifests as some drainage—either a clear fluid or an unsightly mixture of blood and pus. Don't worry; this can be treated simply. Soak a cotton swab in hydrogen peroxide, and gently insert it through the opening in the incision. If the drainage persists, call your physician; you may have infection in the wound that will require a short course of antibiotics.

Urinary Tract Infection

When you have a urinary catheter, bacteria are going to make their way from the skin around the tip of your penis into your bladder. Usually, this is not a problem; to discourage infection, we have our patients take antibiotics around the time the catheter is removed. However, some men may develop a symptomatic infection, with foul-smelling urine and a fever. If you notice either of these symptoms, tell your doctor, who will probably prescribe a more extended course of an antibiotic such as levofloxacin (Levaquin) or ciprofloxacin (Cipro).

When Can I Resume Normal Activities?

Until the catheter is removed, take it easy. You can eat and drink whatever you want, take long (but not strenuous) walks, and make as many trips as you'd like up and down the stairs. You can drive a car once your catheter is removed and resume work two to three weeks after the surgery. Exactly how soon you should resume all activities will depend on how quickly you seem to be recovering, but once the catheter has been removed, most men feel well enough to return to their normal routines (including golf) by four weeks after surgery.

Expect to have some incontinence. This is normal, and it, too, is not permanent. It will go away eventually; don't be discouraged. Also, expect to have some trouble with erections (see chapter 11).

Finally, you'll be encouraged to sit in certain positions, to do leg exercises to boost your circulation, and to walk around. This also is crucial—among other things, it can help reduce your risk of developing blood clots.

Complications

Early Complications

Like all surgery involving anesthesia, radical prostatectomy carries the risk of death, but *this is extremely rare*. In a Johns Hopkins study of more than 4,500 patients, there were three deaths—one man had a heart attack before surgery as the anesthesia was beginning, and two men died after surgery (one at ten days, one three weeks afterward) from a blood clot to the lung. (For important tips on how to recognize symptoms of this, see page 245.)

In the "bad old days" before the anatomical approach, excess bleeding was common. Today, fortunately, the need for blood transfusions is incredibly rare, and usually a result of a blood vessel being injured during the operation. *That's why it is absolutely critical that your surgeon has mastered the techniques for ensuring a bloodless field* (described on page 211). Less common complications during surgery include injuring the rectum or ureters; such injuries can be repaired during surgery with little delay in discharge from the hospital.

Complications shortly after surgery include the following:

Blood Clots

These are among the most common—and potentially most serious—complications of radical prostatectomy. One of the body's most effective defense mechanisms after any trauma is the clotting cascade—a chain of events that causes the blood to coagulate. This can help stop bleeding if you skin your knee or even help save your life if you're in a car wreck, but this helpful system can also be activated when it's least welcome—after surgery—and can do more harm than good. Blood clots that form in the legs' deep veins (this is called deep venous thrombosis) can be, at best, painful. At worst, they can be fatal. The leg veins are, basically, a straight shot to the lungs; the nightmare scenario here is for part of a blood clot in the leg to break free and shoot up to the lungs.

Blood clots in the legs and pulmonary embolism, or blood clots in the lungs, occur in an estimated 2 percent of men. Clearly, the best way to deal with this problem is to *prevent it from ever happening.* Some doctors do this by administering blood-thinning medications such as mini-dose heparin. Some doctors also give their patients compression devices—various forms of heavy-duty support hose—for the legs. One of these looks like a pair of long johns and is designed to force all blood into the deep veins and keep the flow powerful and continuous. (Sluggish blood flow leads to clot formation.) Other hose have special compression chambers that control blood flow and are designed to "milk" blood up the leg.

Important: If you have ever had a blood clot, make sure your doctor knows about it. This could influence the way your anesthesia is administered. Also, men considered at higher risk of developing a blood clot may have a stronger blood-thinning medication administered throughout their stay in the hospital.

These preventive steps are very important, but they're only part of it. The rest, by default, falls squarely on your shoulders. Make sure you and your family members know the warning signs of a blood clot, and *if you think you have any of them, seek treatment immediately.* A blood clot is a problem that can be treated easily with anticoagulants (blood thinners and clot-dissolving medications), if it's caught early. But if diagnosis—and therefore treatment—is delayed, a blood clot can be fatal.

You may have a clot if you have swelling or pain in the leg, especially in the calf; or sudden chest pain—especially if it gets worse when you take a deep breath—or coughing up blood, shortness of breath, the sudden onset of weakness, or fainting. *If you have any of these signs—even if you don't feel anything unusual in your legs—you could have a blood clot in your lungs. Call your doctor immediately!*

CALL YOUR DOCTOR!

Contact your doctor if you have any of the warning signs of a blood clot (see page 244). This is part of being your own advocate. If you have a question or problem during office hours, by all means, go ahead and call; you may not always get the doctor, but you'll get somebody who can help. And if you have a problem that you don't think can wait until morning, call at night.

Most doctors have twenty-four-hour answering services; many doctors have partners who share "on-call" time—they split it up, each taking a certain number of nights, weekends, and holidays a year. They do this because they expect to get some calls at night, because they know from years of training and experience that medical emergencies don't always happen during office hours.

This won't be the first phone call your doctor gets in the middle of the night, and it certainly won't be the last. What would you rather do, wind up in the hospital as a result of a serious complication that should have been treated hours ago, or "bother" your doctor?

Don't wait for your doctor's office hours if this happens in the middle of the night. If you can't get to your doctor, go to an emergency room and tell the doctor there that you need to be evaluated for deep venous thrombosis or pulmonary embolism with ultrasound of the leg veins or a spiral CT of the lungs.

Exercise is another crucial factor in helping to avert blood clots. Walking is good; it pumps blood back to the heart. Walk as soon as you're allowed to after surgery. If you stand up, don't stand still for longer than a few minutes at a time—move around. The only way the blood that's in the veins in your legs gets back up to the heart is by the pumping action of the muscles. Your doctor will probably encourage you to do dorsiflexion exercises—pumping your feet up and down to exercise the calf muscles. Do these often, about one hundred times an hour in between naps. Also, it is essential that you *do not sit upright in a chair* (with your legs hanging down) for more than an hour at a time during the first four weeks. Try to sit with your legs elevated on a sofa, in a reclining chair, or in a comfortable chair with a footstool as much as possible. This accomplishes two goals. Because it raises your feet, it improves the blood flow from the veins in your legs. Also, it protects the area of surgery from bearing your full weight.

Because patients are in and out of the hospital so fast these days, it's likely that any postsurgical trouble you experience will be when you're at home. That's why it's essential that you and your family be aware of the warning signs of a clot in the leg or a clot that has gone to the lung.

Bladder Neck Contracture, or Constriction of the Bladder Neck

This is scar tissue that forms where the bladder neck is sewn to the urethra, and it has been reported in between 1 and 12 percent of men after open surgery; it is less common following robotic surgery. Its symptoms are usually manifested by a very slow or dribbling urinary stream when—this is the tip-off—the bladder is full. Also, it can sometimes appear as a delay in recovery of urinary control, like a sticky faucet that won't open or close completely. Remember, incontinence immediately after surgery is a very common problem. In the early days after surgery, many men who are experiencing incontinence also worry about having a slow urinary stream. But it's hard to achieve a good stream if there's not much in the bladder, and it's impossible to store up urine in the bladder if it keeps leaking out. Bladder neck contracture is different; the bladder is full, but the best you can manage is a dribble, because the scar tissue is blocking the flow, like a stuck washer in a faucet.

If you have a very slow urinary stream or prolonged incontinence, you should be evaluated with a urinary flow rate test and a measurement of residual urine following completion of urination through ultrasound measurement. If your urinary stream is slow and you have residual urine, you have some form of obstruction. This can be confirmed by cystoscopy, and if scar tissue is found, the bladder neck can be reopened in a simple outpatient procedure. The urologist, using a cystoscope (a tiny tube inserted through the tip of the anesthetized penis, through the urethra, and into the bladder) makes a few tiny cuts to relax the tight scar tissue.

To keep the area open, your urologist may recommend that you pass a small catheter through the urethra every day for a month or so after the procedure. This way, the scar tissue won't re-form, and the normal lining of the bladder and urethra will cover the opening as it's supposed to. If the scar tissue is particularly stubborn, your doctor may inject a powerful steroid called triamcinolone into the area of the contracture; this can be effective in preventing the scar tissue from returning.

Inguinal Hernias

Within two years of radical prostatectomy, about 15 percent of men develop an inguinal hernia. Why? It's not clear but we think many men have something called a "subclinical" hernia at the time of their operation. In other words, they already had a hernia but didn't know it. The most durable way to fix an inguinal hernia is by making an incision over the hernia site from the outside. This is typically done as a separate procedure. If you are undergoing extraperitoneal surgery (see page 237), you may elect to have your hernia repaired at the same time. For those undergoing transperitoneal surgery, our general surgery colleagues generally don't recommend a simultaneous hernia operation, because the mesh used to fix the hernia can come in contact with the bowel and cause scar tissue to form.

Long-Term Side Effects

Urinary Continence

Before surgery, many men focus on impotence as the major complication of radical prostatectomy. They're wrong. Recovery of urinary control is far more important and—if it happens slowly or doesn't happen at all—casts a far greater shadow on your life. If something's wrong with your ability to urinate, you'll be reminded of it several times a day—or worse, several times an hour—not just a few times a week or month. And frankly, having to change your adult diaper because you just involuntarily urinated in it can dampen—literally—any romantic thoughts that you do have. Thus, before you go under the knife, you and your urologist need to talk about the risk of incontinence (see page 215).

Why Does Incontinence Happen After Radical Prostatectomy?

Let's take a moment to review the male plumbing. Men are equipped with three separate anatomical structures that control urine—a sphincter at the bladder neck, the prostate itself, and the external sphincter (also called the striated sphincter). Radical prostatectomy knocks out two of these—the sphincter at the bladder neck and, of course, the prostate—leaving only the external sphincter to do the work of three. Because of the powerful structures upstream, this external sphincter is never tested or even used much in most men. Thus, we have no way of knowing before radical prostatectomy how strong this sphincter really is. In some men, it's extremely well developed; in others, it's not. Like the rest of the muscles in the body, this sphincter loses its tone with age, and here's where older men have the disadvantage. Men over age seventy have more problems recovering perfect urinary control after surgery than do younger men. Here, too, is where men differ from women: Women have only this one sphincter. In consequence, they have very thin bladders. Men, in contrast, normally have thicker, more muscular bladders to begin with (see fig. 2.1). Add any element of BPH (benign enlargement of the prostate, which often makes the bladder work harder and become muscle-bound), and a man's bladder can become quite thick. Thus, some men are left with a situation where a burly, thickened bladder is connected to a sphincter that may not have been that effective to begin with.

To make matters worse, at the time of surgery, the sphincter can be damaged, because the major blood vessels that can cause excessive bleeding are intertwined within it. *This is yet another reason why the skill of the surgeon is so important.* One of the first steps in a radical prostatectomy is to divide this complex structure. If too much sphincter is taken out or if the sphincter is injured during the surgeon's attempts to stop bleeding, urinary incontinence can result. Thus, it's vital that your surgeon understand the complicated anatomy and know how to preserve the urinary sphincter and carefully rebuild the urinary tract. Urinary incontinence is a huge quality-of-life issue. You must think about it now, before surgery, and do your best—by choosing an experienced surgeon, and afterward, by following the exercises described below—to minimize trouble later.

The Return of Urinary Control

Some men are lucky. They are dry from the moment the catheter is removed. They can stop their stream on a dime and start it whenever they want to. The great physician Sir William Osler once made a perceptive comment that applies here: "The man who is well wears a crown that only the sick can see." Men who are continent immediately after radical prostatectomy are blessed. Most men, however, have variable amounts of urinary leakage. You may be one of the lucky ones; then again, you may not. Most likely, it will take some time for your control of urine to come back completely. For most men, this process happens in three distinct stages: Phase one is when a man can remain dry when he's lying down. In phase two, you're dry when you're walking around. If you can walk to the bathroom and not urinate until you get there, that's a great sign—it means that the sphincter is intact. And in phase three, you are dry when you stand up (using muscles that put pressure on the sphincter) after sitting.

In young, healthy men operated on by an experienced surgeon, about 80 percent should be wearing no pads—or at most, a security pad to catch the occasional drop—by three months after surgery, and at twelve months, 95 to 98 percent should be continent. Note: We consider any man continent if he wears no pad or if he wears a pad that is dry. Many men continue to wear a small pad just to be safe. Your doctor may have a different definition of continence, which you should find out before surgery. However, most men (even at three months) are not very wet, and when asked in a confidential questionnaire, 96 percent stated that leakage caused little to no bother. It's hard to believe, but urinary control does continue to improve over two years and, in an occasional patient, for even longer than that.

Can you do anything to speed things along and improve your urinary control? First, whatever you do, *do not wear an incontinence device with an attached bag, a condom catheter, or clamp!* If you use any artificial device, you will hurt yourself in the long run. You won't be able to recover your urinary control, because you won't develop the muscle control you need. Until your urinary control returns completely, wear a pad such as a Serenity pad or disposable diaper such as Depends. You can get these at a pharmacy or grocery store.

Some men prefer using a special kind of padded underwear called Sir Dignity briefs; your doctor should have good suggestions and perhaps even some samples for you to try.

Also, until your urinary control has returned to an acceptable level, don't force fluids. When the catheter is in, you're asked to drink a lot of fluids to flush out the system. However, once the catheter is out, you've got to slow the pace considerably. Avoid drinking excessive amounts of fluids, and stay away from caffeine in all forms—coffee, tea, and even soft drinks. Caffeine is a powerful pharmacologic agent that increases the frequency and urgency with which you need to urinate. If you are being treated for high blood pressure with an alpha-adrenergic antagonist such as doxazosin (Cardura) ask your doctor to put you on a different kind of drug. Also, if you were taking tamsulosin (Flomax) for BPH, you should discontinue it. Doxazosin and tamsulosin make the sphincter relax and can make incontinence worse.

Exercises You Can Do

Every time you urinate, do it standing up. You can't practice the following exercises, which strengthen the external sphincter and speed up your recovery of urinary control, while you're sitting down. Start your stream, and once it's in full force, stop the stream by contracting the muscles in your buttocks—not your abdominal muscles, not the muscle up in front around the penis. Tighten your buttocks; imagine you're trying to hold a quarter between your cheeks. Hold the urine back for five or ten seconds, and repeat as many times as you can. *Important:* Perform these exercises *only* when you're urinating; if you keep contracting these muscles throughout the day, you'll overdo it—the sphincter tires easily—and you'll end up wetter than you would be otherwise.

Remember, for many men, the recovery of urinary control is a slow process. The most important thing you can do during this time is not get discouraged. If your doctor told you there is only a 2 percent chance that you will have a long-term, serious problem with urinary control, believe it. This means there's a 98 percent chance that you'll be back to normal someday, even if no crystal ball can say exactly when. It will help for you to discuss your progress at regular intervals with your urologist—even a phone call every so often can make a world of difference in how you see your progress. It may also help for you to take part in a support group so you can talk with other men who are in the same boat, going through the same process of recovery. You can do this online, from the privacy of your own home (this may be better if you are uncomfortable talking about personal matters in front of others), or you can find a local prostate cancer support group. Ask your doctor.

If you are experiencing no progress, it's reasonable to consider whether something else, other than the natural, gradual return of urinary control, could be causing the delay. One possibility is a bladder neck contracture, the formation of scar tissue around the reconnected bladder and urethra (see above).

Incontinence after surgery falls into two basic categories: *stress incontinence* and *urgency incontinence*. Stress incontinence is caused by a weak sphincter; urine leaks out when you cough, sneeze, laugh, or run. Urgency incontinence (also called urge incontinence) is when you know you have to go to the bathroom but can't get there in time, and some urine leaks out. Men with urgency incontinence leak right away, when they have the sudden urge to urinate and can't hold it back.

If you have stress incontinence, there are several medications that may help. For example, decongestants, used to treat allergies and cold symptoms, work by contracting smooth muscle in the nose. The urethra is surrounded by this same smooth muscle. Thus, if you do not have high blood pressure, you may benefit from taking a short-acting decongestant, such as pseudoephedrine (Sudafed), or a long-acting agent combined with an antihistamine, such as loratadine (Claritin-D) and pseudoephedrine. However, some of these drugs can cause drowsiness and a dry mouth, and some men find those side effects worse than the urinary leakage itself. Another drug, called imipramine (Tofranil), works through a two-pronged approach. It relaxes the muscle in the bladder and also tightens the muscle tone of the external sphincter. This drug, too, can cause drowsiness and a dry mouth; however, some men find that if they take just one tablet at night, it lasts well into the next day. (Otherwise, the usual dose is 25 milligrams up to three times a day.)

If you had an enlarged prostate before surgery and experienced a lot of urinary frequency and urgency, you may have urgency incontinence resulting from a hyperactive bladder. Your doctor can check for involuntary bladder contractions with cystometry, a test that measures bladder pressure and sensation by passing a small catheter through the urethra into the bladder. Changes in pressure are monitored as the bladder fills with water.

If you have urgency incontinence, you may benefit from treatment with an anticholinergic medication. A simple, over-the-counter one is diphenhydramine (Benadryl); other choices, available by prescription, are the long-acting drugs tolterodine (Detrol), oxybutynin (Ditropan XL), trospium (Sanctura), and solifenacin (Vesicare), which target mainly the bladder and have fewer side effects (including dryness of the mouth and eyes, headache, constipation, and rapid heart rate) than other drugs of their kind. Anticholinergic drugs have an antispasmodic effect—they can prevent involuntary bladder contractions and help prevent urine leakage. Other drugs, classed as antispasmodics (which means they fight muscle spasms), can help relax an overenthusiastic bladder muscle that contracts too frequently. These include flavoxate (Urispas) and dicyclomine (Bentyl). Antidepressants also may help by strengthening the internal sphincter and relaxing the bladder.

Many doctors advise their patients to undergo something called pelvic floor biofeedback. This includes a forty-five-minute biofeedback behavioral therapy session—a tutorial on how to use your pelvic floor muscles. Patches are placed on the perineal and abdominal muscles to be sure that you're performing these exercises correctly. Most men are able to recover urinary control and learn how to engage their sphincter muscles on their own; however, some men have trouble and find pelvic floor biofeedback helpful.

If It Still Doesn't Get Better

The gains made in recovering urinary control can be incremental, often frustratingly so. But there's a point at which it probably isn't going to get any better on its own. Johns Hopkins urologist E. James Wright is a world-class expert on incontinence. He has found that beyond nine months, men who are wearing more than three pads per day seldom improve enough to be satisfied. In men who have less of a problem, small changes may take place between nine and twenty-four months. Fortunately, there is help for urinary incontinence, including the following:

Urethral Bulking
The sphincter can be bulked up by the injection of a material, in a procedure similar to the one used by plastic surgeons to get rid of wrinkles in someone's face. Collagen was once used, but it is no longer available. The three products in current use are: Hydroxyapatite (Coaptite), Macroplastique, and Durasphere (carbon-coated ceramic beads). Unlike collagen, these materials do not degrade. Before you consider injections, you should be checked with a cystoscope (a lighted tube, inserted into the anesthetized penis and threaded through the urethra into the bladder) to make sure you don't have a bladder neck contracture and to evaluate the anatomy to see whether it's amenable to injection. Injections can be performed as an outpatient procedure. It may take three or four injections at four- to eight- week intervals for you to receive the maximum benefit. Some men feel an immediate improvement, which may ebb over the next few days, then return. It usually takes about a month before the material to settle.

Before you consider it, you should know that this bulking is not for everybody. It is not helpful for men who have had treatment for a bladder neck contracture or for men who have undergone radiation therapy. And bulking agents simply are not adequate help for men who have severe incontinence. Urethral bulking in men is typically a stopgap: something that gets done on the way to doing something better. For patients with mild to moderate symptoms, the perineal sling is a better option. These bulking materials are like sealing wax; their effectiveness is limited. At best, only about 60 percent of men who receive injections have what they consider to be a good result. Also, even if the treatment is successful, it probably won't last forever; you may need repeat treatments every six to eighteen months.

Note: Before you decide on injections, you need to ask yourself some serious questions: Do I really need it? Am I that uncomfortable? The reason we're saying this is that some men have almost perfect control—almost. They wear a small liner in their pants, and they have to change it only once a day. But in an attempt to become perfect, they undergo injections—and wind up wearing adult diapers that they must change two or three times a day. There's an old saying in medicine that perfection may be the enemy of good.

Surgical Options
Slings

E. James Wright, who is an expert in their use, gave me this advice on slings. The first thing to remember, he says, is that slings likely are best suited to men with mild to moderate stress incontinence (who need fewer than three pads a day) and who have not had primary radiation therapy. Slings can often improve incontinence of any severity, but the greatest "cure" rate (needing one or zero underwear liners a day) is seen in men on the favorable end of the spectrum. Evaluation, including measuring the pad weight (to see how much urine is leaking out) and cystoscopy, may help determine if this is the right treatment for you. The slings are made of polypropylene mesh, a durable synthetic material that's well tolerated by the body.

The most common procedure performed today is an adaptation of an incontinence procedure that has been used successfully in women for more than ten years. The transobturator sling threads a band of polypropylene mesh along the inside of the pubic bones to elevate and support the urethra with a postage stamp–sized patch of similar mesh. Instead of compressing the urethra, this sling appears to reinforce sphincter function, reducing the effects of upright posture, gravity, and abdominal pressure on the sphincter, and improving urinary control. (It's the equivalent of sliding a comfy chair under someone who's tired and saying, "Take a load off.") This procedure is most effective in men with only partial impairment of their sphincter (men with mild to moderate leakage). Unlike the artificial urinary sphincter (see below), it does not replace the sphincter; it just helps it work better. The procedure typically takes less than an hour and can be done on an outpatient basis. The mesh acts almost like Velcro at first, and then tissue grows over it, fixing it in place permanently. You will need to limit your physical activity for four to six weeks after this sling is placed to keep it from loosening and losing its supportive effect. Complication rates are generally low, and infection is rare with this mesh. Some men experience decreased penile sensation or numbness, but this is usually temporary and goes away within six to nine months after the procedure. If the sling is not effective at restoring adequate urinary continence, it can be removed and replaced with an artificial urinary sphincter (see below). Both slings and the artificial sphincter are compatible with all forms of therapy for restoring erectile function, including penile implants.

Artificial Sphincter

Men who have severe, prolonged incontinence should undergo placement of an artificial sphincter. This is the gold standard. In this procedure, a soft, silastic (material that's flexible and stretchy, like elastic) cuff is positioned around the urethra and connected by tubing to a reservoir for fluid that's installed in the abdomen. The placement of this reservoir is important. It's designed so that when a man coughs or sneezes, or does anything else to increase the pressure within the abdomen—activities that would otherwise result in stress incontinence—that pressure is instantly transferred to the cuff. This temporarily increases the pressure around the urethra and blocks urine from leaking out. The artificial sphincter features a valve, placed in the scrotum that is used to deflate the cuff and allow urine to pass. The device is somewhat elaborate, but it works very well for men with severe incontinence. The idea is that "the buck stops here"—urine comes out only when you decide it's time.

In the past, artificial sphincters had two main complications—the risks of infection and malfunction. Infection can cause erosion of the tissue that holds the device in place (in the urethra and bladder neck), may make incontinence worse, and may even mean that the device must be removed. If the infection is severe, this tissue damage may limit the success of any replacement sphincter. The device may need to be replaced if, for some reason, the original one is a dud. The good news here is that, as technology evolves, these devices keep getting better, and the odds of malfunction are going down all the time.

Sexual Potency

Chapter 11 is devoted to erectile dysfunction, so you should consider this just an introduction to this difficult subject. The first thing we need to do is make sure we're all talking about the same thing. What do we mean by *potency*? The medical definition is simple—"an erection sufficient for penetration and orgasm." Having said that, it's worth repeating that men who are impotent after radical prostatectomy have normal sensation and normal sex drive, and can achieve a normal orgasm. Their only problem may be in achieving or maintaining an erection.

Potency after radical prostatectomy can be affected by many things: a man's sexual function before surgery, his age, the stage of his cancer, the surgeon's skill, and the extent of tissue removed—in other words, whether one or both neurovascular bundles were removed during the operation.

For men in their forties, potency is similar (about 90 percent) in men who keep both neurovascular bundles intact and in men who have one nerve bundle removed. This suggests that all that's needed for men to achieve erection is *one* of these nerve bundles, and that nature has provided a "spare." Over age fifty, however, sexual potency is better in men who have both neurovascular bundles preserved than in men who lose one bundle. When the relative likelihood of impotence after surgery is adjusted for age, the risk is higher if the cancer has penetrated the prostate wall, if it has invaded the seminal vesicles, or if one neurovascular bundle has been removed. Thus, the men most likely to remain potent are younger, with disease confined to the prostate. These also are the men who will benefit most from surgery.

Continence and Potency: Quality of Life After Radical Prostatectomy

The news is good: Skilled surgeons at three high-volume hospitals (where hundreds of radical prostatectomies are performed each year) reported almost identical results—at one year, 92 percent of their patients wore no pads and 70 percent were potent.

And yet, as surgical procedures go, radical prostatectomy remains one of the most delicate, intricate, and flat-out difficult to perform correctly procedures. Proof of this can be found in the widely varying rates of success of surgeons at hospitals throughout the world—not simply in controlling cancer, but in preserving urinary continence and sexual potency. The unfortunate fact is that when less experienced or less skillful surgeons attempt this procedure, the results can be disastrous. It has taken more than a decade for the results—the good, the bad, and the ugly, if you will—to surface.

Part of the issue is that it's hard to know exactly what happens after a man leaves the hospital, particularly in areas where men feel so vulnerable. Nobody wants to talk about it. It's different when we look at something as black and white as, say, a man's cancer status. All we have to do is follow his PSA tests, and *bingo*—we have all the information we need, a definitive means of knowing whether all of the tumor has been removed. But there aren't such objective ways to tell how a man's doing in the other important areas.

In an effort to be as objective as possible, and out of concern that patients may try to minimize their problems when talking about them directly with their physicians, scientists have determined that the best way to collect information is for patients to fill out a questionnaire and mail it to an independent third party. Scientists create validated questionnaires, score the questions, and assign a number to patients' quality of life. On validated questionnaires, the questions have been tested and retested to avoid ambiguity. However, sometimes these scores have little meaning to patients. I also worry that these results don't always reflect the reality of many men's lives. For example, if a man undergoes a hip replacement and is able to enjoy life without pain, dance with his wife, and walk the dog, he may not be back to the 100 percent level he was at age sixteen, but he has a happy life. However, he certainly wouldn't score 100 on a validated questionnaire. Similarly, after a radical prostatectomy, if a man confidentially reports that he is not wearing a pad and that he and his wife are able to have intercourse more than 50 percent of the time with or without drugs such as sildenafil (Viagra), and he says that he is happy with the result, I believe that this type of information is valuable.

The good news is that there are many skilled surgeons at large referral hospitals and academic medical centers who have excellent results using both open and laparoscopic/robotic techniques. Unfortunately, however, the success of radical prostatectomy is not uniform; patients at some centers report much greater trouble with side effects.

The take-home message here is this: any man who wants a radical prostatectomy and believes it's the best form of treatment for him should seek out centers where experienced surgeons perform many of these procedures, and where the results can be documented through validated, independent outcome studies.

Finally, our work has revealed some interesting things about men in general. It turns out that some men exaggerated their sexual activity before surgery, and on careful questioning, acknowledged that they really weren't potent or had difficulty with erections *before* they had the operation. But after surgery, men did just the opposite. Many of them said they were not potent, but their partners disagreed. In separate questionnaires of the patients' partners, 78 percent reported that the men were potent at the same time the men said they were. But 20 percent of the partners said potency occurred earlier than the men thought it did, and 2 percent thought it occurred later. What accounts for this discrepancy? Often, the women sense their partners are doing better than the men think they are. This is because the men feel that their erection may not be as strong as it was before surgery—and until they have a very strong erection, many men feel any intercourse that occurs "doesn't count."

At many top medical centers, the rates of potency after radical prostatectomy are quite good. But there are still men at those centers, and many men elsewhere, who experience problems. The important thing to remember is that sexual function—potency—can be restored to all men after radical prostatectomy. The main problem for these men is the ability to obtain an erection. But sensation and the ability to achieve orgasm are intact. Many men don't understand this. They think that they can't have an orgasm if they can't have an erection. They forget that half the people in the world have orgasms without erections—women. This is because orgasms occur in the brain. There are many ways to restore sexual function, and these are discussed in detail in chapter 11.

In this chapter, we've covered everything about radical prostatectomy and the complications that can occur in the months after the operation. But what about the long-term outlook and the biggest question of all—has your cancer been controlled? For a detailed discussion of the results of all forms of treatment for localized disease—surgery, radiation, and cryo/thermal ablation—see chapter 10.

9

RADIATION AND CRYO/
THERMAL ABLATION

This chapter was written with expert opinion from Phuoc T. Tran, M.D., Ph.D.

THE SHORT STORY:
The Highly Abridged Version of This Chapter

Radiation therapy is an excellent treatment option for many men with prostate cancer. First and foremost, it requires no surgery. This means there's no risk from anesthesia and no recovery time from a major operation. This is a great advantage for older men as well as for men with other health problems that might preclude surgery. Another bonus: Radiation can be performed on an outpatient basis. Most men who receive external-beam radiation can continue to work during their course of treatment. Men who undergo brachytherapy (implantation of radioactive seeds) usually require just a few days off from work for the procedure and recovery, and can return to most normal activities within a week.

Traditionally, radical prostatectomy has been considered the gold standard of treatment for prostate cancer. But external-beam radiation therapy is proving to have equivalent cure rates, and is showing excellent long-term outcomes. The two major approaches are external-beam radiation therapy, sending radiation into the tumor from the outside; and brachytherapy, implanting radioactive seeds directly into the tumor (doctors also refer to this as interstitial radiotherapy).

Cryoablation and thermal ablation—killing prostate cells by freezing or heating them—are also available as less-invasive forms of treatment for localized prostate cancer. These techniques are enthusiastically endorsed by their advocates, who point out that because they require no surgery, they offer a minimally invasive outpatient treatment with few side effects. However, guidelines from the National Comprehensive Cancer Network (NCCN), the most authoritative, independent, up-to-date source of information for patients on the management of localized prostate cancer, state that "cryotherapy or other local therapies are not recommended as routine primary therapy for localized prostate cancer due to lack of long-term data comparing these treatments to radical prostatectomy or radiation." In other words, don't bet your life on cryotherapy or thermal ablation.

With PSA testing, many prostate cancers are still being diagnosed at a very early stage, and many men with cancer that has been caught so early do not like any of the options they are given: active surveillance, surgery, or radiation. They don't want any side effects, and for them the solution seems simple—why not just treat the tiny area where the biopsy is positive with *focal cryotherapy* or *HIFU*? The major problem is that there is great uncertainty about the effectiveness of these approaches, and they are not free of side effects. Unfortunately, the men who are actually the best candidates for this form of treatment are the ones who probably require no treatment in the first place. They are older, with small tumors, and are ideal candidates for active surveillance.

In this chapter, we cover everything about radiation and cryo/thermal ablation and the complications that can occur in the months after the procedure. But what about the long-term outlook and the biggest question of all—has your cancer been controlled? For a detailed discussion of the results of all forms of treatment for localized disease—surgery, radiation, and cryo/thermal ablation—see chapter 10.

Radiation Therapy for Prostate Cancer

Like radical prostatectomy, radiation treatment for prostate cancer is not a new idea. In fact, it wasn't too long after the urologist Hugh Hampton Young did that first radical prostatectomy in 1904 (see chapter 8) that he and another colleague at Johns Hopkins were among the first to pioneer radiation therapy in this country. (It had been developed a few years earlier in Europe.) The treatment was primitive by today's standards, involving special radium applicators placed in the tissue surrounding the prostate—the urethra, bladder, and rectum.

But the next few decades laid the groundwork for some of today's highly effective radiation therapies: X-ray treatments were introduced, followed by treatment with radium "seeds" that could be inserted into the prostate tumor. Compared with today's technology, the low-energy X-ray beams produced throughout the 1930s were imprecise and lackluster. Radiation treatment, in those days, was not much more than palliative; it could shrink the prostate and relieve pain and symptoms, but it often could not completely eradicate the cancer.

In the 1940s, the impact of hormones on the prostate was discovered (see chapter 12), and radiation was all but abandoned in favor of castration and hormonal drugs. But radiation's exile was not long, thanks largely to scientists who revolutionized the field using an exciting new machine called a linear accelerator. This produced penetrating, high-powered beams that could target radiation doses to a specific site with much less harm to surrounding tissue than previously had been possible. And suddenly, radiation was back in the game as a major player—a treatment that actually could cure localized cancer, not just relieve the symptoms of advanced disease.

Since then, radiation therapy has been refined and made even more powerful. There are two standard approaches: sending radiation into the tumor from the outside with external-beam therapy, and implanting radioactive "seeds" directly into the tumor (this is called interstitial radiotherapy, brachytherapy, or simply seed implantation). The 1990s saw an exciting mini revolution in external-beam therapy, thanks to the development of a new technique called three-dimensional conformal radiation therapy (3-DCRT), followed by intensity-modulated radiation therapy (IMRT). Most recently, image-guided radiation therapy (IGRT) is bringing about yet another revolution in radiation treatment.

Conformal Radiation Therapy

How does an X-ray machine work? The simplest way to think of it is to imagine yourself getting a suntan. The difference here is that you can't feel or see the X-ray energy hitting your body, and the "sunburn" occurs internally. Actually, what happens is that the radiation particles destroy DNA, causing targeted cells to die. Scientists have long known that not all cells respond to radiation in exactly the same way. The effects of DNA damage on a cell are complex, but the cells most susceptible to radiation are the ones that are constantly undergoing division—cancer cells, for example.

Early in the twentieth century, scientists learned that single, whopping doses of radiation did more harm than good; they were more toxic to normal tissues than to cancer. But, they discovered, incremental radiation—smaller daily doses spread out over a period of weeks—worked much better on cancer (although this

conclusion is now being reevaluated; see the section on hypofractionated radiation therapy later in this chapter). They also found
that this was the most effective way to minimize long-term damage to normal cells. That's why today, radiation doses are spread
out over several weeks—usually delivered Monday through Friday,
leaving weekends free, for six to eight weeks. Each treatment lasts
about twenty minutes. That's it. Then you go home and come back
the next day.

In the era before PSA testing and before today's improved radiation technology, the only way to determine the response to treatment was by evaluating whether men developed local recurrence
(cancer that could be felt in a rectal examination, or development
of urinary or other symptoms) and whether men developed distant
metastases. Under these circumstances, early radiation methods
appeared to be quite effective. However, once PSA testing became
available and began to be used as a way to track the success of cancer treatment, scientists realized that only 20 percent of men with
T1 and T2 disease who had been treated with external-beam radiation had low PSA levels after ten years. A study from Toronto, using
multiple biopsies, found that even at four years after conventional
radiation treatment, 38 percent of men who were believed to be
cured turned out to have active prostate cancer. It became all too
clear that conventional external-beam radiation therapy wasn't
doing the job. In a substantial number of men, it failed to eradicate
all of the cancer.

What was happening—or not happening—was that *men weren't
receiving enough radiation.* The problem in some men, we know now,
was similar to what happens when a speaker with an inadequate
sound system tries to make himself understood to an audience of
one hundred thousand people in a vast amphitheater. Some, maybe
even most, of the crowd can hear him, but that still leaves hundreds or even thousands who aren't getting his message. In traditional radiation treatment for prostate cancer, scientists discovered,
this inadequate coverage meant that many men who suffered local
relapses of prostate cancer did so because they were underdosed.

In recent years, radiation oncologists have found that the dose
of radiation received has a lot to do with who gets cured and who
doesn't. In other words, men who receive higher doses of radiation

have lower relapse rates than men who receive less radiation. However, in traditional radiation treatment, delivering a higher dosage almost always meant more, and worse, side effects, particularly to the bladder and rectum.

Three-Dimensional Conformal Radiation Therapy (3-DCRT)

Enter the high-tech advances. (Note: Many of these go by abbreviations, and they all seem to end in "RT," which can make it difficult to tell them apart.) Also, just as surgeons talk of procedures, radiation oncologists speak in terms of personalized "treatment plans," of which the radiation is just one part. One of the most important parts of the plan is making a detailed map of a man's pelvis.

The first high-tech breakthrough was conformal, or three-dimensional conformal, radiation therapy (3-DCRT), which involved having the patient undergo CT scanning ahead of time. Before this, radiation oncologists planned a man's radiation treatment field based on X-rays of the prostate and surrounding area; these usually were two images taken at 90-degree angles to each other. Radiation oncologists relying on these two-dimensional X-ray images had to incorporate enough of a safety margin of normal tissue around the prostate to make sure they did not inadvertently miss the target. The by-product of this was that a substantial amount of surrounding tissue was receiving the same amount of radiation as the prostate, leading to side effects such as bladder irritation, diarrhea (from treatment of the rectum), and even skin reaction.

The CT scans showed a three-dimensional (3-D) view of the prostate and surrounding terrain—which, in turn, allowed for a much more accurate treatment design. Faster computers, intricate software, and imaging systems could lay out the treatment and calculate the radiation dosage per millimeter (or even smaller areas) of tissue. Amazing technological advances made it possible for doctors to custom-design a 3-D model and treatment plan, so each patient's prostate tumor could get the most precise and thorough radiation coverage possible.

Intensity-Modulated Radiation Therapy (IMRT)

The development of 3-DCRT was just phase one in the evolving world of radiation therapy for prostate cancer. Next-generation technology came quickly, in the form of intensity-modulated radiation therapy (IMRT).

As good as 3-DCRT was, it had certain limitations—particularly on how finely the radiation dose could be shaped to fit or avoid key structures in the radiation field. For instance, the radiation could be shaped to approximate a cube around the prostate, but it couldn't reproduce the actual shape of the gland.

Imagine, on a much grander, more sophisticated level, attempting to trace a curved outline with an Etch-A-Sketch. Previously, with external-beam radiation, this meant unavoidably including some normal tissue within the high-dose area. But ideally—because the prostate generally has an irregular shape to start with, and because, like a fingerprint, each man's prostate is unique—treatment should be custom-tailored to fit each man. Another problem: Even with 3-D planning, the coverage was inevitably uneven, with "hot" and "cold" spots—small areas of too much or not enough radiation.

IMRT is the difference between using a rigid Etch-A-Sketch and a fluid paintbrush. It creates a much more sophisticated treatment plan. Instead of using four beams to treat the prostate, it uses multiple beamlets—sometimes hundreds—generated at multiple angles to "paint" the radiation dose to the prostate while avoiding surrounding tissues, especially the rectum. This approach relies on as many as sixty pairs of movable tungsten "leaves"—slim, rectangular-shaped plates that open and close like little shutters. These allow the machine to sculpt the radiation beam, molding it to fit the individual contours of each man's prostate and pelvic region. (See fig. 9.1 for a visual comparison of IMRT and 3-DCRT.)

IMRT treatment planning, like all radiation therapy, is a team effort. Together, the radiation oncologist and physics team use complex, computerized algorithms to fine-tune the treatment and craft the optimal plan.

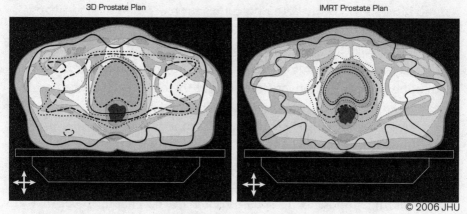

3D Prostate Plan   IMRT Prostate Plan

© 2006 JHU

FIGURE 9.1   A Side-by-Side Comparison of 3-DRT and IMRT Plans

Like a topographic map, the patterned lines show areas receiving different doses of radiation. Note how the IMRT plan spares the rectum and more closely matches the shape of the prostate, keeping to a minimum the normal tissue contained in the high-dose region. The versatile tungsten leaves, a breakthrough in radiation technology, also block the radiation from areas that aren't supposed to receive it—much like the lead drape you wear in the dentist's office when you get an X-ray. Image © 2006 Johns Hopkins University.

Proton-Beam Radiation Therapy

Proton-beam radiation therapy uses charged particles (protons) instead of electromagnetic waves. The difference here is that the proton beam shoots in a straight line, penetrating tissue with very little effect until it reaches a predetermined distance, at which point it suddenly "detonates," discharging all of its tumor-killing energy. Precise targeting is crucial.

Note: When you're reading about it, *pro*ton-beam therapy looks confusingly like *ph*oton radiation (the kind that's used in IMRT, discussed above), and in terms of cancer-killing effectiveness, the results between these two forms of treatment are pretty similar, notes Johns Hopkins radiation oncologist Phuoc Tran. Photon radiation is much more common, he adds. There are no completed randomized studies comparing advanced photon radiation, such as IMRT, directly to proton radiation for prostate cancer. "However, because IMRT has high rates of controlling the disease and low rates of severe, toxic side effects, it seems unlikely that proton radiation will offer significantly better outcomes for most men with localized prostate cancer." Radiation oncologist Anthony Zietman, of Massachusetts General Hospital's proton center, sends patients a letter that says, "Though proton beam has shown considerable benefit in treating tumors in more critical parts of the body, such as the brain or eye, *no one has yet demonstrated a clear benefit in the prostate....*"

Proton-beam radiation therapy "is not a zero-risk approach, and there are men who experience some urinary urgency or rectal bleeding, though these are usually temporary," says Zietman. "Unfortunately, it is no more effective than other kinds of radiation in avoiding impotence (discussed later in the chapter). Approximately 50 percent of our patients will ultimately suffer from this problem." But that has not stopped the growth of this more expensive technology. There are at least twenty-one proton radiation centers in the United States that are treating prostate cancer, and at least another ten in the planning stage or under construction.

What to Expect During Radiation

In all conformal approaches, preparation is key. Like generals masterminding a strategic attack, the radiation oncologists who design your treatment begin by studying the map. Treatment planning begins several weeks ahead of time, with a series of CT images that give enough cross-section views of the prostate, seminal vesicles, and surrounding territory (including the bladder wall, rectal wall, small bowel, bony structures, and skin) to create a detailed, three-dimensional chart of your pelvic region.

Dosage, and its distribution area, can be calculated and fine-tuned plane by plane, millimeter by millimeter. Each radiation beam—the IMRT approach allows more segments of treatment than traditional external-beam therapy does—is automatically shaped by a computer so the energy focuses on the tumor alone (in the prostate as well as tissue outside the gland to which cancer has spread), rather than on its entire neighborhood. This is important, because again, *when it comes to dosage, more is definitely better.* It takes high doses of radiation to kill prostate cancer—higher doses than used to be possible in the years before these newer techniques evolved. But delivering more radiation usually means triggering more side effects. It also makes it more challenging to achieve the right balance—killing the cancer but *not* killing healthy tissue right next door, thereby keeping side effects to a minimum. Here's where the tungsten leaves come into play with the intensity-modulated approach, allowing higher-than-ever levels of radiation to be delivered safely to targeted areas while sparing as much of the surrounding tissue as possible. The advanced technology has allowed doctors to increase the standard dose of radiation, measured in units called gray (abbreviated Gy and named in honor of Louis Harold Gray, an English radiobiologist), from about 65 Gy to about 81 Gy. Before-the-fact dose checks verify that the radiation went to the right spot for the right length of time to help guarantee the most successful treatment possible.

The precision of conformal radiation would be reduced if the patient couldn't keep perfectly still—and frankly, nobody can keep *that* still. Imagine one good sneeze, for instance, or a coughing fit, or even a case of nervous fidgets. Oops—and the bladder gets more radiation than planned while the prostate gets less. To help prevent this, men are fitted for their own custom-built body casts, which keep the pelvis immobilized on the table for the few minutes it takes to receive the daily dose of radiation. The cast also makes sure the same body position can be reproduced every time.

Image-Guided Radiation Therapy (IGRT)

The challenge of keeping still, continued: Even if you were able to lie in exactly the same position every day, there is no guarantee that your *prostate* would cooperate and do the same. This is because the prostate is not fixed to your skin, pelvic bones, or external body contours—the traditional signposts used to align patients for their daily treatment. Research has shown that the prostate can move around within the pelvis beyond a centimeter and the location of your prostate during the treatment planning session represents only a snapshot image of its location during that particular session. At many facilities, patients are told to come for treatment with a full bladder and an empty rectum (a full bladder, so that more of the bladder stays away from the prostate; an empty rectum, because it is easiest for the treatment staff to reproduce this position).

However, even then, the prostate can vary enough to cause occasional errors in targeting. Here is where image-guided radiation therapy (IGRT) can help. Tran says, "Using IGRT, we check the location of your prostate every day after you are placed in the treatment position. Small adjustments can be made based on the location of the prostate *that day*, ensuring that the entire prostate receives the intended treatment—and also that the normal tissues are not in the way."

There is more than one way of performing IGRT. One method is to incorporate a linear accelerator and CT scanner into one machine. The patient lies on the table, a scan is performed, and the images are reviewed and compared with the original CT scan (see fig. 9.2a and 9.2b).

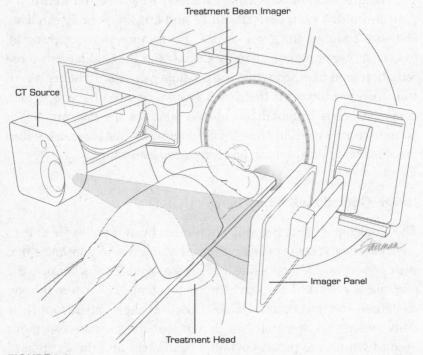

FIGURE 9.2a

A patient undergoes scanning on the linear accelerator just before treatment. This unit contains components for both CT scanning (shown with the beam passing through the man's pelvis) as well as high-energy treatment beams (shown underneath the patient). These components rotate around the patient during scanning and treatment. Image adapted from D. Bolinsky.

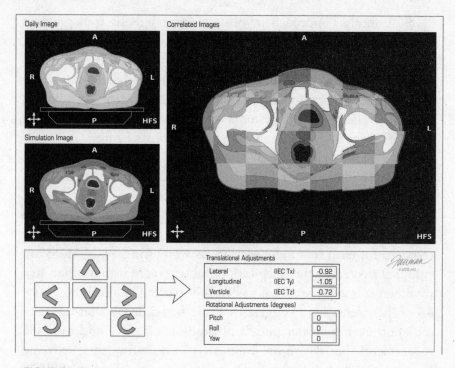

FIGURE 9.2b

Images taken during the CT scan on the day of treatment are "fused" with those from the initial planning CT and compared. Then, the position of both the patient and the table may be shifted slightly so that the treatment is delivered precisely where it needs to go, and healthy, normal tissue is protected.

If, as the images are scrutinized, someone notices a tiny shift in the location of the prostate, the patient's position is adjusted before treatment ever starts. Another method uses an ultrasound device to view the prostate through the skin between the anus and scrotum while the patient is on the treatment table. A small amount of lubricating jelly is placed on the ultrasound device and live images of the prostate are converted into a 3-D image and correlated to the images from the planning CT. Adjustments in the position of the treatment table are made as needed.

Another approach is to place *inside the prostate* small metallic markers or coils (usually, these are made of gold), which are then visible on X-rays taken in the treatment room. The markers appear as beacons, spotlighting the position of the prostate.

Still another approach involves electromagnetic transponders that are permanently implanted in the prostate before treatment begins. Like tiny transistor radios, they transmit "the prostate channel"—safe radio frequency waves that relay the prostate's precise position and any movement—to an image guidance system.

One well-advertised system, the CyberKnife, uses implanted metal markers in conjunction with a pair of cross-firing X-ray imagers for visualization and real-time tracking of the tumor. A small linear accelerator on a robotic arm then follows the tumor as it moves (when the patient breathes, for example).

Hospitals using the CyberKnife tend to limit treatment to no more than five sessions. This is likely related to the length of time required for each treatment session, as well as to an odd Medicare rule that decreases the hospital's reimbursement if more than five treatment sessions are given with this particular machine. Studies of this technology suggest that this schedule—longer doses of radiation over a shorter period of time—is effective and safe. We recommend that if you are interested in pursuing this "extreme hypofractionated or stereotactic body radiation therapy (SBRT)" that you exercise caution and only go to a center with ample experience in these techniques that ideally follow their results in an open clinical trial (see page 297).

Take the Time to Find the Right Doctor

It's more than a question of who's got the best technology. Deciding on treatment, and the doctor to perform it, can be especially confusing when there are so many similar-sounding sets of initials. "A good way to think about IMRT and IGRT," explains Johns Hopkins radiation oncologist Daniel Song, "is that IMRT allows the high-dose region to be individually shaped to 'fit' the prostate, while IGRT enables us to direct that high dose of radiation precisely to the intended location." Ideally, he adds, both techniques are used to achieve the best outcome with the least toxicity.

Although many centers offer these technologies, when you're deciding where to undergo radiation therapy—or any treatment, for that matter—it is important to consider the physician's level of experience and the volume of prostate cancer patients treated at that facility. Tran puts it this way: "You wouldn't consider two surgeons equal just because they happen to use the same instruments. Yet some people believe that one radiation oncology center is equivalent to another if they are using similar technology." In fact, recent findings suggest that patients treated at higher-volume centers actually have better outcomes than those treated at lower-volume centers. There's no magic minimal yearly number of cases to indicate a radiation oncologist's level of expertise, but "I often suggest one hundred cases a year," says Tran.

More advice: Doing it right is not a quick, fly-by experience; it takes time to come up with the best treatment plan. So much work goes on behind the scenes—on the part of the radiation oncologist, medical physicists (physicists specially trained in the use of radioactive materials and technology), medical dosimetrists (people trained in the use of treatment-planning software), and radiation therapy technicians. They don't just plan the treatment; they monitor it exhaustively along the way, performing many checks and double-checks, making sure that the treatment you're receiving each day is correct. *Your goal here is to cure the cancer.* As we discussed in chapter 8, taking a few weeks or even months to find the right doctor and medical center is not going to mean you miss your window for being cured. The cancer has been there for years. Taking a little extra time now to seek therapy at centers with significant expertise, a high volume of patients, and high-end technology may well be the best investment you will ever make.

Complications

For the first few days or even the first couple of weeks of external-beam radiation therapy, men may feel nothing out of the ordinary; it takes a while for the cumulative effect of radiation to manifest itself. They can continue all of their normal activities—driving, working, exercising, and having sex. (Unlike seed implantation, discussed below, this form of radiation does not make men temporarily radioactive). But by the third to fifth week, many men react with symptoms that can range from mild to moderate. Symptoms generally go away on their own, days to weeks after the course of treatment is over.

Fatigue

This is a common complication and is usually mild to moderate. Most men with full-time jobs are able to keep right on working eight hours a day; rarely does the fatigue become severe enough for them to take off work completely. Exercise on a moderate basis, for men already accustomed to it, may help with radiation-induced fatigue.

Urinary Symptoms

During radiation treatment, men may experience an increase in nocturia (waking up from sleep at night to urinate). They may also need to urinate more frequently during the day or experience urinary urgency (inability to suppress the need to urinate). Although these symptoms of urinary tract irritation are temporary, in 25 to 30 percent of men, they become acute enough to require medication, such as terazosin (Hytrin), doxazosin (Cardura), alfuzosin (Uroxatral), or tamsulosin (Flomax), during the treatment course.

Rectal Symptoms

Fortunately, with the use of IMRT and IGRT, symptoms involving the rectum have become much less common and are much less severe. About one-third of men experience a mild increase in the number of daily bowel movements (this usually means two to three per day) or experience more loose and gassy stools than normal. Diarrhea is rare. If needed, a doctor may suggest a reduced-fiber diet or medications such as loperamide (Imodium) or diphenoxylate (Lomotil).

Late Symptoms

Sometimes, men develop what are called late symptoms six months or more after treatment. In one study of 1,100 men, between 1 and 2 percent of men needed minor surgical intervention for urinary symptoms—primarily urethral stricture or bladder neck contracture. Urethral strictures seem to develop mostly in men who have previously undergone a transurethral resection (TUR) procedure for benign prostatic hyperplasia (BPH). A bladder neck contracture can be reopened in an easy outpatient procedure. A urologist, using a cystoscope, makes a few tiny cuts to relax the tight scar tissue. Most urethral strictures respond well to dilation—stretching the urethra in one or two sessions—but stubborn strictures also may be treated with tiny incisions, like those done to ease bladder neck contractures. Note: Many of the men in these studies were treated using older techniques. With today's radiotherapy, late rectal effects have generally been minimized. In a study from the RTOG Foundation (a research group formerly called the Radiation Therapy Oncology Group) of 257 men treated with 79.2 Gy IMRT, just a little over 2.5 percent of the men experienced severe late rectal problems, including rectal inflammation and rectal bleeding. *Important:* If you are on a blood-thinning medication, rectal bleeding can be much higher following radiotherapy (see page 277).

Sexual Function

Radiation can take a gradual toll on a man's ability to achieve an erection. This is thought to be a result of damage to the small blood vessels and/or the neurovascular bundles that control erection; radiation causes them to shrink or become scarred over time. "Controversy still exists over whether radiation-induced impotence is due to the dose to the penile bulb, which sits just below the lower portion of the prostate, or to the nerves," notes Phuoc Tran. In a study from Fox Chase, investigators reported that in men younger than sixty-five, 73 percent were potent at three years, and 59 percent were potent at five years. Another study surveyed 1,187 men five years after they were treated with either surgery or external-beam radiation. Overall sexual function declined in both groups to approximately the same level, but erectile dysfunction was slightly more prevalent in the radical prostatectomy group than in the external-beam radiotherapy group (79 percent compared to 63 percent).

Sexual potency is difficult to measure; age, stage of disease, and a man's sex life before treatment all play a role in his ability to have an erection afterward. Men younger than sixty who are sexually active and who are treated when the cancer is in the earlier stages (when it is confined to the prostate) are most likely to remain potent after radiation treatment. However, many men treated with radiation are older and more likely to have problems with impotence anyway—either because they're taking medications that can interfere with sexual function or simply because of their age (discussed further in chapter 11).

One fact you should know about radiation therapy is that its effect on potency is slower and much more incremental than radical prostatectomy's more immediate impact. Radiation seems to cause a man's ability to have an erection to diminish over time (months to years); about half the men who receive it are impotent at seven years after radiation treatment. This is probably because radiation's effect on the blood vessels results in an eventual decrease in blood flow to the penis. One Australian study found that 62 percent of 146 men who were potent before they began radiation therapy were potent one year afterward; but by two years after treatment, this number had dropped to 41 percent. (This doesn't mean a man who undergoes radiation therapy can't still have a normal sex life. Viagra and other erectile dysfunction drugs can improve sexual function in men after radiation therapy, particularly in men who can achieve partial erections. See chapter 11 for more information.)

I Have Some Health Issues—What Should I Do?

With IMRT and IGRT, more men—including those with other medical conditions—are able to receive curative treatment with minimal side effects, even with very high doses of radiation. However, radiation is not for everybody, and with the perfectly good alternative treatment of surgery, men should be aware of certain conditions that may predispose them for higher risks of radiation-related side effects. Indeed, some men need special precautions, and a few men are just not good candidates for radiation therapy.

If you have a vascular disease, such as diabetes or inflammatory bowel disease (Crohn's disease or ulcerative colitis), or if you are on a blood-thinning medication, you fall into the category of needing extra precautions. Based on clinical experience and retrospective analysis of patients in clinical trials, radiation oncologists have developed dose-volume thresholds—basically, the highest dose of radiation that is safe for nearby organs, particularly the rectum and bladder. If you have one of these conditions or take a blood-thinning medication, your safe maximum dose is going to be lower, because in your body, these fragile tissues are more vulnerable and need extra protection. Scientists at the University of Chicago reported that nearly 16 percent of men on blood-thinning medications (warfarin [Coumadin], clopidogrel [Plavix], and others) are likely to have long-term moderate to severe bleeding in their stool or urine; other studies have produced similar findings.

Currently, radiation is not a good option for men who have a collagen vascular disease such as scleroderma or lupus. These men have a much greater likelihood of developing severe late side effects, even when extra precautions are taken to protect their nearby tissue.

Adding Hormonal Therapy to Radiation

It used to be that doctors would give a man a full radiation treatment and *then*, only if the treatment was not successful months or years down the road, start androgen deprivation therapy (ADT)—shutting off his supply of male hormones such as testosterone (also called androgens; this is discussed in detail in chapter 12). But what if a man takes a temporary course of ADT—for a few months—and *then* begins radiation? This idea, called neoadjuvant hormonal therapy, has been shown in several studies to be beneficial. How much ADT does a man need? Does hormonal therapy make the cancer more vulnerable to the radiation? And will the short-term promise hold up in long-term studies? The answers are not yet clear. One study performed by the Radiation Therapy Oncology Group compared four months of hormonal therapy with two years and four months of hormonal therapy, with both groups of men also receiving radiation. They found that the men who received the hormones longer, particularly those with very high-grade cancers (a Gleason score of 8 or higher) had better results on their follow-up PSA tests and were less likely to die from prostate cancer.

What is it about hormones that makes radiation more effective? For one thing, they shrink the volume of the prostate, which means that radiation has less ground to cover—and this, in turn, can lower the risk of side effects to healthy tissue in the rectum and bladder. For another, hormones make radiation more efficient. Experimental studies have shown that with hormonal treatment, a lower dose of radiation (fewer Gy) is needed to kill the cancer, in part because the body's repair systems—which cancer cells use to fix radiation damage—are suppressed by hormone treatment, and also because there are fewer cancer cells that need to be killed. This combination of hormones and radiation also shifts cancer cells from an active to a resting phase, making them much more like the proverbial sitting ducks—and much easier to kill.

In brachytherapy (treatment with implanted radiation seeds, discussed on page 283), when hormones reduce the size of the prostate, it's easier to place the seeds accurately and to make sure they're reaching the entire gland. This is not always an easy task if a man has a very large prostate that extends under the pubic arch. Taking a three-month course of hormones before brachytherapy also may reduce the likelihood of complications such as urinary retention or incontinence in men with large prostates.

The first study that provided encouragement for using hormones with radiation therapy was reported in the *New England Journal of Medicine* in 1997, and updated in 2010 in *Lancet Oncology*. Researchers found that men with locally advanced prostate cancer who received conformal radiation therapy plus three years of hormonal therapy were more likely to be disease-free at ten years than were men who received radiation alone. Most important, this study showed a *20 percent improvement in prostate cancer survival.*

However, some physicians wondered whether hormones alone would have provided these same results. This question has recently been answered by three international studies, together involving thousands of men with prostate cancer. In all of them, compared to men who received hormonal therapy alone, the men who received *both* radiation and hormonal therapy had fewer instances of PSA failure; there was also an increase in survival among men with locally advanced (high-risk) prostate cancer. Side effects were slightly higher in the men who received both treatments. These studies strongly suggest that men with locally advanced prostate cancer do better with both treatments than with either alone.

Over the last decade, several studies have suggested that for men with intermediate- or high-risk cancer—the men currently treated with combined hormonal therapy and radiation—the *radiation dose matters.* Results from four Radiation Therapy Oncology Group studies showed that among men with high-grade (Gleason 8 to 10) disease, receiving a higher dose made a significant difference in PSA control (discussed more in chapter 10), and also in survival. At least seven high-quality, randomized studies have examined whether receiving a higher dose of radiation improves prostate cancer outcomes. One of the first, from MD Anderson Cancer Center, compared the effects of using 70 versus 78 Gy of radiation on patients with a PSA level greater than 10 ng/ml. The study's investigators found that the men who received higher doses not only had better PSA control but were less likely to have distant metastases.

At the heart of the discussion regarding the importance of radiation dosage in men with high-risk prostate cancer is whether the disease is contained within the prostate, or whether tiny bits of cancer have already spread elsewhere (these are called micrometastases), beyond the local area. Research from Harvard analyzing the relationship between local control and distant metastases sheds some light here. In a study of more than 1,400 men treated with radiation, local failure (the return of cancer within the prostate or in nearby tissue) was the strongest predictor of future distant metastases. This study had a very interesting finding: the risk of developing distant metastases increased with time *after* local failure occurred— suggesting that these metastases were not present at diagnosis, but that they occurred *because of the local failure.* As we'll discuss in chapter 12, hormones alone cannot cure prostate cancer, which is why for patients with intermediate- or high-risk prostate cancer (discussed on page 177), it is necessary to double-team: using radiation plus hormones, not just hormones alone.

Although no study has shown across the board that all patients who receive radiation benefit from getting hormones, in most studies there have been subsets of men who seemed to do better— particularly men with positive lymph nodes, large tumors, and high Gleason scores.

How Long Should I Take the Hormones?

A man with advanced disease (for example, a bulky T3 tumor), a high Gleason score, or positive lymph nodes who undergoes external-beam radiation therapy should also receive hormonal therapy for at least two or three years. There is good evidence, says Phuoc Tran, that short-course hormonal therapy (given just around the time of radiation therapy) may be enough for men with intermediate risk cancer—a tumor of moderate size or a midlevel Gleason score (see page 195). Investigators from the RTOG Foundation studied men who received a short course of hormonal therapy before and during their radiation treatment. They found that after ten years, in the men who had both treatments, there was not only an improvement in cancer control but in overall survival. This short course of hormonal therapy was of greatest benefit to men with intermediate-risk cancer. In another study, scientists at Harvard found similar benefits to a short course of hormonal therapy added to radiation therapy in this same group of men.

Hormonal Therapy and Your Body: Some Things to Consider

Before you commit to hormonal therapy, you should consider another very important issue: quality of life and the potential for an increase in cardiovascular, cerebrovascular, and metabolic complications. There are some definite downsides to the use of hormone-suppressing drugs. In some men, testosterone production doesn't always return promptly after these drugs are stopped. The side effects of hormonal therapy can be profound. Even with a short course (two or three months), men experience the loss of libido and potency, plus "hot flashes" and weight gain. With long-term treatment (two years or longer), there are the additional risks of osteoporosis (and fractures that result from this bone degeneration), anemia, fatigue, loss of muscle mass, depression, diabetes, colorectal cancer, cognitive impairment, and perhaps even cardiovascular trouble, including a higher risk of heart attack.

There is now evidence that hormonal therapy can increase the risk of death in men who have already had heart trouble—a heart attack, coronary artery disease, or congestive heart failure. For this reason, if you have heart failure, or if you have had a heart attack, you should discuss the risks carefully with your internist, cardiologist, or endocrinologist before you begin long-term treatment with hormone-suppressing drugs. This is also true for older men who have multiple health problems. Also, depending on the particular kind of hormone suppressors you are prescribed, this treatment can be very expensive. (A detailed discussion of hormonal therapy can be found in chapter 12.)

Will It Be Worth It for Me?

To sum up, *starting hormonal therapy is a serious step.* Will the benefits outweigh the risks? It depends on your cancer. For most men—those diagnosed with early-stage, low-risk cancer (Gleason 6, PSA less than 10, and clinical stage T1c or T2a)—radiation therapy alone is enough, says Johns Hopkins radiation oncologist Ted DeWeese. "These men rarely experience a clinical recurrence of cancer after treatment. But some men," he continues, "are diagnosed with more aggressive disease and are at greater risk for recurrence."

At five years after treatment, men with intermediate-risk disease have a likelihood of biochemical recurrence—the return of PSA—of about 40 to 50 percent. The odds of recurrence for men with high-risk disease is 65 to 75 percent. "Clearly, for patients with intermediate- and high-risk disease, we need better therapeutic approaches."

Men at high risk of recurrence: For men with localized prostate cancer in the high-risk category (Gleason 8 to 10, or PSA level greater than 20, or clinical stage T2c or T3), evidence from a number of studies shows that taking hormone-suppressing drugs for three years after radiation treatment provides a significant advantage in controlling the cancer locally, limits the risk of developing metastatic disease, and prolongs life. A number of studies strongly argue for this combined approach in high-risk men. To avoid the side effects of hormonal therapy, there is the option of increasing the dose of external radiation with a brachytherapy boost (see page 283). However, this increase in dose comes at an increased risk of rectal and urinary toxicity.

Men with perineural invasion: Other men who may require more than radiation alone are those found to have prostate cancer that invades the spaces around the nerves of the prostate. This is called perineural invasion (PNI) on the biopsy specimen. Recently, scientists at Johns Hopkins studied 657 men who received radiation and found that men with PNI had a higher chance of PSA failure and were more likely to die of prostate cancer. Similar results have been confirmed by other groups. At Hopkins, men with PNI on their prostate cancer biopsies who choose radiation therapy are typically offered more aggressive treatments that may include hormonal therapy and an increased dose of radiation.

Men at intermediate risk: Men with an intermediate risk of recurrence have stage T2b disease, or a Gleason score of 3 + 4 or 4 + 3 (Grade Group 2 or 3), or a PSA level between 10 and 20 ng/ml. "The latest evidence suggests that temporary hormonal therapy can help these men, too," says Phuoc Tran. Earlier in this chapter, we talked about the results for men with intermediate-risk cancer in two studies; the men were treated with either a short course (four to six months) of hormonal therapy plus radiation or with radiation alone. Both studies showed that the short course of hormonal therapy can improve overall survival. However, there is emerging evidence that men with "low intermediate-risk" prostate cancer, Gleason 3 + 4 or PSA 10 to 20 ng/ml alone, particularly men with other serious health conditions or men who otherwise do not expect to live more than ten years, *may not benefit from a short course of hormones.* Furthermore, adds Tran, "The jury is still out, because studies with hormones for intermediate-risk men used lower doses of radiation than we currently use today." Could this mean that hormonal therapy is helpful only with lower doses of radiation? A RTOG Foundation study, currently underway, is attempting to figure out whether short-course hormonal therapy plus high-dose radiation therapy is better than high-dose radiation therapy alone for intermediate-risk patients. Finally, as DeWeese points out, the field of radiation therapy is constantly evolving. "As we are able to deliver significantly higher doses of radiation with unprecedented accuracy and precision, whether all patients will ultimately require hormonal therapy in the future is not clear."

SPACEOAR: PROTECTING THE RECTUM

Although radiation techniques have become increasingly more sophisticated with IMRT and SBRT/SABR, the physics of radiation cannot be broken. In some men, the rectum, which sits just behind the prostate, actually rubs up against the prostate. This makes it impossible to spare the rectum completely from radiation damage.

A recent—and temporary—solution that shows great promise is the injection of a biodegradable hydrogel between the prostate and rectum. The procedure is very similar to a prostate biopsy. Many of the initial studies for this were conducted at Hopkins under the lead of Ted DeWeese. Commercially known as SpaceOAR, this procedure has now been tested in a Phase III randomized study of 222 men with prostate cancer treated with radiotherapy: seventy-three men to a sham procedure and 149 on the SpaceOAR arm before radiation treatments. The results from the two groups can only be described as "a space" apart. Men who underwent the SpaceOAR procedure experienced significantly less late rectal toxicity (2 percent) and declines in quality of life compared to the men who had the sham treatment (9.2 percent). SpaceOAR is FDA-approved, and although it is not yet covered by Medicare or insurance, it is likely to be covered in the near future. Because of the many advancements in radiation therapy, SpaceOAR is not needed in all men; ask your doctor whether it is something that might benefit you.

Interstitial Brachytherapy
(Implanting Radioactive Seeds)

Brachytherapy is basically hand-to-hand combat, implanting tiny sources of radiation directly in the cancerous tissue instead of launching missiles from a distance. (The term *brachy* comes from the Greek word for "short," as in a short distance away from the malignancy. Confusingly, doctors often use the terms *brachytherapy, interstitial radiotherapy,* and *seeds* interchangeably.) The concept is not new. Pierre Curie thought of it a century ago, even before external-beam radiation treatment came onto the scene, and doctors in New York tried it several years later. They inserted thin glass tubes containing a radioactive substance called radon directly into tumors. The treatment killed tissue, but the results were uneven; some of the targeted tissue was devastated, while other tissue remained unscathed. In the next decades, scientists improved the technique, but its popularity waned as hormonal treatment developed and external-beam radiation therapy improved (see page 263). In the 1950s and '60s, however, improvements in dosages and radioactive materials helped foster a comeback for brachytherapy: doctors implanted radioactive gold "seeds," or tiny chunks of radioactive material, in men with prostate cancer. This was combined with external-beam radiation therapy. A few years later, doctors began using radioactive iodine seeds to fight prostate cancer.

Over the years, several other radioactive materials, including palladium, have been tested, and the means of implanting them have evolved from a subjective, freehand technique (which required surgery to give the doctor access to the prostate) to state-of-the-art, ultrasound- and CT-guided systems involving templates. Doctors have become highly sophisticated in targeting and placing these tiny pellets—at 4.5 millimeters long, they're the size of a grain of rice—and monitoring the dosage.

Who Should Get This Treatment?

Brachytherapy alone (the use of seeds without something else, such as external-beam radiation therapy) is not ideally suited for men with a large, bulky tumor; a high-grade (Gleason score 8 or above) tumor; or lymph node metastases. Most implantation regimens don't include the seminal vesicles or tissue outside the prostate, so if there's the slightest risk that cancer has spread to these areas, implanting radiation seeds *within* the prostate won't do anything to fight the cancer *outside* it. (Although, because the radiation dose can extend a few millimeters beyond the wall of the prostate, some men with extracapsular penetration may still be candidates for brachytherapy.) If there is a risk that cancer has spread beyond the prostate, men are also treated with supplemental external-beam radiation therapy.

The clinical research committee of the American Brachytherapy Society and the Prostate Brachytherapy Quality Assurance group recently published recommendations for selecting patients who are best suited to brachytherapy alone, brachytherapy plus external-beam radiation therapy, and brachytherapy in conjunction with hormonal therapy. *Radiation seeds are not recommended for men who have had a previous TUR procedure.* For one thing, because they've had significant amounts of tissue around the urethra removed, there's not a lot left to hold the seeds in place. (Think of a bulletin board riddled with holes from too many thumbtacks.) Men who have had a TUR are also much more likely to develop urinary problems such as urethral stricture and incontinence from brachytherapy. Men with urinary problems (who score higher than a 14 on a symptom score questionnaire such as the one in chapter 2) are not ideal candidates for brachytherapy. Also, men who are in otherwise poor health, men who have a life expectancy of less than five years, and men with distant metastases should not undergo this procedure.

The American Brachytherapy Society also notes that some men who are not ideal candidates for brachytherapy can be implanted successfully if the procedure is performed by a physician with expertise in handling cases that present "technical difficulties." The problem here is the risk that the radiation coverage may be inadequate or uneven. Men in this group include men with prominent median lobes of the prostate (detected by ultrasound), men with severe diabetes, men who have had previous pelvic surgery or radiation treatment, and men with obstructive urinary problems resulting from BPH. Men with very large prostates (greater than 60 cubic centimeters) are not ideal candidates for brachytherapy. This is because the larger the prostate, the more seeds it takes to kill the cancer, the greater the likelihood of complications and the larger expanse of rectum exposed to radiation; also, a very large prostate may intrude on anatomical structures, such as the pubic bone, which may interfere with seed placement. As we discussed above, some men with large prostates may be able to have this treatment if they have a course of hormonal therapy first (lasting three to six months) to shrink the prostate.

The Ideal Patient for Brachytherapy Alone

The ideal patient for this treatment is a man with localized disease who is also ideally suited for external-beam radiation therapy and radical prostatectomy—early-stage cancer (T1 to T2a), Gleason score 6, and a PSA level less than 10 ng/ml. Men with stage T2b cancer and higher, with Gleason scores of 7 or higher, or a PSA level greater than 10 will likely be given external-beam radiation therapy, too, as a "boost" to brachytherapy. Some men with low-volume, low intermediate-risk prostate cancer can also be considered candidates for brachytherapy alone.

As with conformal external-beam therapy, the technology here is continually improving. Before the development of sophisticated guidance systems, major problems arose from seeds being either too far apart or too close together, resulting in an uneven distribution of radiation throughout the prostate; some cancer cells were killed, but some weren't. In many cases, the cancer returned or never completely went away in the first place. Better placement, thanks to three-dimensional scans like those used to design conformal therapy, may change this picture.

As a treatment choice, brachytherapy has many attractive features: There's no hospitalization; it's a simple outpatient procedure. There's hardly any recovery time and no lengthy time away from work or normal activities. And very high doses of radiation can be concentrated within the prostate, with hardly any damage to surrounding tissue.

Brachytherapy as a Boost

Several years ago, when brachytherapy was becoming established as a treatment for localized prostate cancer, some radiation oncologists worried that the seeds alone would not prevent cancer at the capsule of the prostate from spreading outside it. So they decided to hedge their cancer-killing bets, adding low-dose (45 to 50 Gy) external-beam radiation to brachytherapy. This practice continues in many centers. Some physicians prefer to start with external-beam radiation; others put the seeds in first. To minimize side effects, the two treatments are often separated by a three- to five-week break (see also page 168). This combined approach has been used for many years for intermediate-risk and high-risk men, often with shorter courses of hormones (usually less than a year), and sometimes without hormones at all.

This combined approach is a reasonable option to consider—but there are still many unknowns. The ASCENDE-RT trial, conducted in Canada, offers the most promising evidence in favor. Nearly four hundred men were randomly assigned either to the standard eight-week course of external beam radiotherapy or to a five-week course of external-beam radiotherapy plus a brachytherapy boost. "Outcomes for high-risk men suggested an improvement by 20 percent in PSA control over nine years of follow-up," says Phuoc Tran. "However, we still don't know over the long run whether this improvement in PSA control will ever turn into an improvement for preventing death from prostate cancer." As you might expect, this increase in dose comes at an increased risk—18 percent, compared to 5 percent from brachytherapy alone—of rectal and urinary toxicity (particularly of significant late urinary issues like urethral stricture).

What to Expect

Before beginning interstitial brachytherapy, you should undergo an extensive physical examination. The physician will estimate the volume of your prostate based on the rectal exam and a CT scan or the ultrasound performed at the time of biopsy. You may need to undergo a cystoscopy (in which a tiny, lighted tube is inserted through the anesthetized penis and threaded through the prostate into the bladder to evaluate your particular anatomy (especially to see whether your prostate has a large middle lobe that protrudes into the bladder) and make sure the cancer is contained within the prostate. Next is the treatment-planning session, which is usually performed several weeks before the procedure (but it can also be done during the procedure; this is called intraoperative treatment planning). With the help of transrectal ultrasound, CT scans, and a computerized guidance system, doctors can create a template that marks exactly where the seeds should go, plus determine how many seeds you need, how deeply they should be inserted, and how strong their radiation should be. You may need other tests to make sure your body can tolerate anesthesia; these may include blood tests (to check for bleeding problems), an electrocardiogram (EKG), or a chest X-ray.

To Prepare

Starting two days before the procedure, eat a low-fiber diet (fiber is found in fruits and vegetables and in whole grains such as oatmeal and most cereals). After midnight, drink clear liquids only, and try not to drink anything for six hours before the procedure. Note: If you are on medications that must be taken regularly or with food, or if you have other dietary needs, don't worry; this is very common. Plan ahead by discussing this problem with your doctor. Do *not* simply stop taking any medication just because you're not supposed to eat or drink anything. Because it's essential that the bowels are clear (so that nothing blocks or interferes with the ultrasound image of your prostate), you will be asked to give yourself an enema on the morning of the procedure.

During the Procedure

A combination of antibiotics (to minimize the risk of infection) will be administered intravenously. Anesthesia varies; you may be given general or regional anesthesia. At Johns Hopkins, general anesthesia is usually preferred because the patient is asleep and less likely to move during the procedure. In spinal anesthesia, a tiny needle is used to inject a local anesthetic into the small of the back through the dura, the membrane lining the spinal cord, and into the spinal fluid. Within minutes, the patient feels numb, relaxed, and heavy from the waist to the toes. Afterward, the patient will be asked to lie flat in bed until the numbness goes away and he can move his legs again. Epidural anesthesia is like having an intravenous (IV) tube hooked up to the back instead of to a vein in the arm. A local anesthetic enters the body through a tiny plastic tube inserted near the small of the back, and temporarily numbs the nerves in the lower body. Unlike spinal anesthesia, which comes in one dose, epidural anesthesia can be given continuously. The area of numbness can be adjusted; so can the degree of pain relief.

The procedure is performed with the patient on his back in the lithotomy position—this gives the best access to the perineum, the area between the rectum and scrotum—with his legs raised in knee

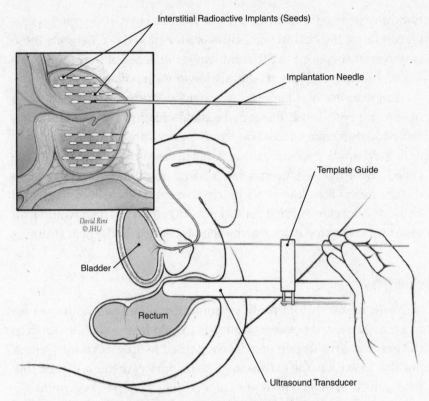

Interstitial Radioactive Implants (Seeds)

Implantation Needle

Template Guide

David Rini
© JHU

Bladder

Rectum

Ultrasound Transducer

FIGURE 9.3   Implanting Radioactive Seeds (Brachytherapy)

Radiation oncologists use advanced-guidance ultrasound systems, three-dimensional treatment planning, and templates to ensure the precise placement of seeds. This approach also helps guarantee an even distribution of radiation throughout the prostate.

stirrups, hips elevated, and buttocks at the end of the table (see fig. 9.3). Your doctor will probably use transrectal ultrasound during the procedure to guide seed placement and stabilizing needles to help keep the prostate as still as possible. Depending on the size of your prostate and the radioactive material your doctor is using, you will probably receive between fifty and eighty seeds.

At some centers, the needles are inserted under CT or MRI guidance; some centers also use fluoroscopy (an X-ray image that appears live on a TV screen instead of as a still photograph). The choice of radioactive isotopes (seed material) also varies; some doctors prefer iodine, others palladium. Palladium has a shorter duration of effect but puts out a higher initial dose of radiation. Its half-life (the time it takes for half the material to disintegrate) is seventeen days; the half-life of iodine is fifty-nine days. Because these isotopes emit energy in different ways, the doses of iodine and palladium used are different (slightly lower with palladium).

Innovations in imaging have helped doctors do a better job of spacing both kinds of seeds to avoid creating "hot spots," areas receiving too much radiation—particularly around the urethra—and "cold spots," where cancer is not treated. A refined technique called the modified peripheral loading method also helps keep dosage even. The American Brachytherapy Society looks forward to the development of real-time, online dosimetry, which would provide immediate feedback during the procedure, in the near future.

Afterward

You will be taken to a recovery room for about two hours; an ice bag may be placed between your legs to help keep swelling down in the perineal area. When you have regained feeling in your legs (and are able to walk to the bathroom), the urinary catheter will probably be removed. (In some men, the catheter may be left in overnight.)

You will probably be given a round of antibiotics to take for about five days and some form of pain medication and anti-inflammatory medication, although the vast majority of men do not feel the need to take any pain medication. If you do require medication, an OTC drug such as ibuprofen (Motrin, Advil) or acetaminophen (Tylenol) works well; however, if you are in severe discomfort, your doctor may prescribe a stronger medication (one containing codeine or morphine).

Although brachytherapy is an outpatient procedure, you may feel some fatigue and drowsiness afterward due to lingering effects of the anesthesia. Plan on having someone drive you home, and don't try to drive for at least twelve hours afterward. Note: *Most doctors will refuse to perform the procedure or may want you to stay in the hospital overnight if you do not have a ride home.*

There are no dietary restrictions; after you are out of the recovery room, you can eat and drink whatever you wish. For the first two days, avoid heavy lifting or strenuous exercise. To minimize the risk of blood clots, avoid sitting or standing in the same position for a prolonged period. Drink plenty of fluids (at least six to eight large glasses) to keep your urine clear; eat extra servings of fruits and vegetables (to help prevent constipation), take it easy, and rest often. Because men are basically radioactive after brachytherapy, you will probably be advised to avoid close contact with children (letting them sit on your lap or come within two feet of you) and pregnant women for a few weeks to months after the implantation, until the radioactivity wears off (the length of time depends on whether you have received iodine or palladium).

Guidelines vary, but you will probably be told it's okay to sleep in the same bed as your spouse or partner. Studies have shown that people living in Denver, Colorado, for a year receive more radiation (due to the sun) than the partner of a man who has had brachytherapy. There has never been a published account of a man ejaculating a seed into his partner, and the risk of radiation damage from a single seed is minimal. But to be on the safe side, some doctors advise men to abstain from intercourse for as long as two months and to wear condoms for a similar period of time. There is also a minimal risk that a seed might migrate to the lung. Although this does not cause any symptoms or harm to the lung, you may be scheduled to have a chest X-ray at your first follow-up visit. Some doctors perform cystoscopy after surgery to remove any blood clots and stray seeds from the bladder or urethra.

Call your doctor immediately if…

- You pass blood clots larger than a dime, either through your penis or rectum;
- You are unable to urinate within four hours of drinking two large glasses of liquid;
- You have a temperature greater than 100.5 degrees Fahrenheit or shaking chills;
- You are in pain and pain medication doesn't help; or
- Your Foley catheter falls out of your bladder.

Complications

Remember, any form of radiation—or any treatment, for that matter—is operator-dependent. In other words, it's only as effective as the doctor performing it. Seed implantation takes skill and practice. If you choose to undergo brachytherapy, you should have it done at a center where at least several procedures are performed a month. In addition, make sure your radiation oncologist performs a CT scan or some other form of imaging "quality check" after the procedure. Your doctor should also follow the course of brachytherapy patients afterward to check for any side effects or complications. Knowing what happens to you is (at least, it should be) essential for your doctor and treatment team. It gives them valuable feedback and can help them fine-tune their methods to achieve the best results. Unfortunately, not all centers perform these necessary quality-assurance tasks.

One major consideration to keep in mind when evaluating complications of brachytherapy is that the placement of the seeds has changed dramatically over the last decade. In recent years, with better understanding of dosimetry and with the help of ultrasound imaging, physicians have begun placing the majority of the seeds toward the outer edges of the prostate rather than uniformly throughout. With this technique, called peripheral loading, the center of the prostate still receives adequate radiation, but the dose to the urethra is no longer overwhelming. "Much of the earlier published literature on complications after brachytherapy was done on patients who received uniformly loaded rather than peripherally loaded implants," notes Daniel Song.

Here are some of the complications you can expect from the implantation of radioactive seeds. The risk of death is extremely rare and generally is linked to anesthesia. There is a great variation in the incidence of late (not immediately after the seeds are implanted) complications—ranging from 0 to 72 percent—depending on which study one chooses to quote; the most common range is from 5 to 10 percent.

Urinary Retention

The major immediate complication of brachytherapy is urinary retention, the inability to empty the bladder completely. This happens when the tissue surrounding the implants begins to react— with bleeding, swelling, and inflammation—to the trauma of having a needle stuck in it repeatedly (just as, on a smaller scale, the prostate swells after a biopsy). Most but not all men will experience some degree of urinary retention during the first few days after seed implantation. Some radiation oncologists start all of their patients on alpha-blockers such as doxazosin (Cardura), terazosin (Hytrin), alfuzosin (Uroxatral), or tamsulosin (Flomax) prior to the implantation. Patients may continue to take them for two or three months after the procedure and then taper them gradually as the symptoms resolve. Other radiation oncologists also administer low doses of steroids as a preemptive strike before and during the procedure to combat swelling of the prostate.

Urinary retention may have a delayed onset as well, peaking between two weeks and three months after brachytherapy. The symptom is the same, but the cause is different—irritation in the urethra and prostate, which develops as the radiation's effects begin to be felt. This, too, is only temporary; it gradually improves and usually goes away within about two months. In the most severe cases of urinary retention, some men (about 5 percent) may need an indwelling Foley catheter (usually for a week or so) or may choose to insert a catheter several times a day to drain the bladder. Rarely, men may need a TUR of the prostate, if urinary retention does not improve with time. Several studies have found a high rate of incontinence in men who have had a TUR *before* receiving the seeds (see below). There is less information on the risk of incontinence in men who undergo a TUR *after* seed implantation, but the risk may be as high as 17 percent; it is probably lower if a more conservative TUR is performed.

Bowel Problems

Brachytherapy, in theory, has better rectal-sparing properties than external-beam radiation. Overall, 10 to 15 percent of men experience rectal symptoms, including loose stools, diarrhea, rectal bleeding, or rectal urgency after seed implantation. A study of 825 men treated at Memorial Sloan-Kettering Cancer Center with brachytherapy (140 also received some external-beam radiation) found that 9 percent of men reported mild rectal symptoms that didn't require medication or treatment, and 7 percent had symptoms that did require medication such as suppositories or steroid enemas. Symptoms tended to peak in incidence at eight months and had resolved in all patients by three and a half years. In other studies, rectal bleeding has been reported in between 5 and 20 percent of men. Men treated more aggressively (for example, men with larger stage T3 or T4 tumors who also got external-beam radiation) or men who had larger tumors (and therefore got more seeds or a higher dose of radiation) tended to develop more severe rectal problems such as ulcers. Stool softeners, steroid enemas, and anti-inflammatory drugs may help rectal ulcers go away, but more serious ulcers that destroy tissue may require further intervention. In the Memorial Sloan-Kettering study, four patients (0.5 percent) developed rectal ulceration (confirmed during a colonoscopy), but in three of the men, this went away on its own. None of these men required hospitalization or surgical intervention. In many cases of rectal bleeding, healing eventually occurs with time and supportive care such as steroid enemas, but if the bleeding is persistent, further measures may be needed. New evidence suggests that argon plasma coagulation or hyperbaric oxygen therapy (this involves sitting in a pressurized oxygen chamber for several sessions) may be effective treatment for rectal ulceration caused by radiation. Note: If you have rectal bleeding after brachytherapy, there is also the chance that it is caused by something else—perhaps polyps in the colon or colorectal cancer. See your doctor; you may also need to be examined by a gastroenterologist to rule out other causes.

Prostatitis

In one study of 115 patients who had radioactive seeds implanted, five men developed prostatitis (for more on prostatitis, see chapter 2) and reported severe irritative urinary symptoms. The investigators suspected that in these men, the seeds became infected.

Urinary Problems

From 10 to 37 percent of men in several studies had urinary problems including urethral stricture, bladder neck contracture, and damage to the urethra that caused irritative urinary symptoms. Most of these occurred in men who had already experienced such problems (from BPH, for example) or who had undergone a TUR procedure. Incontinence, which occurred in 5 percent of men, was not a problem for men who had not had a TUR. As many as half of men who have had a TUR who undergo brachytherapy develop incontinence, sometimes months after the procedure. In rare cases, severe, prolonged bleeding may also occur, requiring treatment with hyperbaric oxygen (see page 293). As we discussed earlier, a major factor in the development of urinary problems seems to be placement of the seeds. In the past, trouble was more likely to develop when seeds were implanted too close to the urethra. Such complications have become less common as doctors have moved to the peripheral loading approach, and as brachytherapy has been increasingly ruled out in men who have undergone a TUR or other surgical intervention involving the urethra.

How do the side effects of brachytherapy compare with those of other forms of treatment? A recent multicenter study from Spain monitored, for up to three years, the side effects in men who had undergone brachytherapy. Researchers found that men who had undergone brachytherapy initially had worse irritative-obstructive symptoms, but these improved over the next three years.

Sexual Problems

The major sexual side effect after brachytherapy is impotence, although ejaculatory pain, pain in the testicles, and blood in the semen may also occur. In several studies, impotence was found to affect at least 40 percent of men—although not immediately after implantation. A man's ability to have an erection appears to diminish over time after brachytherapy, finally reaching a plateau, just as it does in men who get external-beam radiation treatment, probably because of gradual damage to small blood vessels. This can be helped by erectile dysfunction drugs such as sildenafil (Viagra), which are discussed in chapter 11.

Much of the information on the recovery of sexual function after brachytherapy is anecdotal. However, a recent study from the University of Pennsylvania used a validated quality-of-life questionnaire in men who underwent seed implantation between 1992 and 1998. In general, the patients were older than men who undergo radical prostatectomy; the average age was sixty-nine. Before treatment, eighty-one men said that they had erections sufficient for intercourse. Two years after treatment, 49 percent of these men remained potent. As with every form of treatment for prostate cancer, younger men fared better: 52 percent of men younger than seventy remained potent, compared with only 45 percent of men over age seventy. The study also found that short-term (for three to six months) treatment with hormones before brachytherapy did not increase the likelihood of erectile dysfunction. More favorable results have been reported by others who noted that at three and six years, 80 and 60 percent, respectively, were potent. The major factors that influenced this were a higher dose of radiation and whether sexual function was normal or marginal before treatment. A large study of 992 men compared brachytherapy with external-beam radiation. Men who received brachytherapy reported greater sexual function and the least change in sexual function overall, and those who had both external-beam radiation and brachytherapy reported the greatest decline in sexual function.

Despite the fact that most men have infertility (from either partial or complete loss of semen) after brachytherapy, there has been a report of three patients impregnating their partners. To be on the safe side, it is advisable to use contraception while the seeds are still active as well as two to three months afterward to minimize the potential risk of conceiving with sperm affected by radiation.

Temporary Seeds: High-Dose-Rate Brachytherapy

A variant of brachytherapy, usually given along with external-beam radiation, is high-dose-rate (HDR), or temporary, brachytherapy. As its name suggests, the seeds don't stay in; they're removed at the end of each treatment session. These temporary seeds, used more frequently in Europe and at a few centers in the United States, are made up of highly radioactive iridium-192. They are inserted (and removed) with the help of a robotic arm through plastic tubes, or catheters, at precise locations throughout the prostate. Most centers performing HDR brachytherapy use several treatment sessions. Typically, after the catheters are placed, two or three treatments are delivered, with at least six-hour intervals in between treatments. Patients are usually admitted to the hospital while they wait between treatment sessions, and pain medication is given to minimize discomfort from the catheters. At some centers, the catheters are removed, and the men go home and then come back a few weeks later for another round of treatment (which requires another visit to the operating room for catheter placement). Most recently, some centers have explored single-fraction, large-dose HDR implants; early results have been promising, but longer follow-up is needed.

In general, temporary brachytherapy has been used for men with more aggressive cancer or with cancer that extends slightly beyond the prostate. Most studies have evaluated the use of HDR as a "boost" during or after external-beam radiation, a means of getting higher doses of radiation to the prostate. The results of these studies are somewhat difficult to interpret because of significant variations in the characteristics of the patients treated, but when compared with the results of external-beam therapy alone, the cancer control rates are about the same or better. No randomized studies have been performed comparing HDR treatment with high-dose external beam radiation. A few centers in the United States are using HDR alone, mainly for men with low-risk prostate cancer.

Hypofractionated Radiation Therapy and Stereotactic Ablative Radiotherapy (SABR)

As we discussed earlier in this chapter, radiation oncologists have long believed that the best way to balance killing tumor cells with protecting normal tissue is to spread the radiation dose out over many weeks. This idea is called *fractionation*. However, new laboratory and clinical evidence suggests that this may not necessarily be true for prostate cancer—that prostate cancer may be particularly vulnerable to larger daily doses of radiation, much more so than other tumor cells. As a result, there has been interest in hypofractionated radiation, in which higher doses of radiation are delivered over a shorter time period—four to five weeks instead of eight weeks; this is "moderate hypofractionation." Some centers even offer an ultra-short or "extreme" regimen of as few as five daily treatments over the course of one week. In the past, giving such large doses of radiation on a daily basis would have increased the risk of damaging normal tissues. However, with today's new targeting and treatment-planning methods, it is possible that hypofractionated radiation can be safely administered.

Clinical results from multiple investigators in primarily low-risk patients with localized prostate cancer have conclusively shown that moderate hypofractionated is an equally good option to the standard seven- to eight-week course of radiotherapy. A study from the RTOG Foundation randomly assigned 1,101 men with low-risk prostate cancer to either an eight-week or a five-and-a-half-week course of radiotherapy and found no significant differences in cure rates. There was a slightly increased risk of urinary and rectal toxicity, but this was not found to be clinically meaningful.

What about extreme hypofractionation, also called stereotactic body radiotherapy (SBRT) or stereotactic ablative radiotherapy (SABR)? A seminal study from Stanford of forty-one low-risk patients who received the five high-dose treatments has shown this ultra-short regimen to be safe and effective, with PSA failures similar to those of conventional eight-week radiotherapy. Numerous published studies of SBRT for localized prostate cancer since have shown very similar results. Unfortunately, we just don't have long-term results yet. SBRT is generally covered by Medicare. If you decide on this approach, Phuoc Tran advises "enrolling in a clinical trial if you can, and choosing a center with heavy experience in prostate SBRT."

A NEW WAY TO ATTACK EARLY METASTATIC PROSTATE CANCER

In the blockbuster movie *Independence Day*, terrifying space aliens invade Earth. From one mother ship, dozens of smaller but equally deadly ships spread out around the planet. But these evil aliens are beaten by a tiny home force who attack the mother ship. Without its protection, the smaller ships are vulnerable.

This is a pretty good model for what Johns Hopkins radiation oncologist Phuoc Tran wants to do with metastatic prostate cancer in its earliest stages. He believes that by eliminating the bigger sites of cancer, tiny new ones won't be able to flourish. It's an idea that has shown success in the treatment of breast cancer, "where improved local control decreases metastatic as well as local relapse," Tran says. "This local treatment model is true for prostate cancer, too. Better control of localized cancer by adjuvant radiation to the area around the prostate (called the prostatic bed) lowers the risk of other metastases and improves overall survival. We believe that sites of *macroscopic* disease—visible on MRI or other images—support the maturation of *microscopic* spots of cancer into future metastases." Going after the cancer that can be seen "has substantial clinical implications" for the cancer too small to be seen, he adds. "This is hardly ever performed in prostate cancer."

In the spectrum of cancer from localized to advanced meta-static disease is a kind of midpoint called an *oligometastatic* state. There are bits of cancer that have spread, or metastasized, beyond the prostate—but not that many, and not to very many locations in the body. Cancer in this state is still vulnerable, and still responds to treatment. For example, "Local radiation treatment to the primary tumor for oligometastatic sarcomas and colorectal cancers and radiation to iso-lated metastases, together with chemotherapy, can result in long-term disease-free survival in between 25 and 40 percent of patients," says Tran. "Our own clinical experience suggests an oligometastatic state exists in a subset of prostate cancer patients who benefit from local radiation treatment to all sites of macroscopic metastatic disease." Oligometastatic refers to patients who have three or fewer metasta-ses to bone.

Picture, if you will, the bloodstream. It goes throughout the body, flowing in one direction. Cancer cells that make their way into the blood, like seeds floating on a river, leave the original tumor—the mother ship—and drift for a while, eventually coming to rest at a dis-tant site, where they may start to grow. This is the generally accepted model of how cancer spreads. But Tran suspects that these circu-lating tumor cells (CTCs) get homesick—that they pay an occasional visit back to the original tumor, or maybe visit one of their siblings that has struck out on its own and built a home. These visits are invigo-rating: "The CTCs become more robust," he says, "and this cyclical process of CTCs interacting with more established cancer results in the release of signals that foster tumor growth." Like a domino effect, then, tumor growth leads to angiogenesis—the paving of new roads, made of blood vessels, to supply the tumor. Angiogenesis is followed by immune evasion—the cancer mutates to dodge the body's militia of immune cells—and ultimately, "the formation of new, macroscopic metastases." This theory of macroscopic metastases being self-seeding communal sanctuaries is supported by recent genomic data from studies of human prostate cancer cells, Tran says.

What's the best way to target these little blots of cancer? Tran believes the key is stereotactic ablative radiation (SABR), "a highly focused, localized, high-dose radiation delivered in a hypofractionated course," meaning in several large doses, spread out over several days. "It's ideally suited for treatment of oligometastatic patients, and has shown high local control rates with minimal toxicity," he says. "SABR effectively targets the microenvironment of tumors, and in melanoma patients, has been shown to have antitumor effects on the irradiated tumor and an abscopal effect"—think of a shock wave, affecting areas not part of the original blast—"on distant metastases when combined with other immune system-stimulating agents." Tran is starting a multi-institutional study aimed at killing oligometastatic cancer through SABR and immune system-targeting agents.

Cryo/Thermal Ablation (Freezing or Heating the Prostate)

Before we even begin this section, I would like to review the recommendations from the National Comprehensive Cancer Network (NCCN), the most authoritative, independent, up-to-date source of information for patients on the management of localized prostate cancer. These guidelines, formulated by world-renowned experts from twenty-seven approved cancer centers in the United States, state that, "Cryotherapy or other local therapies are *not recommended as routine primary therapy for localized prostate cancer* due to lack of long-term data comparing these treatments to radical prostatectomy or radiation." And yet, these techniques are enthusiastically endorsed by their advocates, who point out that because they require no surgery, they offer a minimally invasive outpatient treatment with few side effects. What could be better?

Well, actually, what could be better would be radical prostatectomy or radiation therapy, and the reason is the urethra. The
prostate, as we learned in the beginning of this book, is strategically
located between the urethra and the bladder. When it is removed
surgically, the bladder is mechanically reconnected to the urethra.
With radiation therapy, although the cancer cells are eliminated, the
shell of the prostate remains behind, like the ribs and timbers of
an old shipwreck, as a scaffolding to link the bladder and urethra.
With cryoablation (also called cryotherapy, cryosurgery, or cryosur-
gical ablation) or thermal ablation, the prostate is physically heated
or cooled to extreme temperatures, causing all of the cells to die.
If this truly happened and the entire prostate were destroyed, the
urethra would be zapped right along with it. Then there would be
no connection between the bladder and the distal urethra (the part
of the urethra on the other side of the prostate), and you could not
urinate. Instead, with cryotherapy the urethra is protected, kept at a
normal temperature while the surrounding prostate is frozen. With
thermal therapy, the urethra is not protected, and for this reason,
strictures may develop later.

But this is where the multifocal nature of prostate cancer, which
we've talked about earlier, presents a problem. A study from the
Mayo Clinic found that 66 percent of prostate cancers were located
within 5 millimeters of the urethra, 45 percent were within 1 millimeter, and 17 percent actually touched the urethra. *This means, theoretically, that as many as 83 percent of men could have their cancer spared
right along with the urethra.* Any man with localized prostate cancer
who is otherwise healthy and can expect to live for many more years
should consider this fact very carefully before choosing cryoablation.

Cryoablation

Who is a candidate for cryoablation? If you ask the doctors who
perform this treatment, they will tell you that the ideal candidate is
a man with a high-grade or high-volume tumor who is not potent
or interested in maintaining potency, or a man whose cancer has
returned after radiation therapy. In addition, cryoablation is also
being offered to men with localized prostate cancer, especially men

who are not candidates for radical prostatectomy because of obesity, cardiac disease, or inflammatory bowel disease. However, the most recent guidelines from the American Urological Association state that it is not recommended for men with high-risk disease, outside of a clinical trial. Further, cryoablation advocates believe that any man who has no evidence of metastatic disease and at least a ten-year life expectancy can be considered a candidate, as well—if, after reviewing all the information, he believes that watchful waiting, radical prostatectomy, and radiation therapy are not options for him.

Who is probably not a candidate? Men who have undergone a TUR procedure for BPH (especially if a lot of tissue was removed), men with a very large prostate, and men who do not have a rectum or whose rectum is not easily accessible because of rectal stenosis or other major rectal problems. Men who have had a TUR are more likely to develop sloughing of the urethra (passing bits of dead tissue during urination) and urinary retention; for men with prostates larger than 50 cubic centimeters, the pubic bone may interfere with complete freezing of the prostate. (However, a short course of hormonal therapy may shrink the prostate to a more treatable size.)

The technology for cryoablation has come a long way since the 1960s, when freezing was accomplished through the urethra. Today's cryoablation technique involves the placement of multiple 17 gauge (1.5 millimeter) needles, through which pressurized argon gas is used to freeze the prostate. Then helium is used to thaw it. The placement of the needles varies, but the physician, using a template similar to that used in brachytherapy, places eight to twenty-five needles into the prostate through the perineum without making an incision. This is done under anesthesia, with the patient placed in the dorsal lithotomy position (as in brachytherapy), with his legs in stirrups. Transrectal ultrasound helps guide the needle placement and also helps the doctor monitor the degree of freezing until an "ice ball" has been created. Multiple thermocouples (temperature change–measuring devices made up of two different metals) are placed throughout the prostate—at the sphincter, over the rectum, and adjacent to each neurovascular bundle. The thermocouples at the external sphincter and rectum are sentries, on guard to minimize the risk of causing incontinence or a fistula (a hole in the rectum). The thermocouples in the middle of the gland and near the neurovascular bundles are there to make sure that the temperature goal of -40 degrees Celsius is reached. But even if the target temperature is not reached, the freezing process is stopped when the edge of the "ice ball" has extended just beyond the capsule of the prostate.

Before the freezing begins, a warming catheter is placed through the urethra into the bladder. Heated (to 43 degrees Celsius) saline is continuously circulated through this catheter by a water pump. Your doctor will probably perform two 10-minute freezing sessions, allowing the prostate to thaw passively between sessions. After these freeze-thaw cycles, the urethral warmer will be left in place for a few minutes to minimize the risk of urethral sloughing. And then it's over. The needles are removed, pressure is applied to the perineum, the urethral warmer is removed, and a Foley catheter is inserted; this catheter will be removed in two or three days. You may be allowed to go home that same day, or you may spend the night in the hospital. You will probably take antibiotics, an oral pain medication, and an alpha-blocker for several days.

Although with modern techniques, incontinence rates are low (2 to 4 percent), patients may develop sloughing of necrotic material from the urethra (6 percent or fewer) or a fistula between the prostate and rectum (1 percent or fewer).

Previously, in theory, doctors thought that all men should be impotent after cryoablation because, in an attempt to destroy all the cancer, the prostate tissue closest to the neurovascular bundles was deliberately frozen. (For more on these neurovascular bundles, see chapter 8.) In practice, however, because these nerve bundles have an abundant blood supply, it was more difficult to reach a low temperature in this region. Recently, some doctors have worked to limit the amount of freezing in a technique known as a "male lumpectomy"—in which the prostate is frozen only on one side or even in just a few spots (see page 306).

Thermal Ablation

It's the opposite approach taken in cryoablation—applying heat instead of cold—but the idea is the same. Tissue-destroying heat is delivered to the prostate. Currently, doctors are exploring several different sources of heat, studying their potential to eradicate the tumor, minimize complications, and shorten recovery time. These include:

- High-intensity focused ultrasound (HIFU)
- Photodynamic therapy (PDT)
- Microwave energy
- Radio frequency interstitial tumor ablation (RITA)
- Irreversible electroporation

Currently, the most popular technique uses the Sonablate system and the Ablatherm HIFU device. During this procedure, done with a man under general or spinal anesthesia, an ultrasound probe is placed in the rectum, inside a balloon-shaped latex cooling device that keeps the temperature of the rectal wall at less than 37 degrees Celsius. Guided by ultrasound imaging, the doctor determines the boundaries of the treatment area and marks the distance between the rectum and the wall of the prostate. The procedure itself sounds like an artillery drill: Once the coordinates have been set, the computer places the firing head in the target region, and treatment begins automatically. A beam of focused ultrasound waves is emitted intermittently. Each shot lasts three to five seconds, with a gap in between. The treatment continues, layer by layer, until the entire area is covered. It takes less than three hours to treat a small prostate. As in the case of cryoablation and brachytherapy, men with large prostates may undergo hormonal therapy ahead of time to shrink the prostate.

There is a new approach to HIFU that is currently undergoing investigation. Here MRI is used in real-time to identify the outlines of the prostate, and thermal energy is delivered through the urethra using ten ultrasound transducers. An endorectal (inside the rectum) cooling device is used during the procedure to provide cooling and prevent the unwanted destruction of nearby tissues.

There is contradictory information in the literature on the side effects and complications of HIFU. In some reports, it sounds as if the treatment is entirely complication-free, as close to the proverbial "walk in the park" as one could get. However, overall, the range of men who have urinary retention is reported as between 1 and

9 percent; urethral strictures, between 5 and 15 percent; incontinence, between 1 and 15 percent; erectile dysfunction, between 13 and 53 percent; and a fistula between the prostate and the rectum, between 0 and 3 percent. Advocates of this form of treatment state that if it fails, no problem—you can just have it again. But with repeated treatments comes a greater likelihood of side effects. Some doctors who perform thermal ablation advocate sparing the neurovascular bundles in an effort to preserve potency. This may help avoid impotence, but it may also leave a few cancer cells behind.

Is HIFU FDA approved? Yes and no. The FDA failed to approve HIFU for whole-gland treatment of localized prostate cancer or salvage therapy for recurrent prostate cancer following radiation therapy, because the manufacturers failed to prove that the devices were reasonably safe and effective for that use. So the manufacturers took another tack. They applied for and received FDA approval for prostate tissue ablation. This is similar to the approval of a scalpel, a tool to cut tissue but not approved to treat specific diseases, so don't be fooled if you are told otherwise.

Most of the other thermal ablation techniques are still investigational. PDT involves administering a photosensitizing drug intravenously and then shooting light at a certain wavelength at the targeted area. This causes a photochemical reaction that is highly toxic to tissue. The trick here is to produce enough illumination to penetrate the prostate.

In theory, all of these forms of therapy—although promising and effective in treating BPH—suffer from the same Achilles' heel as cryoablation does: the urethra. Sparing even some prostate tissue means that some cancer cells may sneak past treatment as well. Also, the nature of the prostate—its irregular shape and its proximity to vulnerable structures just a few millimeters away—provides further challenges. How can a physician eliminate the prostate's peripheral zone, where cancer often grows, without injuring the rectum, the neurovascular bundles, or other important organs? For a detailed discussion of the *results* of all forms of treatment for localized disease—surgery, radiation, and cryo/thermal ablation—see chapter 10.

Focal Therapy: The "Male Lumpectomy"

Earlier, we discussed the downside of PSA testing: the fact that it picks up some cancers that never needed to be detected, because they were never going to become dangerous. There are men in this boat who hear all the treatment options we've discussed for localized prostate cancer—active surveillance, surgery, or radiation—and say, "None of the above." These men feel perfectly normal; they don't want any side effects, and don't feel that they ought to have any side effects, because they barely have cancer to begin with. For them, the solution seems simple—why not just treat the tiny area where the biopsy is positive? Well, this does seem like a reasonable suggestion. The trouble is that infuriating word, *multifocal* (see chapter 5). Remember the image of the strawberry with a bunch of tiny seeds throughout? One reason why prostate cancer is such a formidable enemy is that there are usually three to eight separate tumors in each radical prostatectomy specimen. So if only one biopsy core—which samples 1/1,000th of the prostate—shows cancer, this doesn't mean that the rest of it is as pure as the driven snow. If the conditions were ripe for cancer to begin in one tiny spot, and prostate cancer usually forms in several tiny spots, do the math: the odds are good that more cancer—even just a few cells—is in there somewhere.

Johns Hopkins scientists Jonathan Epstein and Alan Partin examined the prostate specimens that were removed at surgery from one hundred patients whose original needle biopsy suggested limited disease. From the biopsy, these guys looked great: fewer than three cores showed cancer; each positive core had less than 50 percent cancer; the Gleason score was 6; 66 percent of the men had only one positive core; and on average, only 14 percent of each of those positive cores had tumor cells. All of these men were ideal cases for a "male lumpectomy." Then they had surgery, doctors got to look at the entire prostate instead of just few specks of it, and their surgical specimens told a different story. The average number of separate tumors within the removed prostates was three; 65 percent of the men turned out to have cancer on both sides of the prostate—and in 23 percent of these men, the tumor on the opposite side was *larger* than the tumor on the side of the positive biopsy. Most disturbing was that 13 percent of the cancers turned out to be Gleason 7 or greater.

What about visualization of these tumors with imaging? Multiparametric MRI (mpMRI) has been improved in recent years, and this has emboldened advocates of focal therapy to declare that they can now map the prostate and detect and eliminate the microscopic lesions within the prostate. Yes, it has been improved, but there are several limitations. It is effective in finding many high-grade lesions, but still misses about 25 percent of Gleason 3 + 4 (Gleason Group 2) or greater tumors. Also, as tumors become more aggressive, it becomes more difficult to define their boundaries for targeting because they send out tentacles infiltrating surrounding tissues.

Further, these experts agree that they still are unable to identify most of the low-grade lesions (Gleason 3 + 3; Gleason Group 1), but argue that these lesions are not aggressive enough to require treatment. There are several reasons that this is incorrect. At Hopkins we studied the autopsy findings on a man with widespread metastases who had undergone a radical prostatectomy seventeen years earlier. Tracing the cancer's genetic family tree, we found that the clonal origin (the particular mutation that is the "bad seed" ancestor of cancer) of the disease that killed him was a 2mm focus of Gleason pattern 3 disease—an innocent-looking group of "good" cancer cells. Given the long natural history of the disease, Gleason pattern 3 can evolve into more aggressive disease. Young men who are the most interested in preserving their quality of life are the ones at highest risk for this event. Finally, genetic alterations in benign tissue resemble the cancer more than they resemble normal cells in prostate glands without cancer—indicating a field effect, in which nearby cells have already started down a molecular pathway toward becoming cancerous.

Some experts advise a "saturation biopsy"—with the patient under general anesthesia, taking up to sixty-four cores of tissue 5 millimeters apart, with the help of a template like the one used in brachytherapy. The problem here is that these techniques are not reliable; in fact, they may even be harmful. If a man needs a radical prostatectomy after one of these biopsies, it is difficult to preserve sexual function because the neurovascular bundles can be stuck to the prostate by scar tissue. I operated on a man who had undergone five biopsies, in which a total of 132 cores of tissue were removed; one of these was a saturation biopsy, performed by the pioneer of the technique, in which 83 cores were taken. Only one core was positive, and even this had only a tiny focus of cancer, with Gleason 6 disease. And yet his radical prostatectomy specimen showed Gleason 3 + 4 cancer on both sides at the apex, involving the anterior (top) portion of his prostate, with extensive tumor extending outside the prostate. Fortunately for him, because he underwent an open operation by an experienced surgeon, it was possible to save both neurovascular bundles, to obtain negative surgical margins, and he is cancer-free many years later. But who would have expected this, based on so many reassuring biopsies? Clearly, this demonstrates the limitation of biopsies to identify potentially lethal disease. Even so, many patients see focal treatments as the easiest way out and are opting to have them—zapping just a part of the prostate with HIFU aimed at the dominant lesion, or undergoing focal nerve-sparing cryotherapy, in which only one lobe of the prostate is frozen.

I also want to make it clear that focal therapy for prostate cancer is not the equivalent of a male lumpectomy. This analogy is often used because lumpectomy is the most common treatment for breast cancer, which is also characterized by its multifocal nature. So what is involved with lumpectomy in women? Treatment of the dominant lesion is more complete. The dominant lesion is surgically removed and sent to a pathologist for immediate examination. If the surgical margins are positive, more tissue is removed. Plus, radiation is routinely performed to eliminate small spots of cancer in the residual normal breast tissue; if radiation is not used, local failure is higher. Many women are then placed on anti-cancer drugs like tamoxifen for the next five or ten years. In contrast, focal therapy in prostate cancer is monotherapy, where there is uncertainty if the dominant lesion has been completely destroyed and where there is no treatment of the microscopic tumors left behind. This analogy is misleading and should never be used.

Sadly, the men who have the greatest interest in the "male lumpectomy," cryotherapy, and HIFU are also younger men who have the most to lose because of the long-term potential for cancer to come back—either in areas where the tumor was inadequately treated, or in brand-new spots, where cancer crops up in the normal prostate tissue that's left behind. There is no massive long-term follow-up here; for these forms of treatment, results are limited to the short-term, and only available in small numbers. In chapter 10, we will discuss the results of cryotherapy and HIFU in terms of cancer control. Who are the best candidates for these forms of treatment? The ones who probably don't need treatment in the first place—older men with small tumors, who are also ideal candidates for active surveillance.

10

HOW SUCCESSFUL IS TREATMENT OF LOCALIZED PROSTATE CANCER?

THE SHORT STORY:
The Highly Abridged Version of This Chapter

Will my cancer be cured forever? Out of a massive amount of information about a complicated, confusing, infuriating disease, we have only two incontrovertible facts about a cure: If you are going to be cured of prostate cancer, your disease must be diagnosed at a stage when it is curable, before the cancer has established itself in a distant site. And the treatment has to work.

What's the best form of treatment for localized disease? This is a moving target. There are multiple surgical options; several forms of external-beam radiation therapy, plus brachytherapy with or without external-beam radiation and all of these with or without hormonal therapy. Worse, there are many definitions of success, and study results can vary widely, depending on the stage of the disease when a man is treated.

No one form of treatment is best for everyone, but there are two good options for the cure of localized prostate cancer: surgery and radiation. We have followed the results of surgery for decades; we'll discuss our long-term findings in this chapter. And with recent advances in state-of-the-art imaging and high-dose delivery techniques, it is possible with today's radiation therapy to make certain that all prostate cancer cells are killed.

The next step is up to you. Your task now is to take all this information, decide on the treatment that is best for you, put yourself in the hands of the right expert, get past this disease, and start living the rest of your life.

Curing Localized Prostate Cancer

Will my cancer be cured forever? This question is the bedrock of this book, what everyone wants to know, and what every man with localized prostate cancer has the right to expect.

Out of a massive amount of information about a complicated, confusing, infuriating disease, there are two incontrovertible facts: If you are going to be cured of prostate cancer, your disease must be diagnosed at a stage when it is curable, before the cancer has established itself outside your pelvis. And the treatment has to work.

Remember what we've said throughout this book—*prostate cancer is multifocal*. It's not like an isolated dandelion that springs up and (if the seeds haven't blown elsewhere) can be dug up and eliminated. It's more like clover, which crops up in more than one spot at the same time. Prostate cancer starts in many places throughout the prostate simultaneously. The same factors that cause cancer in one area of tissue cause it to develop a few millimeters away, and a few millimeters away from that. *The average number of separate tumors in prostates removed in surgery is three to seven.* This is why surgeons must work very hard to remove the entire prostate and avoid positive surgical margins, and why radiation oncologists must deliver high doses of radiation precisely to the prostate. It also explains the Achilles' heel of cryo/thermal ablation—because, in order to avoid side effects, it is very difficult to achieve the goal of total prostate coverage.

Now, how do we know we've scored a bull's-eye? Which forms of treatment mark a direct hit in the target, and which fall short? Our greatest judge of the success of treatment is PSA.

Until PSA testing, the possibility of being cured of prostate cancer was unlikely, because for most men, even at the point of diagnosis, it was already too late. Now, thank goodness, *most men who are diagnosed with prostate cancer have potentially curable disease*—all the more reason why it's so important to identify the best way to cure them. The disease can be cured if the treatment works.

Cancer Control After Radical Prostatectomy

There is no better way to cure cancer that is confined to the prostate than total surgical removal. This is what all other forms of treatment attempt to accomplish. Thus, it's important that you understand the results of radical prostatectomy—what it can and cannot do—and the fine points in interpreting these results, before you can make an informed evaluation of other treatment approaches.

Surgical Margins

Again, *for any form of treatment to cure prostate cancer, the cancer must be curable in the first place.* Is your disease curable? We can learn almost everything we need to know about where you stand before surgery from the Han tables (see page 151)—the next best thing to a crystal ball—using your *clinical stage, PSA level, and Gleason score*. After surgery, other information helps fine-tune this picture. The pathologist can learn more about your cancer—the Gleason score of the *entire prostate*, for example (as opposed to the educated guess made by examining just a few cores of tissue). From the pathologist, we can learn whether the cancer was organ-confined, whether there was capsular penetration with negative surgical margins (also called specimen-confined disease), whether the margins were positive, and whether the seminal vesicles or lymph nodes were involved. All these factors have a profound impact on predicting the success of treatment. In some cases, molecular testing of the specimen can add additional information.

What Are Surgical Margins, Anyway?

This is a confusing point for many men. When the prostate is removed, it should be covered by several layers of tissue. It may help to think of the cancerous prostate as a gift in a box (although it's not much of a present) and the tissue surrounding it as wrapping paper. After radical prostatectomy, your prostate goes to the pathologist, who immediately coats the outside of the entire specimen—outlining the wrapping paper—with India ink. The prostate is then put in formalin for twenty-four hours before it is sectioned, stained, and examined under the microscope. The India ink creates a landmark so the pathologist can figure out exactly how far the cancer has spread. If the cancer is all contained within the box, we call it *organ-confined*. Even if the cancer penetrates the box (this is called *capsular penetration*), it can still be completely covered with the wrapping paper. We call this *specimen-confined*. In both of these cases, the men are considered *margin-negative*. If the cancer has penetrated the box and the wrapping paper as well, this is called a *positive surgical margin*. The pathologist can see cancer cells at the edge of the India ink, and this suggests that there may be cancer beyond the outermost edge, where the surgeon removed the prostate. In chapter 8, we talked about men who had positive margins with organ-confined disease. How does this happen? To continue our box image, imagine the package has been damaged; there is a tear in the wrapping paper and the box.

Some of the box may even be missing. This is how a man can have a positive margin even if his cancer is still confined inside the prostate.

When Surgical Margins Are Positive or Too Close to Call

In an ideal world, the pathologist would immediately send a triumphant report to the surgeon: "I've looked at the prostate tissue you removed from Mr. Jones, and all the edges are clear. Congratulations! You've removed all the cancer!"

Fortunately, it often happens that way. At Johns Hopkins, fewer than 10 percent of our patients are found to have cancer at the margins, the edges of the removed tumor. Sometimes, however, the pathologist's report is more ambiguous. The report states that the margins are *close*, meaning that cancer is just a hairbreadth away from the edge of the specimen.

Close Margins Are Almost Always Negative

Johns Hopkins pathologist Jonathan Epstein has good news about these margins. He studied men whose tumors were particularly close—less than 0.2 millimeter—to the surgical margin. Even though there wasn't a comfortable cushion of tissue between the tumor and the edge of the prostate, "those patients do just as well as if there's more separation between the tumor and the margin."

Even if the surgical margins are positive, cancer has not necessarily been left behind. How can this be? "There are several different explanations why, when the margins are positive, the tumor may still be cured," says Epstein. "One is that, literally, you cut across the last few tumor cells," and what appears to be remaining cancer is actually a cross-section of the perimeter of the tumor. "Even though it looks like it's a positive margin, there's really no cancer left in the patient."

Another explanation is that the *act of surgery itself* finishes the job, killing any remaining cells. No cut or injury to tissue happens in a vacuum; the area around the cut is affected, too. Think of lightning striking a tree; the tree dies, but so does a ring of grass around it. "When the surgeon cuts across tissue, the blood supply is cut off, there's dead tissue, and that can kill off the last few tumor cells that might have been left behind," Epstein says.

There's also the potential, "and this probably accounts for a lot of cases," says Epstein, that it's an "artifact"—basically, a false positive margin. Sometimes, "since there's so little tissue next to the prostate, when the surgeon tries to dissect it from the body and hands it to the nurse, and the nurse hands it to the pathologist, everyone's touching the gland. If you're talking about 0.2 millimeter of tissue, that tissue can be disrupted very easily. It can appear that the tumor is at the margin—but in fact, there was some additional tissue there that just got disrupted during all the handling." In other words, a few good buffer cells got rubbed off.

And Then There's the Sticky Cell Phenomenon

When cancer reaches beyond the prostate to invade nearby tissue, it produces a dense scar tissue that acts like glue. As a surgeon removes the prostate, this thick scar tissue sticks to the surrounding cancer cells—picking them up like a lint brush. So in some cases, although the pathologist may see cancer cells at the margin and make a judgment of positive surgical margins, there are no cancer cells left inside the patient. The sticky scar tissue took them all away.

Epstein has extensively studied instances in which the surgeon removed the prostate, looked at it, suspected that some cancer cells were left behind, and went back and cut out more of the surrounding tissue. "In pathology, we got two separate specimens," says Epstein. "One was the prostate, and one was this extra tissue, the neurovascular bundle that the surgeon was thinking of leaving in the patient but decided to remove." Even when there appeared to be a positive surgical margin at the edge of the prostate, in 40 percent of these patients, there turned out to be *no cancer left behind* in that adjacent tissue.

PSA After Radical Prostatectomy

The best way to determine whether all the cancer has been removed in a radical prostatectomy is to check for the presence of PSA. Many men are surprised by this; they reason—and rightly so—that if the prostate has been removed, there should be no PSA. Indeed, after a radical prostatectomy, the PSA level should be undetectable. If it is not, this suggests that some prostate cancer cells managed to escape the prostate before it was removed.

But don't have your PSA tested too soon. PSA has a lengthy half-life in the bloodstream (two or three days)—which means it takes quite a while for PSA levels to go down after a radical prostatectomy. For example, if your PSA level before surgery was 10 ng/ml, it would take seven half-lives before the PSA fell into the undetectable range (less than 0.1 ng/ml). If you had your blood tested the day after surgery, your same level of PSA would pop right up, suggesting that the operation hadn't done any good. This is misleading, of course. To avoid having to deal with such unnecessary stress, you should not have your PSA tested until about six to twelve weeks after surgery—when PSA should be at rock bottom. After this point the PSA level should be tested every six months in men with positive margins, seminal vesicles, or lymph nodes. For most other men, a PSA measurement is only necessary once a year.

What kind of PSA measurement do you need? A simple, total PSA. You don't need a free PSA test. To determine if you should have an ultrasensitive PSA, see Ultrasensitive PSA Tests, page 326.

Do you need any other tests? No. PSA is extremely sensitive—so much so that if your PSA is undetectable, there is no other test—no rectal exam, bone scan, CT scan, MRI, or other blood test—that could find any residual tumor. For many men, this is good news.

Results of Radical Prostatectomy at Johns Hopkins: What We Have Learned About the Probability of Cure

How do we measure the success of radical prostatectomy? What is failure? Surgeons like their evidence in black and white. Therefore, we have a strict cutoff: after radical prostatectomy, we believe that the PSA level should be undetectable—less than 0.2 ng/ml, although some urologists use a cutoff of 0.4 ng/ml.

Using long-term follow-up data on 10,600 men who underwent a radical prostatectomy at Johns Hopkins from 1978 to 2009, we can estimate a man's probability of keeping an undetectable PSA at ten years, based on his Gleason score and the pathologic stage of his prostate specimen (see Table 10.1). Among those who

TABLE 10.1

WHOSE PSA IS UNDETECTABLE TEN YEARS AFTER SURGERY?

This table shows the results of more than 10,600 men who underwent a radical prostatectomy at Johns Hopkins and did not receive radiation therapy or hormonal therapy. The numbers are percentages. We can use these results to predict, with 95 percent accuracy, the likelihood that a man will have an undetectable PSA level at ten years after surgery. For example, 96 percent of men whose Gleason score was 3 + 3 (Grade Group 1) and whose pathological specimen showed that their cancer was organ-confined, with negative surgical margins, had an undetectable PSA level ten years after surgery. If the margins were positive, 76 percent had an undetectable PSA level at ten years. The numbers in the parentheses indicate that only 5 percent of patients will fall on either side of these limits, and the "N" numbers tell how many men were in each category.

	Organ-Confined + Negative Surgical Margins (N = 6,399)	Organ-Confined + Positive Surgical Margins (N = 282)	Capsular Penetration + Negative Surgical Margins (N = 2,199)	Capsular Penetration + Positive Surgical Margins (N = 881)	Seminal Vesicle Invasion (N = 446)	Lymph Node Metastases (N = 331)	Total# (N = 10,538)
Gleason 6 (Grade Group 1)	(N = 4,911) 96.4 (95.4–97.2)	(N = 173) 76.4 (63.1–85.4)	(N = 944) 86.4 (83.2–89.1)	(N = 378) 71.7 (64.9–77.4)	(N = 60) 48.7 (30.8–64.3)	(N = 18) 28.7 (9.8–51.1)	(N = 6,484) 91.5 (90.4–92.5)
Gleason 3 + 4 (Grade Group 2)	(N = 1,069) 83.3 (79.0–86.8)	(N = 82) 57.9 (38.9–72.9)	(N = 778) 61.7 (56.7–66.3)	(N = 285) 44.9 (36.0–53.4)	(N = 164) 33.4 (23.9–43.2)	(N = 101) 22.5 (13.7–32.6)	(N = 2,479) 64.8 (62.0–67.5)
Gleason 4 + 3 (Grade Group 3)	(N = 260) 71.0 (61.6–78.5)	(N = 17) 70.6 (26.0–91.4)	(N = 274) 41.8 (33.2–50.1)	(N = 126) 24.1 (14.2–35.5)	(N = 92) 11.9 (3.9–24.8)	(N = 79) 0	(N = 848) 38.4 (33.5–43.3)
Gleason 8–10 (Grade Groups 4 and 5)	(N = 159) 55.1 (41.3–66.9)	(N = 10) 100	(N = 203) 38.9 (30.5–47.2)	(N = 92) 14.5 (6.5–25.5)	(N = 130) 10.9 (5.3–18.8)	(N = 133) 1.0 (0.1–4.9)	(N = 727) 25.9 (21.7–30.2)

TABLE 10.2

IF YOUR PSA IS UNDETECTABLE AT TEN YEARS, WHAT DOES THE FUTURE HOLD?

What happens after ten years—can you just stop having your PSA measured? Along with New York University urologist Stacy Loeb and her colleagues, I recently studied 1,580 men who had an undetectable PSA level at ten years and who were followed for up to *another* eighteen years to determine what percentage subsequently developed an elevated PSA level or a positive bone scan. We can predict with 95 percent accuracy the likelihood that a man in this situation will (a) develop an elevated PSA level or (b) metastasis at twenty years after surgery. The numbers in the box are percentages, and the parentheses indicate that only 5 percent of the patients will fall on either side of those limits. Keep in mind, too, that many of these men were operated on just as PSA testing and early screening were beginning to become widespread, and that most men today have their prostate cancer detected when it is at a much earlier stage.

(A) LIKELIHOOD OF DEVELOPING AN ELEVATED PSA 20 YEARS LATER

	Organ-Confined	Positive Surgical Margins	Capsular Penetration	Seminal Vesicle Invasion	Lymph Node Metastases
Gleason 6	(N = 754)	(N = 95)	(N = 373)	(N = 9)	(N = 3)
(Grade Group 1)	3.9	30.1	17.9	20.0	66.7
	(2.1–7.3)	(18.5–46.7)	(13.0–24.4)	(3.1–79.6)	(22.6–99.1)
Gleason 3 + 4	(N = 123)	(N = 40)	(N = 166)	(N = 15)	(N = 10)
(Grade Group 2)	12.2	16.7	7.6	–	–
	(3.6–36.7)	(7.1–36.5)	(3.6–15.3)		
Gleason ≥ 4 + 3	(N = 44)	(N = 14)	(N = 66)	(N = 8)	(N = 1)
(Grade Group 3)	14.1	37.3	25.7	46.7	–
	(3.6–46.8)	(11.7–82.8)	(13.1–46.5)	(13.7–93.2)	

(B) LIKELIHOOD OF METASTASIS 20 YEARS LATER

	Organ-Confined	Positive Surgical Margins	Capsular Penetration	Seminal Vesicle Invasion	Lymph Node Metastases
Gleason 6	(N = 754)	(N = 95)	(N = 373)	(N = 9)	(N = 3)
(Grade Group 1)	0	0	0	0	0
Gleason 3 + 4	(N = 123)	(N = 40)	(N = 166)	(N = 15)	(N = 10)
(Grade Group 2)	2.2	0	0	0	–
	(0.3–14.7)				
Gleason ≥ 4 + 3	(N = 44)	(N = 14)	(N = 66)	(N = 8)	(N = 1)
(Grade Group 3)	0	14.3	2.0	20.0	–
		(2.1–66.6)	(0.3–13.1)	(3.1–79.6)	

These results are encouraging. Men with an undetectable PSA level ten years after surgery have a low risk of developing an elevated PSA level or metastasis, and only one man who had an undetectable PSA level at ten years died from prostate cancer within twenty years after surgery. Furthermore, these results suggest that annual PSA testing may be safely discontinued after ten years for men with a prostatectomy Gleason score of 6 or lower, or a man who has other health issues that could affect his life expectancy.

had an undetectable PSA at ten years, some men continue to be at an increased risk of PSA failure over the next ten years (see Table 10.2)—but beyond twenty years, the risk is minimal. Of the 732 men with an undetectable PSA at twenty years, a decade later seventeen (2.3 percent) had developed an elevated PSA, sixteen (2.2 percent) had local recurrence of cancer, one (0.1 percent) had developed metastatic disease, and no one died due to prostate cancer. Based on these findings, twenty years is a reasonable time to discontinue PSA testing.

What about the risk of cancer death? In a study of 11,500 men treated with radical prostatectomy at five academic centers including Johns Hopkins, Memorial Sloan Kettering, Cleveland Clinic, Baylor, and the University of Michigan, urologist Scott Eggener reported that the presence of Gleason 8 to 10 disease (Gleason Groups 4 and 5) and seminal vesicle invasion on the radical prostatectomy specimen were the prime determinants of prostate cancer death.

Later in this chapter we will discuss the probability of metastases to bone, and death from prostate cancer, for men with a rising PSA.

The Pathology Report Suggests My Cancer Might Return: What Happens Next?

One of the major advantages of radical prostatectomy is that it gives some early, definitive answers. In contrast, when men undergo radiation therapy, there is no pathologic specimen to evaluate, and many patients find this unnerving. They say, "You mean I just have to sit around and wait to see what happens?" Well, yes. But for men who undergo radical prostatectomy, the removed prostate is a walnut-sized crystal ball that contains a lot of information about the future. If the cancer is organ-confined, you know there was no better way to completely eliminate the local cancer. If there is capsular penetration with negative margins, again, the surgery did the best job any form of treatment could do.

RADICAL PROSTATECTOMY IN MEN YOUNGER THAN FIFTY

In the past, very few men diagnosed with prostate cancer—only around 1 percent—were younger than fifty. However, with the widespread use of PSA testing as well as improved public awareness of prostate cancer, that number has gone up to around 4 percent. And with more men to study, we have learned something very important. We used to believe that if a younger man was diagnosed with prostate cancer, he must have a much more severe case or more advanced disease. It turns out that this was true—but only because no one ever checked for prostate cancer in these men, especially in its earliest stages. This "old man's disease" wasn't on doctors' radar for younger patients. We now know that just the opposite is true—that *younger men are more curable*, for several reasons.

Recently, we studied 2,900 men who underwent a radical prostatectomy between April 1982 and September 2001. In this study, 341 men were younger than fifty. We found that these men had a greater chance of having organ-confined disease and that they were more likely to be cured than older men (age seventy or older). We believe that the operation is also more successful because these men have smaller prostates. There is more tissue surrounding the prostate, and the margins of resection (the surgical border between healthy tissue and cancer) are wider. Finally, in younger men, the neurovascular bundles are located farther from the prostate and are easier to preserve. This provides a win-win situation—an excellent chance for cure with improved quality of life.

But what if the margins are positive, or if cancer was found in your seminal vesicles or pelvic lymph nodes? What should you do? Will any other form of treatment help right now? Let's say, for example, that you've had your first PSA test after surgery, and it was undetectable. But from studying the pathology report, you can see that the probability that your PSA level will *stay* undetectable is not that high. Is it possible that you can act now to get rid of any remaining cancer cells? Should you have radiation therapy to the prostate bed, the area where the prostate used to be?

Adjuvant vs. Salvage Radiation Therapy After Surgery

Who's at higher risk of developing an elevated PSA after surgery? Men with "adverse pathology"—that is, cancer that extends outside the prostate with or without positive margins, or involvement of the seminal vesicles or pelvic lymph nodes. These men may benefit from further treatment—radiation—to the pelvis.

When should they do this? Three randomized trials of men with adverse pathology and negative lymph nodes have compared getting radiation immediately—this is called *adjuvant radiation*—to observation. However, no studies have looked at getting radiation later, when PSA begins to go up; this is called salvage radiation.

PROSTATE CANCER IN THE PELVIC LYMPH NODES FOLLOWING SURGERY

*W*hat do I do if cancer is found in my pelvic lymph nodes? This used to be the case in as many as 40 percent of men in the pre-PSA era. As PSA screening became widespread, it dropped to the single digits. But surgeons are operating on more men with high-risk, localized prostate cancer; regrettably, we are also seeing more men with node-positive cancer who did not have PSA screening because the U.S. Preventative Services Task Force (USPSTF) did not recommend it (see page 86). The standard treatment, based on an older, randomized study, has been ADT following prostatectomy. But a number of studies now suggest that adjuvant salvage radiation may work better and improve survival.

In all three trials, investigators agreed that immediate adjuvant radiation therapy reduced the future risk for developing an elevated PSA. However, it is unclear what impact adjuvant radiation had on survival or on the risk of local recurrence of cancer. The only trial that showed an improvement in overall survival was the one carried out in the United States by SWOG (formerly the Southwest Oncology Group). Although that study showed that fewer men who received early radiation therapy died, 72 percent of these deaths occurred in men without metastases, and there were only five more cancer deaths in the observation group. Thus, this study did not prove that adjuvant radiation prevented death from cancer. In contrast, the largest study, which was carried out in Europe by the EORTC (European Organization for Research and Treatment of Cancer), failed to demonstrate any improvement in freedom from metastases, local recurrence, or overall survival. Notably, it did demonstrate a significant *decrease in survival* in two groups who received radiation: men over age seventy, and men who had penetration of cancer though the capsule but negative margins.

Given these results, there are many patients for whom I recommend holding off on adjuvant radiation until they have their first elevation of PSA. First, *many men with adverse pathology will never develop an elevated PSA*. At Hopkins, ten years after surgery in patients who did not receive radiation, men who had extension of cancer outside the prostate but negative surgical margins had a 90 percent chance of an undetectable PSA if their Gleason Group was 1 and a 62 percent chance if their Gleason Group was 2. If they had a positive margin with Gleason Group 1 disease, their likelihood not to have a rising PSA was a very encouraging 75 percent. These men are ideal candidates for close observation, with salvage radiation at the earliest sign of PSA recurrence. Second, there is good evidence that men who have adjuvant radiation are likely to have more problems with rectal bleeding and incontinence.

Even though there are no randomized trials that evaluated salvage radiation, there are observational studies that are encouraging; two of the best come from Hopkins and Harvard/Duke. Both studies demonstrated improved cancer-specific or overall survival in men who were treated with salvage radiation at the time of PSA relapse. The one from Hopkins showed that the men who had a survival benefit all received radiation within two years of PSA recurrence. It also showed that if PSA dropped to the undetectable range following radiation—even if it later came back up—these patients had improved odds of survival.

Based on all of this information, this is what I tell my patients: You should *not* receive adjuvant radiation if:

- You have capsular penetration with negative margins; or
- You are more than seventy years old, unless you are otherwise very healthy and have high-grade or positive margins; or
- You have a bladder neck contracture or significant incontinence and marginal indications.

You should strongly consider adjuvant radiation if:

- You have Grade Group 2 or greater pathology and positive margins; or
- Genomic testing like Decipher suggests that your risk for developing metastases is high; or
- You have positive seminal vesicles or pelvic lymph nodes (see page 321).

CAN GENETIC TESTING HELP?

For decades, prostate cancer treatment has been determined by what we can see: pathologic findings, anything that shows up on the physical examination, imaging, and lab tests. But we have also known for a long time that these factors aren't enough to help all men. It's like reading a map where only the big streets are marked—but maybe what you're looking for is a small street. We have needed better guidance, and within the last few years, we've gotten it in the form of gene-based tests.

This is personalized medicine, a treatment based only on your cancer, not on what works best for other people. The Decipher test by GenomeDx is done on your surgically removed prostate tissue. It looks at the activity of twenty-two genes known to be involved in the development and progression of prostate cancer to predict the cancer's aggressiveness and your likelihood of metastasis. The test has been validated in more than two thousand patients by institutions including Johns Hopkins, the Mayo Clinic, and Thomas Jefferson University.

Not every man needs genomic testing. In some men, the need for post-operative radiation is clear-cut, based on pathologic findings alone. But in some men, the decision is not as clear, and Decipher can be very helpful.

What Should I Do If My PSA Comes Back After Surgery?

PSA is a very sensitive marker for the recurrence of prostate cancer. In fact, it's probably the most sensitive marker there is for any cancer. Because PSA is made only by prostate cells, when PSA levels become elevated after a radical prostatectomy, this suggests that some cancer cells are still present (although in a rare case, it is possible that some benign tissue was left behind, and is causing PSA to show up in the blood).

But before we talk about this, let's make sure you're not having it tested too soon. You should not have your PSA tested until *two to three months after surgery*. If your PSA is elevated more than three months after surgery, the first thing to do is have it checked again. Some laboratories are not able to measure PSA at its lowest levels (see page 326). For most men, an elevated PSA level means that cancer is present. If you repeat the test and it, too, is elevated, the next question is, where is the cancer? Is it still localized to the prostate area, or has it spread elsewhere? Were there some cancer cells that slipped outside the prostate—but are still hanging around the old neighborhood, the prostate bed—that were not removed at the time of surgery? Or have the cells escaped to a distant site? (See Better Molecular Imaging, below.)

BETTER MOLECULAR IMAGING

One thing we can say about advanced, prostate cancer-specific imaging: There have never been more options! Also, it's confusing! There's radiolabeled choline, and acetate, and FACBC (fluciclovine). These are all molecules called radioactive analogs that mimic fatty acids and amino acids that prostate cancer cells use—which means that using them as radioactive tracers can help show where prostate cancer is lurking in the body. It would be really helpful if they could help us find prostate cancer when PSA comes back after salvage radiotherapy, but at PSA levels lower than 1.0, these agents are not very good.

Fortunately, new imaging agents that target the prostate-specific membrane antigen (PSMA) have shown great promise in breaking the very low PSA barrier. A PSMA-imaging agent called DCFPyL, developed by Martin Pomper, M.D., Ph.D., at Johns Hopkins, produces images that are stunningly clear and is currently undergoing testing for FDA approval. Pomper has shown that when used prior to a radical prostatectomy, this PSMA-targeting agent can predict the presence of cancer in lymph nodes with high accuracy if the scan is positive, but cannot rule out the presence of cancer if the scan is negative. He has also shown that in many men with a rising PSA after treatment, he is able to detect the source of the cancer—raising the very exciting possibility that in the future, we may no longer be left shooting in the dark. If we can target cancer cells, we are well on our way to being able to kill them. There are other PSMA-imaging agents available in Europe and Australia. In the future, PSMA-targeting agents will likely change the way we direct salvage radiation and other treatment decisions.

My PSA Is Elevated: Should I Get Radiation?

Could salvage radiation therapy eradicate any remaining prostate cancer cells? Or would it just cause new complications by needlessly treating an area that's already free of cancer? This is not an easy question to answer—in part because PSA is so very sensitive, and when a few cancer cells are present, they can't be seen by any of the usual imaging studies, such as MRI or CT. However, two important studies have shed some light on the helpfulness of salvage radiation.

In one study, first published in the *Journal of the American Medical Association* and recently updated in the *Journal of Clinical Oncology*, scientists studied more than 2,400 men, patients at ten academic centers who underwent radiation therapy after radical prostatectomy. More than 60 percent of these men were free from disease for at least five years if they started radiation before their PSA level was above 0.5 ng/ml. This disease control appears to be long-lasting; only a small percentage of men who were free from disease longer than six years were found to have a return of their prostate cancer.

ULTRASENSITIVE PSA TESTS

One advantage of surgery is that your PSA should fall to the undetectable range and remain there unless the cancer returns. The question is, what is "undetectable"? Despite what the lab reports, there is actually no such thing as zero PSA. In immunoassays, there is always a level lower than the assay can measure—it's like trying to count the number of angels dancing on the head of a pin. That's why the reports say "less than 0.1" ($<$0.1). Always look for the "less than" sign ($<$) before the number. How low can the laboratory accurately measure your PSA? One definition of an undetectable PSA is $<$ 0.2. This is the level above which additional treatment with radiation therapy is often advised.

Ultrasensitive assays can measure PSA as low as $<$ 0.01. Is this a good thing? Should you have an ultrasensitive PSA? Some laboratories offer two assays, one for screening and the other to monitor the success of treatment. The doctor who orders your PSA needs to know which one to select. The one used for screening makes no effort for accuracy below 0.1; the other is the ultrasensitive one. In this case, you must have the ultrasensitive one because you will worry if your PSA is 0.1—take my word for it.

For more than thirty years, I have personally entered in my database the PSA results of the 4,569 men I operated on and weekly I have conversations with patients who are fretting over this. However, if the laboratory has only one PSA assay and it measures PSA to $<$ 0.1, then I would choose that one; this is what we do at Hopkins.

What is the advantage of the ultrasensitive test? If your pathology report suggests that not all the cancer has been removed—if it shows positive margins, seminal vesicles, or lymph nodes, and you are being considered for postoperative salvage radiation or other treatments—then this information can be helpful. Lori Sokoll, professor of pathology and associate director of clinical chemistry at Johns Hopkins, carried out a study of ultrasensitive PSA in 750 men who had a PSA $<$ 0.1 three months following surgery. If the ultrasensitive PSA was $<$ 0.03, only 14 percent of these men had an elevated PSA a decade later. However, if it was greater than ($>$) 0.03, the PSA became elevated in 78 percent. These patients need to be followed more closely, and they need ultrasensitive testing.

Note: Not all laboratories have the same quality control. For example, patients write to me saying that their PSA is going up: "Last year it was 0.006, and this year it's 0.007." But both of these numbers are $<$ 0.01, and there is no way to measure a difference. A more common problem is a fluctuation in a man's yearly PSA values from the same laboratory—one year it's 0.02, then 0.03, then 0.01. These laboratories do not have ideal quality control, but since the numbers are not rising, I tell patients not to worry.

Finally, if your PSA report is really 0.1 and last year it was < 0.1, you need to have it measured again in the same laboratory as last year, and also consider going to a major reference laboratory at a university to confirm it. This approach has saved many patients from worry and unnecessary radiation.

In this study, radiation therapy was less likely to be successful in men with Gleason scores of 8 or higher, men who had higher PSA levels before they underwent salvage radiation, men who did not also receive hormones with salvage radiation (see page 328), and men whose prostate cancer had reached their seminal vesicles. (It may be more successful in these men today; see page 328.)

What about ADT? In chapter 9, we discussed how temporary hormonal therapy—often for just a few months—can make radiation more effective. What about men who have salvage radiation? Do they need these hormone-suppressing drugs, too? At Hopkins, we generally reserve ADT for the treatment of patients with Gleason scores of 7 to 10, men whose PSA level begins to go up sooner than three years after surgery, men with a rapid PSA doubling time, men with high pre-salvage radiation PSA levels (> 0.7), or very young men (see page 328).

In the second study of salvage radiation, Johns Hopkins epidemiologist Bruce Trock studied more than six hundred men who had radical prostatectomy and compared those who received salvage radiation—about one-third—to those who did not. Overall, the study demonstrated a threefold improvement in survival for the men who underwent salvage radiation. The investigators noted that this survival advantage was limited to men who received radiation within two years of their first PSA elevation, and to those in whom the PSA became undetectable after treatment. Further, Trock found that if PSA became undetectable following salvage radiation—even if it later became detectable—these men still experienced improved survival.

HORMONES WITH SALVAGE RADIATION

*I*f I'm getting adjuvant salvage radiation after surgery, do I need hormonal therapy, too? Several studies from institutions including Stanford, Memorial Sloan Kettering, MD Anderson, the University of Michigan, and Ghent University Hospital suggest that a short course of ADT given along with adjuvant salvage radiation therapy helps high-risk men.

A French trial recently confirmed the benefit of six months of ADT with salvage radiation therapy for "failure-free survival." The results, published in *Lancet Oncology*, showed an 18 percent benefit at five years.

A randomized trial, conducted by the RTOG Foundation and published in the *New England Journal of Medicine*, showed that hormonal therapy can improve overall survival with salvage radiation. However, men in the twenty-year-old RTOG trial received high-dose bicalutamide (Casodex)—a drug that is neither commonly used nor currently approved for use in the United States—for two years. The study showed no benefit with high-dose bicalutamide in men whose PSAs were < 0.7 ng/mL before salvage radiation. So basically, we don't know for certain whether adding a course of ADT to adjuvant or salvage radiation will help. Fortunately, we expect the results of several trials soon, and these should help guide us in the future. Until that time, the best thing to do is to talk about the relative *potential* benefits, and the side effects, with your surgeon and radiation oncologist.

Finally, with today's salvage radiation, there is much greater cause for real hope—because the technology is better and the doses of radiation are higher. In the studies we have just discussed, men were treated with doses between 64 and 66 Gy, which are considered low by today's standards. An analysis of salvage radiation data from Stanford researchers suggests that *doses of at least 70 Gy* may be required to cure the cancer. With today's conformal radiation techniques, it is now possible to give higher radiation doses with more precision, and with greater probability of disease control.

In almost all studies of men receiving radiation therapy after a radical prostatectomy, one message stands out: *the lower the PSA level at the time of treatment, the better.* "Although no one has determined an absolute cutoff beyond which radiation does not work, most studies have shown differences in outcome once PSA rises beyond the 0.5 ng/ml range," advises radiation oncologist Phuoc Tran. "Because of this, at Johns Hopkins, we encourage patients to seek an evaluation sooner rather than later to see if they are an appropriate candidate for salvage radiotherapy."

Although salvage radiation has possible side effects, with better CT-based radiation treatment planning, these are much less severe than they used to be. A study published in the *Journal of Clinical Oncology* reported the side effects seen in men receiving salvage radiation therapy. In this study, men who had full urinary continence *before* radiation had it afterward. Only about 1 in 10 men required medication for rectal side effects (intermittent light bleeding and passing mucus or loose stools). A similar percentage of patients required treatment for a urethral stricture, but these were found in men who had already experienced a urethral stricture before radiation therapy, or they were related to a local recurrence of cancer.

Ultimately, it comes down to two things: One is the likelihood of success. The other is the possibility that your prostate cancer—even if you have a detectable PSA level—may not cause significant problems for the rest of your life. *The good news is that for many men with PSA recurrence after surgery, it may take a long time for problems to develop—if they ever do.* (For more on this, see page 330.) If you can otherwise expect to live for many years or have the unfavorable prognostic factors mentioned above, you should strongly consider undergoing radiation therapy.

Before You Undergo Radiation After Radical Prostatectomy

Your doctor may want you to undergo some further tests. If there is a slight chance that the cancer may have spread beyond the local area, your doctor may suggest a bone scan, chest X-ray, and pelvic CT scan or MRI (all of these are discussed in chapter 6). The main reason for these tests is *not* because your doctor expects them to be positive, but to establish a baseline of information. Note: You probably do *not* need a biopsy of the prostate bed. If you are going to have radiation therapy after prostatectomy, it's because all signs point to a local recurrence of cancer. It might be tiny—so tiny, in fact, that a biopsy might be falsely negative. If local recurrence is likely (based on the criteria described above), even if the biopsy were negative, radiation would still be your best course of action. So why put yourself through a biopsy you don't need? Similarly, if all evidence suggests that the PSA is coming from distant metastases, a biopsy is not necessary—because even if it were positive, radiation therapy to the prostate bed will not cure you, and it can cause side effects. Imaging tests that are more sensitive and specific for prostate cancer are now available, and even better tests are being developed (see page 324).

My PSA Is Elevated: What's Going to Happen to Me?

How much time have I got? When is my bone scan going to become positive? If you're in panic mode, the first thing you need to do is take a deep breath, calm down, and read the good news in this section. The return of PSA is a possibility that strikes terror in the heart of every radical prostatectomy patient. In fact, for many men, the dreaded PSA tests after surgery can be almost worse than having the operation itself. Although radical prostatectomy provides excellent cancer control in most men with clinically localized disease, in the past, 20 to 30 percent of men have experienced a detectable PSA level within ten years of surgery. So what will you do if your PSA is no longer undetectable? *The good news is, you may not need to do anything for years.*

In a landmark paper, the results of the largest, most complete study of the return of PSA after radical prostatectomy were published by Johns Hopkins doctors, who have laid out guidelines to help patients and doctors know what to do if PSA comes back. They have produced a simple chart that accurately predicts a man's risk of developing metastatic cancer. This chart has the potential to be of great help as doctors and patients make decisions about what to do next (see page 331).

IF MY PSA BEGINS TO RISE AFTER SURGERY, WILL MY BONE SCAN BE NORMAL?

This chart estimates the likelihood that a man with an elevated PSA level will remain free of metastatic prostate cancer (seen on a positive bone scan) at three, five, and seven years from the time of his initial increase in PSA after a radical prostatectomy. It is based on three factors: when his PSA first went up after radical prostatectomy (was it more or less than two years?), his Gleason score on the radical prostatectomy specimen (was it greater than or less than 8?), and the time it took for his PSA level to double during the two years after the first elevation (was it more or less than ten months?).

If you have a Gleason score of 5 to 7 and your time to first PSA recurrence was greater than two years:

If your PSA doubling time was greater than ten months, your chance of *not* developing metastasis (having a positive bone scan) in

Three years = 95 percent
Five years = 86 percent
Seven years = 82 percent

If your PSA doubling time was less than ten months, your chance of *not* developing metastasis in

Three years = 82 percent
Five years = 69 percent
Seven years = 60 percent

If you have a Gleason score of 5 to 7 and your time to first PSA recurrence was less than two years:

If your PSA doubling time was greater than ten months, your chance of *not* developing metastasis in

Three years = 79 percent
Five years = 76 percent
Seven years = 59 percent

If your PSA doubling time was less than ten months, your chance of *not* developing metastasis in

Three years = 81 percent
Five years = 35 percent

Seven years = 15 percent

If you have a Gleason score of 8 to 10 and your time to first PSA recurrence was greater than two years, your chance of *not* developing metastasis in

Three years = 77 percent
Five years = 60 percent
Seven years = 47 percent

And if your time to first PSA recurrence was less than two years, your chance of *not* developing metastasis in

Three years = 53 percent
Five years = 31 percent
Seven years = 21 percent

As we've discussed, PSA is very sensitive in detecting any recurrence of cancer. That's because only prostate cells make PSA—so if the PSA level goes up after a radical prostatectomy, it means prostate cells are still present somewhere. Basically, it means the cancer has come back, and that can be a scary thought. The first thing many patients want to know is, "How long am I going to live?" And the first thing many doctors want to know is, "When should we begin second-line treatment, and what's the best approach?" Does the man have a local recurrence of cancer that would respond to radiation, or are there micrometastases to lymph nodes and bone?

For many years, there was no way to tell. However, two studies from Johns Hopkins, whose results were published in the *Journal of the American Medical Association*, have helped unravel the mystery. In the first study, published in 1999, we evaluated 315 men who developed an elevated PSA level (defined as being higher than 0.2 ng/ml) after radical prostatectomy. This study included men in whom radiation therapy—given at the time PSA increased—failed to control the disease. We set out to answer some important questions: For patients who had metastases, how long would it take before these became visible on a bone scan? And once that happened, how long would they live? The news was actually quite good: *Most men did very well for a long period of time.* On average, it took *eight years* from the time a man's PSA first went up until he developed metastatic disease—which suggests *there is no need to panic at the first sign of a rise in PSA level.* Even better, at fifteen years after surgery, 82 percent of men were still free from metastatic disease. Even after developing metastatic cancer (detected by bone scans), men still lived an average of five years—and if the metastases showed up more than seven years after surgery, men had a 70 percent chance of being alive seven years later.

"When men see their PSA levels rise again, they think that means the cancer is back and they need to get treated right away," says Johns Hopkins oncologist Mario Eisenberger, a coauthor of the study. "But men often live for years without having the cancer spread. This information will better equip doctors and their patients to decide what treatment—if any—is most appropriate."

Who Needs Aggressive Treatment?

The second landmark Johns Hopkins study, published in 2005, found that not all recurrence is equal and that not all men need aggressive treatment—or any treatment right away if cancer comes back. In this study, spearheaded by urologist Stephen Freedland, we looked at the long-term outcomes of 379 radical prostatectomy patients (out of the five thousand men who underwent this procedure at Johns Hopkins between 1982 and 2000) who, after surgery, developed an elevated PSA level. Some of these men underwent radiation therapy to the prostatic bed, but their PSA level either did not go down or continued to rise. Our goal was to see who had died from the cancer and who was alive and well, and to try to understand what made the difference in these men.

From this study, we developed reference tables for physicians and patients that help determine which men are going to be in trouble and in need of more aggressive treatment, and which men have a slow-growing cancer that may not cause trouble for years—those who are relatively safe and can be carefully watched. Table 10.3 estimates the chances that a man will die from prostate cancer five, ten, and fifteen years from the time his PSA first goes up after surgery.

TABLE 10.3

IF MY PSA BEGINS TO RISE AFTER SURGERY, WHAT IS THE LIKELIHOOD THAT I WILL *NOT* DIE FROM PROSTATE CANCER?

Estimate of the risk of not dying from prostate cancer in men who have an elevation of PSA following radical prostatectomy. The numbers in parentheses are the 95 percent confidence limits (the likelihood that 95 percent of patients would be between these two numbers).

Before looking at this table, you must realize that this is the worst-case scenario. All these men were treated more than five, ten, or fifteen years ago, at a time when prostate cancer was typically diagnosed at a more advanced stage. Also, the many new and upcoming tools for the management of advanced disease that you will receive were not available to them. *Your outlook will undoubtedly be much better.*

A: FIVE-YEAR ESTIMATE

PSA doubling time (in months)	Recurrence > 3 years after surgery		Recurrence ≤ 3 years after surgery	
	Gleason sum < 8	Gleason sum > 8	Gleason sum < 8	Gleason sum > 8
15 or more	100 (98–100)	99 (98–99)	99 (96–100)	98 (90–100)
9.0–14.9	99 (70–100)	98 (75–100)	97 (76–100)	94 (63–99)
3.0–8.9	97 (81–100)	94 (74–99)	91 (67–98)	81 (46–95)
Less than 3	92 (70–98)	83 (52–96)	74 (37–93)	51 (19–82)

B: TEN-YEAR ESTIMATE

PSA doubling time (in months)	Recurrence > 3 years after surgery		Recurrence ≤ 3 years after surgery	
	Gleason sum < 8	Gleason sum > 8	Gleason sum < 8	Gleason sum > 8
15 or more	98 (96–100)	96 (93–98)	93 (80–98)	86 (61–96)
9.0–14.9	95 (75–99)	90 (58–98)	85 (49–97)	69 (30–92)
3.0–8.9	84 (62–94)	68 (37–89)	55 (25–82)	26 (7–62)
Less than 3	59 (29–83)	30 (10–63)	15 (3–53)	1 (< 1–55)

C: FIFTEEN-YEAR ESTIMATE

PSA doubling time (in months)	Recurrence > 3 years after surgery		Recurrence ≤ 3 years after surgery	
	Gleason sum < 8	Gleason sum > 8	Gleason sum < 8	Gleason sum > 8
15 or more	94 (87–100)	87 (79–92)	81 (57–93)	62 (32–85)
9.0–14.9	86 (57–97)	72 (35–92)	59 (24–87)	31 (7–72)
3.0–8.9	59 (32–81)	30 (10–63)	16 (4–49)	1 (< 1–51)
Less than 3	19 (5–51)	2 (< 1–38)	< 1 (< 1–26)	< 1 (< 1–2)

The difference between high- and low-risk recurrence can be a matter of years. Some men in the low-risk group lived more than sixteen years after their cancer returned, with no sign that the cancer had spread to bone. We found that the severity of recurrence depended on three risk factors:

- *PSA doubling time.* Based only on the PSA values during the first two years after PSA reappeared, how long did it take for the PSA level in the blood to double? Less than three months, between three and nine months, from nine to fifteen months, or more than fifteen months?
- *Gleason score.* Is it 7 or lower, or Gleason 8 to 10? And
- *Time from surgery to the return of PSA.* Was it within three years or afterward?

If a man's PSA doubled in less than three months, his risk of dying from prostate cancer was much higher than that of a man whose PSA doubling time was more than a year. The same holds true for the time from surgery to the return of PSA. If PSA appears on a blood test within three years after surgery, that man is at higher risk than is a man whose PSA returns in five years.

The differences in risk turned out to be great. If you are a man who has all the low-risk features—if your PSA doubling time is greater than fifteen months, your Gleason score is below 8, and your PSA comes back after three years—your odds of being alive fifteen years later are 94 percent. Best of all, you do not need further treatment, because if you're alive and well fifteen years after surgery with no further treatment, anything we do to treat you is unlikely to improve on that and probably would only affect your quality of life.

In contrast, if you are a man at highest risk—if your PSA doubling time is less than three months, your PSA returns within three years, and your Gleason score is 8 or higher—your odds of being alive fifteen years after surgery *without further treatment* are less than 1 percent. This means that you *do* need further treatment, including joining clinical trials and starting more aggressive therapy.

The estimates in these tables represent the outcome of patients who did not have the benefit of the remarkable recent advances in the treatment of advanced disease (Chapter 13). Because these new treatments have prolonged survival, the estimates should be considered the worst case scenario.

Where Do I Go from Here?

The above information can help you and your doctor decide whether you would benefit from immediate treatment if your PSA comes back after radical prostatectomy. In chapter 12, we will talk about all the options that men in this situation should consider.

Cancer Control After Radiation Therapy

How many meters in a mile or yards in a kilometer? Comparing the cancer control results of radical prostatectomy and radiation therapy is not always as easy as you might think. For surgeons, the definition of success after radical prostatectomy is simple: A PSA level of 0.1 ng/ml or lower is considered undetectable. A PSA level of 0.2 ng/ml or higher signals a recurrence of cancer, because there should be no remaining prostate tissue to make any PSA. But with radiation, it's more complicated, for several reasons. There is no definitive PSA cutoff point between success and failure, and although PSA is still useful as a marker, PSA levels require some interpretation. This is because the killing effect of radiation is directed at cancerous prostate tissue, not at normal prostate tissue. The entire prostate is not eliminated; some tissue remains behind, and PSA usually doesn't go away completely.

To understand why this happens, let's take a brief look at radiobiology—the biology of radiation therapy. As we discussed in chapter 9, radiation isn't like a machine gun, blasting indiscriminately at good and bad tissue and destroying everything equally. Instead, radiation's effect is different on normal tissue than it is on cancer. Low, regular doses of radiation do a better job of killing cancer cells, and normal cells are not as easily damaged by this gentle approach. At larger doses, however, the opposite is true. Normal cells are more susceptible, and cancerous cells somehow are able to hang in there and withstand the assault. This is why, traditionally, radiation oncologists have used multiple treatments of radiation instead of one single, large blast. However, Phuoc Tran reports that this idea is "very actively being questioned for prostate cancer." (Hypofractionation, a short course of higher-dose radiation, is discussed in chapter 9.)

For many men who have completed radiation therapy, then, some normal prostate tissue survives and continues to make small amounts of PSA. This presents radiation oncologists with a difficult challenge when interpreting PSA scores after radiotherapy: Is this "good" PSA, pumped out by the remaining normal tissue, or is it "bad" PSA, still being made by a few renegade cancer cells that somehow survived the radiation? Right now, there is no way to tell (although it's possible that new assays, such as those described in chapter 4, might one day be able to say, "This PSA comes from normal cells. Not to worry!" or "This PSA is being made by cancer"). Instead, the most common strategy has been to watch the *trend* of PSA—to see what it does over time, with the idea that if it's coming from benign tissue, the PSA level should remain stable, but if it's coming from cancerous tissue, the PSA will creep back up as the cancer cells multiply.

In 2005, a panel of radiation oncologists met in Phoenix to discuss replacing an older definition of PSA failure after radiation. They decided to define treatment failure as a PSA level that has risen 2 ng/ml higher than a man's PSA nadir (the lowest level it reached following treatment). This definition has been correlated more accurately with long-term results in all patients, and it takes into account such factors as hormonal therapy and the benign PSA "bounce" (see below). Failure is now considered to occur when the PSA level reaches the nadir + 2 value. This is called the Phoenix definition. Still, it takes time to determine this value, so this equation should not be used to gauge the success of treatment in men with less than two years' worth of PSA tests after radiation therapy. Furthermore, the consensus panel that developed this definition cautions, "Physicians should use individualized approaches to managing young patients with slowly rising PSA levels who initially achieved a very low nadir and who might be candidates for salvage local therapies" (see page 343).

Lastly, there's the phenomenon of PSA "bounce"—and this, too, can confound results using older definitions of PSA failure. Say you've had your radiation therapy, you're feeling good, and your PSA is going down. Then, all of a sudden, it goes up. What just happened? Think of it as PSA's last fling. This bounce is transient and has been studied using a variety of definitions. It is generally described as a sudden rise of at least 0.1 to 0.5 ng/ml, followed by a decrease. This usually occurs within the first two years after treatment, and may happen in as many as 40 percent of men after either external-beam radiation or brachytherapy. In most studies, it seems more likely to occur in younger men. *This does not mean that you are not ultimately headed for a healthy, low, stable PSA level.* The largest study to look at this phenomenon, involving nearly five thousand men who were treated with external-beam radiation alone, found that the PSA bounce did not seem to raise the risk of local failure or distant metastases. Preliminary research using magnetic resonance spectroscopy imaging (MRSI) suggests that the bounce may actually be caused by inflammation of the prostate after radiation.

Cancer Control After External-Beam Therapy

As you've just read, one problem for radiation oncologists and patients is simply figuring out how success and failure of treatment should be measured. Another is that we always desire to use the most mature data we have—but studies involving older radiation techniques are no longer accurate. It is unfair and illogical to compare the results from decades ago with those achievable in the past ten years. Years ago, many men who received radiation were what doctors call "adversely selected" for this approach, because their cancer was too extensive for them to be cured by surgery. Unfortunately, this means that many men who received radiation in the past probably did not have curable disease to start with. Plus, the technology today is markedly better than it was a few years ago. And finally, one of our best markers for determining the extent of disease, PSA level, was not measured until when most of these men were treated.

All these issues have plagued oncologists and prostate cancer patients for many years. Fortunately, an important new study from the United Kingdom called ProtecT has given us some clarity on this issue (see chapter 6). ProtecT had an average follow-up of ten years and showed clearly that the cancer control for surgery, the gold standard for localized prostate cancer treatment, and more modern radiation combined with a short course of ADT are essentially equivalent. Although we still have much to learn from this study in the coming years, this is tremendous news. Many of us suspected this, but now it's confirmed with highest level of scientific evidence: *Men with localized prostate cancer can feel comfortable that cure is just as possible with radiation as it is with surgery. The best information we have suggests that surgery and high-dose radiation plus a short course of ADT are likely equivalent for men with low-risk cancer, as well as for most men with intermediate-risk disease, at least after ten years of follow-up.*

How about high-risk and very high-risk prostate cancer? Results from more recent studies, in which men with intermediate- and high-risk cancer received high-dose conformal radiation along with hormonal therapy, report "freedom from PSA failure" (using the Phoenix definition; see page 337) of *90 percent or greater at four to five years* of follow-up. In addition, says Phuoc Tran, "For those men with the most unfavorable, very high-risk disease, consideration should be given to using brachytherapy as a boost" (see chapters 6 and 9). "The early results with this combined external beam and brachytherapy approach are highly encouraging, but we will feel more comfortable when longer follow-up information is available."

What About Proton-Beam Radiation?

Of the forms of external-beam radiation available, is proton beam better than the more commonly used photon beam at controlling cancer? "There is little reason to believe so," comments Tran. "Cancer cells respond the same way to both." In published reports detailing PSA nadirs, cancer control, and side effects, there are no significant differences seen between proton-beam radiation and other modern radiation techniques.

Cancer Control After Brachytherapy

How effective is brachytherapy? Modern brachytherapy involves sophisticated, high-tech guidance systems, working with ultrasound or CT and crafting a custom-designed template for each patient, placing the radioactive seeds more accurately and effectively than ever before. The ideal patient for brachytherapy is someone with a moderate-sized prostate, few urinary symptoms (minimal urgency or frequency and with a strong stream), and organ-confined disease.

How do the results compare with those of external-beam radiation or surgery? According to Johns Hopkins radiation oncologist Daniel Song, there is no straightforward answer. "This question is frequently a source of spirited debate between radiation oncologists and surgeons, and the issues involved are complex."

One problem, again, is that the definitions of success after prostatectomy and radiation are different, and the Phoenix definition (see page 337) is not perfect. Then there's that PSA bounce we talked about earlier (see page 338), which can affect up to 40 percent of men who undergo brachytherapy and which likely confused the results of older reports. Another issue is patient selection. "Consciously or unconsciously, it has been noted that urologists often select for surgery those patients who are likely to do well regardless of treatment," comments Song, "referring the less-favorable patients for treatments such as radiation. It's akin to having the first pick of the litter." The bottom line, he adds, is that in low-risk men, multiple studies have shown similar results for brachytherapy, high-dose external beam radiation, and radical prostatectomy. In fact, the National Comprehensive Cancer Network (NCCN) panel has stated that surgery and radiation should be considered effective therapies with somewhat different side effects. Finally and very importantly, a study published in 2010, of 1,656 men who received brachytherapy, echoes the importance of having the procedure performed by a skilled radiation oncologist. In all of these men, the quality of the radiation coverage, as determined by the dose, was excellent, and reached 90 percent of the prostate. More than 95 percent of men with low- and intermediate-risk disease were cancer-free at seven years of follow-up (using a definition of PSA of 0.4 ng/ml or lower).

What About High-Dose-Rate (HDR) Brachytherapy?

High-dose-rate (HDR) brachytherapy uses high-powered, temporary seeds (for more information, see chapter 9). It has been used mostly on men with intermediate- or high-risk disease. So far, there have not been head-to-head comparisons with standard brachytherapy. Some studies have shown that HDR brachytherapy plus external-beam therapy does a better job of controlling cancer than external-beam radiation alone does. However, the doses used in the patients receiving external-beam radiation alone were lower (approximately 66 Gy) than most men are routinely getting today. In general, the current knowledge regarding HDR brachytherapy suggests it is a reasonable option for men with prostate cancer, and that it's comparable to permanent seed implantation. Again, it is critical that your HDR brachytherapy be performed by a skilled radiation oncologist with a high-volume practice.

Which Form of Radiation Therapy Is Best?

This is the $64,000 question. And the answer is...we don't know. Again, no long-term studies are long-term *enough* yet to tell us how men fare with brachytherapy, conformal external-beam radiation therapy, or a combination of the two, with or without the addition of hormonal therapy.

What will the results of these radiation treatments be after ten or fifteen years? This is a crucial question for healthy men under age seventy-five who can expect to live long enough to really need to know the answer. But nobody knows. And in an era of constantly refining techniques and technology, the downside is that when the treatment changes, the results achieved with the outmoded therapy lose their meaning. As you look at the results of a certain form of radiation treatment or a particular hospital's success rate, you have the right to know such criteria as:

- What was the preoperative PSA level, clinical stage, and Gleason score of the patients they treated? (If all the patients were in the elite, low-risk group, then the five-year success rate *ought* to be good.)
- What are the researchers using as an end point? Is it the nadir + 2, or the older ASTRO definition (defined as three consecutive rises in PSA, taken at least three months apart, after PSA reaches its lowest point after treatment), or some other standard?
- In what era were their patients treated? Before or after PSA testing came into widespread use?
- Are they comparing apples to apples—men treated during the same era?

What Happens If My PSA Goes Up After Radiation Treatment?

The purpose of radiation treatment is to disable the prostate, to stop cancer from continuing to grow. Because the prostate is the source of PSA, if PSA continues to be made and its level begins to rise, there are two possibilities. Either the cancer has reactivated locally, within the prostate or surrounding tissue, or a distant metastasis—a tiny bit of cancer that probably escaped the prostate before treatment began—has started causing trouble.

It is sometimes difficult after radiation therapy for a man to know where he stands, because cancer often takes its time in announcing itself; it usually takes several PSA measurements before a man and his doctor can figure out whether treatment has failed. Also, don't forget the phenomenon of the "PSA bounce" discussed above, which can occur in up to 40 percent of men and does not appear to mean much in the long term. Some men worry that this period of uncertainty is a window of opportunity for curing prostate cancer. Here's some good news: most studies have found no difference in cancer control between men who received salvage treatment after radiation therapy and men who did not—as long as men received the extra treatment before their PSA levels reached 10 ng/ml. If you are being closely followed by your doctor and it turns out that the radiation alone has not killed the cancer, this should be evident long before your PSA level reaches that point.

However, it's worth repeating that the consensus panel that developed the Phoenix definition (nadir + 2) advises, "Physicians should use individualized approaches to managing young patients with slowly rising PSA levels who initially achieved a very low nadir and who might be a candidate for salvage local therapies."

If your PSA level continues to rise, what should you do? To determine whether you are a candidate for other treatments after radiation, you will need to have a prostate biopsy to confirm that the cancer recurrence is local; you will also need a bone scan and CT scan or MRI of the abdomen and pelvis to rule out the possibility that cancer has spread to distant sites. The guidelines above (see page 324) may one day be adapted for men who have failed radiation treatment, but the overriding principles can be useful here in identifying the likelihood of metastases. If you have a high Gleason score (8 or greater), or if the PSA level begins to rise early after radiation therapy, or if the PSA level has a rapid doubling time, it is more likely that you have metastases than a local recurrence, and in this case, you should seek systemic therapy (see chapter 13). Fortunately, new imaging techniques are becoming available that may help us with this vexing problem (see page 324).

Salvage Therapy

If the cancer appears to have stayed put—to be still localized to the prostate bed—what are the options? Salvage radical prostatectomy, salvage brachytherapy, HIFU, and cryoablation.

In the past, with standard radiation therapy and less sophisticated brachytherapy, performing a radical prostatectomy on a man who had undergone radiation treatment was a surgeon's nightmare. The prostate was adherent to everything around it and thus very difficult to remove cleanly; in fact, it was often necessary to remove the bladder as well. The side effects were high, particularly the risk of incontinence and rectal injury. With the advent of three-dimensional conformal external-beam therapy, it may be easier to perform surgery as a salvage procedure. There is too little information yet available about salvage surgery after brachytherapy to make a judgment. Under the best circumstances, in men who appear to have no evidence of distant metastases, the likelihood of being cancer-free following a salvage radical prostatectomy at five and ten years is about 50 percent and 30 percent, respectively. The price for this in quality of life, however, is high.

One of the largest studies to look at radical prostatectomy after radiation comes from a multi-institutional study from such hospitals as Memorial Sloan Kettering and the Mayo Clinic. At an average of fifty-two months after salvage surgery, 404 men underwent either prostatectomy or cystoprostatectomy (removal of both the prostate and bladder). At five years after surgery, 48 percent of men remained free of cancer. Other studies of salvage prostatectomy have reported that between 33 and 75 percent of men remained cancer-free. Averaging across many studies that comprise more than 1,300 men, urinary incontinence developed in 50 percent of men, 26 percent had bladder neck strictures, and 5 percent had rectal injury following surgery. The percentage of men who had impotence was not typically recorded, but this is almost inevitable with salvage prostatectomy.

Salvage Cryoablation

Freezing the prostate (discussed in chapter 9) is a good option for radiation-treated patients with rising PSA levels. The largest studies looking at cryoablation for men who have rising PSA and localized disease following radiotherapy are from the aptly named COLD registry: in 279 patients, the five-year PSA control was 59 percent. A PSA less than 0.1 ng/ml following cryotherapy is predictive of treatment success. As it is with radiation therapy, success is difficult to determine following cryotherapy. Nonetheless, the results suggest that salvage cryotherapy can control prostate cancer about as well as salvage surgery can. Although far fewer men have been treated with salvage cryoablation, there appear to be fewer complications compared to salvage surgery. The COLD registry reported that only 5 percent of men developed urinary incontinence and 7 percent had bladder neck stricture/retention; rectal injury was not reported. The average results from other salvage cryotherapy studies suggest a less optimistic view—but one that still has fewer complications than salvage surgery does.

What About Additional Radiation?

This is a third option—another round of radiation in the form of brachytherapy. Current studies suggest that salvage brachytherapy may be as effective as salvage surgery for some men, especially those with PSA levels lower than 10 ng/ml. Note: Salvage prostatectomy has been attempted more often than salvage brachytherapy has, so we're not working with vast amounts of information. The risk of urinary incontinence with salvage brachytherapy has been reported to be as high as 31 percent; however, this was with the older, "uniform loading" technique (see chapter 9), which has been associated with higher incontinence in general. Averaging across thirteen studies encompassing 297 men treated with salvage brachytherapy, only 6 percent developed urinary incontinence, 8 percent had bladder neck strictures, and 5 percent had rectal injury. In one study from Harvard, investigators found that complications were more likely to develop if the time from the initial external-beam radiation treatment to the salvage brachytherapy was less than four and a half years. Note: *If you are considering this option, it is essential that the procedure be performed by someone who is skilled at delivering radiation to an already irradiated area.* The RTOG Foundation is conducting a trial to determine how well brachytherapy works in men with cancer that has returned to the local area (as confirmed by biopsy) after external-beam radiation, but the results will take years to become clear.

Lastly, your doctor may want you to start long-term hormonal therapy only if or when you develop symptoms from local recurrence or metastatic disease. The field of treating advanced disease is constantly changing, and there are many new, exciting, and hopeful advances. These are discussed in chapter 13.

How Well Do Cryoablation and Thermal Ablation Work?

There are two ways in which cryoablation and thermal ablation are used: whole gland treatment as an alternative to surgery or radiation, and as focal therapy (just treating individual spots where cancer has been detected).

Whole Gland Treatment

As we discussed in chapter 9, the NCCN guidelines state that "cryotherapy or other local therapies are not recommended as routine primary therapy for localized prostate cancer, due to lack of long-term data comparing these treatments to radical prostatectomy or radiation." But cryotherapy for prostate cancer has been in use for at least three decades: why don't we know more about its efficacy in cancer control? Cryotherapy is ablative—designed to eliminate the prostate, like surgery does. There should be data on how often cryotherapy results in a sustained PSA of < 0.1 or even < 0.6. These findings are difficult to find, possibly because this endpoint is not reliably achieved—because cryotherapy may not achieve long-term prostate ablation.

So instead, cryotherapy investigators have used the ASTRO or Phoenix definitions—but these were designed for the evaluation of radiation therapy, which is not ablative. Worse, after thirty years there is zero evidence that cryotherapy reduces the risk of metastases or death from prostate cancer.

Well, what about HIFU? The FDA failed to approve it for whole-gland treatment of localized prostate cancer, or for salvage therapy for prostate cancer that has come back after radiation therapy—because the manufacturers failed to prove that the devices were reasonably safe and effective for that use.

To sum up, there is lack of evidence that these technologies produce long-term cancer control, plus cryotherapy and HIFU have side effects, as well.

Focal Therapy

This section will focus on the results with the two techniques that are used most commonly, HIFU and cryotherapy, but as you will see, there is lack of good, prospective, long-term randomized data.

We've discussed some of the issues with cryotherapy and HIFU in treating the entire prostate gland. But how well do they work as focal, or "spot," treatment for prostate cancer? Let's start by asking who is being treated: in many cases, it is older men with small tumors—men whose cancer probably doesn't need to be treated—and it's no surprise that they are the ones who do the best.

What yardstick is being used to measure success? Often, it's repeated needle biopsies after treatment. Although some studies suggest that up to 90 percent of men who undergo HIFU have negative biopsies afterward, the problem is one that you have already heard—each needle biopsy samples only one one-thousandth of the gland. Furthermore, in one high-quality study in which twenty-five men underwent extensive needle biopsies six months after treatment with HIFU, residual cancer was present in 44 percent, and in 28 percent, there was no evidence of any significant effect on the normal tissue.

What is the definition for PSA failure?

Here the problem is more complex; there is plenty of prostate tissue left behind. How much of the PSA is coming from this normal tissue, and how much is coming from cancer? The definitions of PSA failure are inconsistent, too, and many authors use the definitions used to measure the success of radiation therapy. As we discussed above, these definitions are not appropriate for evaluating ablative procedures. The most appropriate definition should be the PSA nadir—which, ideally, should be very low (PSA less than 0.2 ng/ml). Even using inappropriate definitions, PSA failure rates as high as 75 percent have been reported. And don't believe that MRI will be able to determine whether the cancer has been eliminated.

Why doesn't HIFU work better?

One reason is that there is no real-time monitoring while the treatment is being performed. Another is that although intense heat is generated, it is usually in very small areas, and when the focal point moves to the next location, "skip lesions"—places where a few cells are missed here and there—can be created.

What happens when HIFU fails, even after it is repeated?

Both salvage radiotherapy and surgery have been performed after HIFU. In a study from France, men whose cancer returned after HIFU were treated with radiation therapy, and after five years,

75 percent of the patients were considered successfully treated based on the ASTRO definition. In a Canadian study of fifteen men who underwent salvage surgery after HIFU had failed, 64 percent had capsular penetration and 27 percent had positive surgical margins; at one year, only 60 percent were continent, and all were impotent. The authors concluded, "The pathology results are alarming, given the number of cases with extraprostatic extension. These results should be factored in when counseling men who wish to undergo primary high-intensity focused ultrasound."

With cryotherapy, it is possible to monitor the ice ball in real time to determine how the treatment is progressing. The most common techniques involve either hemiablation (treatment of one entire lobe), in cases where there are positive biopsies on only one side, or what is called a "hockey stick" ablation (one entire lobe with a small extension of the iceball into the opposite side). Unfortunately, as with whole-gland treatment, there are no long-term results. What we do have are reports of biochemical-free survival using the flawed endpoints discussed above. Two studies—one of focal cryotherapy and the other of focal HIFU—are due to be reported soon and will provide information on biopsy results at three years.

The most comprehensive study of focal therapy was recently published. This was a large, randomized trial of photodynamic therapy versus active surveillance in men with low-risk prostate cancer that involved four hundred patients at forty-seven European centers. The authors' published conclusion was that focal therapy was a safe, effective treatment for low-risk disease. What was the real story? At two years, cancer had progressed in more than a quarter of the treated men; 51 percent still had cancer in their prostate, and 30 percent had suffered serious side effects.

If focal therapy's results came anywhere close to matching the hype, the truth wouldn't need to be masked.

Final Thoughts on Treatment for Localized Prostate Cancer

Which has better results, surgery or radiation therapy? The answer, today, is that both are excellent. For many years, before we had long-term outcomes and before both techniques were refined to reduce side effects, surgeons and radiation oncologists would argue which was best. Comparisons of short-term PSA results were confusing and unreliable. The only way to know was to perform well-conducted, randomized trials and then wait for a long time to see if there was a difference in cancer control (defined as a reduction in the development of metastases and death from cancer).

Over the years, while we waited, we learned that the outcome of both forms of treatment in men with low- and intermediate-risk disease was excellent. And now we have the first results from the ProtecT trial—which randomly assigned men with low- and intermediate-risk disease to active monitoring, surgery, or radiation plus short-term neoadjuvant hormonal therapy. At ten years, both surgery and radiation therapy proved equally effective in reducing the risk of metastatic disease (for more on this, see chapter 6).

What about high-risk disease? There is no big, helpful, randomized trial waiting in the wings to give us the answer in a few years. All we can do is tell you where we stand today. Once again, both major treatments—radiation therapy plus neoadjuvant and adjuvant hormonal therapy and surgery with or without salvage radiation—have proven to provide good cancer control. Some surgeons claim that if you compare published nonrandomized trials, the outcome in patients treated with surgery is almost always better. But these comparisons are difficult. There are many variables that can't be measured, and these can influence the results; also, it is impossible to measure the effect of selection bias. Surgeons see the patients first and it is likely that they operate on the more favorable cases and refer the ones who will be more difficult to cure for radiation therapy.

What should a man with high- or very high-risk prostate cancer do? Seek out a Center of Excellence with a multidisciplinary approach to the problem—a place where radiation oncologists, surgeons, pathologists, medical oncologists and radiologists can evaluate the facts and help you make the right decision. It may come down to the availability of high-quality surgery or radiation therapy in your region, or the side effects you are likely to face. This is what we know: the goal is complete elimination of the primary tumor in the prostate, and every effort should be made to achieve this.

11

ERECTILE DYSFUNCTION AFTER TREATMENT FOR LOCALIZED PROSTATE CANCER

This chapter was written with expert opinion from Trinity J. Bivalacqua, M.D., Ph.D.

THE SHORT STORY:
The Highly Abridged Version of This Chapter

Men who have trouble with erections after surgery or radiation therapy have normal sensation and normal sex drive and can achieve a normal orgasm. Their only trouble may be in achieving or maintaining an erection. That's the bad news. *The good news is that this problem, called erectile dysfunction (ED), can always be treated.*

Why does ED occur? There are many reasons in addition to the fact that a man has had prostate treatment. Aging is one reason for ED. But ED can also result from medical conditions such as atherosclerosis, dyslipidemia (too much fat or cholesterol in the blood), diabetes, obesity, or hypertension; from certain medications; from the overuse of alcohol, cigarettes, or other drugs; and even from emotional or psychological problems.

The important message here is that for most men, ED does not have to be a permanent situation. If there's a will, there's generally a way. After treatment for prostate disease (except for men who are being treated with hormonal therapy), recovery of sexual function is almost certain. Take heart! You will get through this.

What Is Erectile Dysfunction (ED)?

As its name suggests, erectile dysfunction (ED) is trouble having or maintaining an erection. There's no minimum age requirement for ED; it can happen to any man at any time. It's especially common after treatment for prostate cancer with radical prostatectomy or radiation therapy. Having ED does not mean your sex life is over—far from it. In fact, a man with ED has *normal sensation and normal sexual desire and can achieve a normal orgasm*. He may just need a little help with erections. And this is a problem that can be fixed.

The purpose of this chapter is to let you know two things: First, that you're not alone. By age sixty-five, about half of all men—those who have been treated for prostate cancer as well as men who have never had it—experience at least some ED. In the United States alone, ED affects an estimated ten to thirty million men. (Note: ED is different from the loss of sexual desire that results from hormonal

AFTER RADICAL PROSTATECTOMY, TESTOSTERONE GOES UP

Some men experience a loss of sexual desire after radical prostatectomy. This is different from ED. It's not about having trouble with sex—it's about not wanting to have it at all. Some scientists have theorized that perhaps after surgery, there is a decrease in male hormones (particularly testosterone), and perhaps this accounts for the diminished desire in some men.

But a Johns Hopkins study has found that this is not the case; in fact, it's the opposite of what we suspected. Before we go any further, let's take a quick look at testosterone. The story begins in the brain—in the pituitary gland, which makes a hormone called luteinizing hormone (LH). In the chemical chain of events involved in the production of testosterone, the pituitary is the thermostat, the regulator that controls the testes—the furnace, in effect. The furnace cranks out heat—testosterone—which, in turn, stimulates the prostate. The level of testosterone in the blood is constantly monitored by the brain, which regulates how much LH is needed.

This study showed that when the prostate is removed, LH goes up—and so, then, does testosterone—suggesting that the prostate somehow produces a substance that controls LH secretion. The investigators were studying the effect of radical prostatectomy on these hormones in sixty-three men, wondering whether some change in hormonal makeup might explain the loss of sexual desire experienced by some men after surgery. Normally, the major factors that influence sexual function are blood flow, nerve supply, and hormones. A great deal of attention has been placed on studying how to avoid disrupting the nerve supply and blood flow during surgery—but up to this point, there has been little attention paid to what happens to the hormones.

The discovery that the pituitary gland makes more LH after radical prostatectomy suggests that the prostate is also making an inhibitor that regulates the release of LH from the pituitary, raising the fascinating idea that the prostate itself may influence hormone levels in an effort to modulate its own growth.

The increase in testosterone is not noticeable, but it certainly dispels the theory that a loss of male hormones contributes to a loss of sex drive. Instead, a more likely cause of this diminished interest in sex after surgery is the lack of psychogenic erections. This occurs early on after surgery. Another cause may be depression, and fortunately, treatment can restore the sex drive.

therapy—discussed in chapter 12.) A report from the Massachusetts Male Aging Study suggests that the incidence of ED triples from 5 to 15 percent between ages forty and seventy. Aging (and the general nerve loss that goes along with it; see page 356) is one reason for ED. But ED also can result from a host of medical conditions, including obesity, sleep apnea, atherosclerosis (the buildup of plaque in your arteries), dyslipidemia, diabetes, hypertension, and some emotional or psychological disorders. Certain prescription medications can cause ED; so can the overuse of alcohol, cigarettes, or other drugs. The second point here is that *help is available*. For most men, ED does not have to be a life sentence. If there's a will, there's generally a way.

Some of the advice you will find in this chapter is not available from any other source. You won't hear it anywhere else, because it isn't anywhere else. It has been gleaned from more than 20,000 telephone conversations I have had with my patients over the years, coaching them to recovery. I spoke to every single man on whom I performed the anatomical radical prostatectomy—4,569 men— every three months for the first year, and longer if he had not fully recovered. In this chapter, you will learn what my patients have taught me.

What Happens in Normal Sexual Function?

In medical terms, normal erection in men can be reduced to a neurovascular event. But this seems too simple a description for the delicate, complex interplay between blood vessels (veins and arteries) and nerves. The penis itself is a remarkable structure, made up of nerves, endothelium (cells lining the arteries), smooth muscle tissue, and blood vessels. It has three cylindrical, spongy chambers that are essential to erection; one of these is called the corpus spongiosum, and the other two are called the corpora cavernosa.

When sexual function is normal, this is what happens. A man becomes sexually aroused. A substance called nitric oxide is released by the nerve endings and endothelium, and the smooth muscle tissue in the penis begins to relax. The spongy chambers (also called sinusoids) within the corpora cavernosa begin to dilate. Meanwhile, arteries continue to pump blood, as usual, into these spongy chambers of the penis. As the penis elongates, the veins are stretched; they clamp down against the thick tissue that surrounds the corpora cavernosa—shutting themselves off so the blood can't leave the penis. The chambers become engorged, and this keeps the penis inflated during sexual activity. An erection is born.

After ejaculation, nitric oxide stops being released; the smooth muscle tissue contracts, and the blood flow to the penis is reduced—the veins ease their viselike grip. Once again, blood is allowed to leave the penis, and the erection goes away.

What Can Go Wrong?

There are four components to normal sexual function in men—sexual desire (libido), erection, emission of fluid (ejaculation), and orgasm. All of these elements are regulated separately; there is no centralized sex control center.

Sexual Desire (Libido)

The sex drive is controlled by male hormones, and also by psychological and environmental factors. Testosterone, the main male hormone that affects sexual desire, is made in the testicles. When this hormone supply is shut off—as it is in hormonal therapy (actually, hormone-deprivation therapy) for advanced prostate cancer—testosterone levels fall considerably, to extremely low levels. When this happens, most men on hormonal therapy lose all interest in sexual activity. Men who have undergone a radical prostatectomy or radiation therapy may also experience a loss of libido, but it's not caused by the loss of testosterone, and it's not usually as severe. There is some evidence that radiation therapy may cause a slight decrease in the production of male hormones, although this is unlikely to be significant enough to reduce sexual.

Surprisingly, after radical prostatectomy, testosterone levels actually go *up*. The most likely cause of diminished desire after surgery is the early loss of erections that are brought on by visual and mental stimulation; these are called *psychogenic* erections. As we'll discuss later, most men rely on these signals to increase their desire, and when they are absent, they sense that they've lost interest in sexual activity. (It's like thinking, "The lights aren't on; therefore, nobody is home"—without even knocking on the door to find out!) Other causes may be stress, performance anxiety, discouragement, or depression. Many men find that if they take a vacation and get their mind off their work and other problems, they lose an overlay of stress they may not even have realized they've been carrying around, and their sexual desire returns. It's also common for men to become distracted by fretting about the mechanics of sexual relations rather than the pleasure of intimacy. When a man sits around and broods about whether he's going to have an erection—when he agonizes over the thought of disappointing his partner or even starts to obsess about various blood vessels doing or not doing their jobs right—it probably isn't going to happen. This is known as performance anxiety.

Important to consider: After any major treatment or trauma to the body, depression can occur (this is common in men after a heart attack, for example). Paradoxically, it may be even more acute when the treatment is successful. Depression is one of the body's natural responses to stress, and in many men, treating the depression restores the sex drive to normal.

For all these reasons, after radical prostatectomy, many men may perceive a decrease in their sexual desire. This usually returns over time, as these problems correct themselves one by one. Because it can take as long as two to four years for the quality of the erections to improve, many depressed men feel that their sexual desire is not the same. These men often believe their testosterone levels are low. When the level is actually measured and proven to be normal, this actually helps with their recovery. Again, you are not alone: talk to your urologist. Many clinics have counselors who help couples work through issues of sexual dysfunction and intimacy. They wouldn't offer these services if a lot of men didn't need them—so if you feel you need help, ask to be referred to a sexual health counselor.

Erection

The most common sexual problem for men after prostate treatment is the inability to have an erection sufficient for sexual intercourse. The nerves that lead to and from the penis are extremely important to erection. Particularly essential are nerves in the two bundles that sit on either side of the prostate (see the illustrations in chapter 8). Even if these nerve bundles are not removed during radical prostatectomy, they can still be damaged by the surgery. They also can be injured during radiation treatment and other procedures, including HIFU and cryoablation. But remember, *these nerves are necessary only for erection—not for sensation, and not for orgasm.* The nerves that are responsible for sensation travel *outside the pelvis* for a long distance. These nerves are not close to the prostate and should not be damaged. Loss of erection after radical prostatectomy or radiation is multifactorial—in other words, it's probably not caused by one single problem.

In the most skilled surgeon's hands, if both neurovascular bundles are preserved during a radical prostatectomy, potency should return in at least 80 percent of men in their forties and fifties and in 60 percent of men in their sixties. However, only about 25 percent of men over age seventy are potent after surgery. Why are the numbers so much lower? We think a large part of the problem is something that comes with the territory of aging in general—a gradual loss of all nerves, including those involved in erection. Plus, other health conditions, such as hypertension and diabetes, can affect the vascular system throughout the body and take a toll on erection, as well.

When a younger man undergoes a nerve-sparing radical prostatectomy, it's likely that about 20 percent of the nerves involved in erection are damaged, 60 percent are preserved normally, and 20 percent are *temporarily* disabled but eventually recover. This explains why for most men, sexual potency doesn't just snap back like a coiled spring. For most men, the recovery of erections sufficient for intercourse can take up to a year after surgery, and it may be two years until they have maximal recovery. However, I have seen patients who recovered erections as late as four years after surgery. With radiation therapy, it is just the opposite: initially, things seem fine, but by five years about half of men report having difficulty with erections. (Note: This doesn't mean these men can't have sexual intercourse. Don't despair, and keep reading!)

So at best, a younger man after prostatectomy has about 80 percent of these nerves left for erection. But as we age, we constantly lose nerves. *By age sixty, a man has only about 60 percent of the nerves he was born with*—which means that if 20 percent of them are damaged by treatment for prostate cancer, only about 48 percent remain. This explains why ED is more common in older men after surgery and in men in whom it is necessary to remove one neurovascular bundle.

Erection problems also can result from vascular injury— damage to the blood vessels in the penis. For a normal erection to occur, the arteries that supply blood to the penis must be intact. This blood supply can suffer after radiation treatment; in fact, damage to these arteries is believed to be the main cause of ED after radiation treatment, although recent studies suggest that radiation may also injure the neurovascular bundles. In a few men, this blood supply can also be reduced by radical prostatectomy—even though the major arteries that supply the penis do not normally travel next to the prostate. In these men, for some reason, the major blood supply to the penis runs *inside* the pelvis—instead of outside, as it does in most men, and so these arteries can be damaged inadvertently during radical prostatectomy. At Johns Hopkins, once we recognized this, we modified our surgical technique, and now any major arteries that run on top of the prostate can be saved. The quality of the nerve-sparing procedure matters, too. Recent evidence shows that if nerve sparing does not occur or is not done well, tissue in the penis loses the vital smooth muscle necessary for erection; in fact, this healthy tissue changes to become fibrous, with dense collagen.

Another major problem with erections in men after radical prostatectomy or radiation therapy results from a problem called *venous leak*. Remember, as blood flows into the penis and it elongates, veins stretch and clamp down against the thick tissue that surrounds the corpora cavernosa, shutting them off so the blood can't leave the penis. However, early on after radical prostatectomy, the blood flow into the penis may not be rapid enough to cause these veins to go into their "stretch and automatically close" mode. Imagine a bucket with a hole in it, with water running in and then running out (except in this case, it's blood flowing in but draining back out, because the veins can't dam it up properly). For these veins to clamp down, the penis must be fully engorged. If a man never gets a full erection, there's a constant leak. Also—yet another consequence of aging—as men get older, the fibrous tissues that surround the penis weaken, and this, too, undermines the ability of the veins to hold in the blood.

Emission

In normal ejaculation, several events must take place. Sperm, which are made in the testicles, travel to the epididymis, a "greenhouse" in which they mature. During orgasm, sperm are rocketed from the epididymis through the vas deferens during a series of powerful muscle contractions. They shoot through the ejaculatory ducts and mix with fluid produced by the prostate and seminal vesicles. Simultaneously, a muscular valve in the bladder neck slams shut, forcing this fluid out the only possible exit—through the urethra and penis to the outside world, rather than backward into the bladder.

After radical prostatectomy, there is usually no emission of fluid because the prostate and seminal vesicles, which produce the vast majority of this fluid, are gone, and the vas deferens has been shut off. (Thus the term *dry ejaculation*. A few men, however, do continue to produce a small amount of ejaculate. This fluid comes from the nearby Cowper's glands; like the prostate and seminal vesicles, these are known as sex accessory tissues.)

After radiation therapy, many men also have a loss of ejaculate fluid because the glands responsible for making this fluid are dried up. In any event—no matter what causes dry ejaculation—the lack of fluid should not interfere with orgasm. This is because orgasm doesn't really have much to do with the prostate. Think about it— women don't have prostates, yet they do have orgasms. Here's why.

Orgasm

Orgasm happens primarily in the brain. For orgasm to take place, there must be sensation and stimulation. In men who have ED after radical prostatectomy or radiation therapy, sensation is not interrupted; therefore, orgasm should always be possible, and it should be no different from the way it was before treatment. Many men don't realize that they can have an orgasm without an erection, and they're surprised to hear that half of the people in the world have orgasms without an erection—women. (Again, it's different for men receiving hormonal therapy for prostate cancer; orgasm is not an issue because—although a few can still have erections—the treatment causes a loss of interest in sexual activity.)

A few men experience an inadvertent leakage of urine at orgasm (this is called climacturia). This can be minimized by emptying the bladder before sexual intercourse. This is most common soon after surgery, before urinary continence has returned. Fortunately, this gets better over time. In the meantime, if it is bothersome, some men try condoms. If that is not successful, it may help to take pseudo-ephedrine (Sudafed) before intercourse, which constricts the blood vessels. Note: This is not Sudafed PE, but the original formula that you have to sign for at the pharmacy counter.

A recent study suggested that for some men, up to 14 percent, there is greater intensity or even some pain during orgasm after radical prostatectomy. For most of my patients who experience this problem, it gradually diminishes over time. It may be that there is a spasm of the sphincter at the time of orgasm. For this reason, treatment with an alpha-blocking drug such as tamsulosin (Flomax) can improve the problem or cause it to resolve completely.

What Can You Do About ED?

It's worth repeating: You are not alone! This is a common problem even in men who have not been treated for prostate cancer, so by all means, talk to your doctor about it. The first thing you can expect is to have a detailed history taken and a physical exam performed. The doctor is going to try to pinpoint the exact problem and figure out what's causing it. Is it trouble with sexual desire, erection, ejaculation, or orgasm? Even though it may seem pretty obvious—your erections were just fine before prostate cancer treatment and inadequate or nonexistent afterward—the doctor needs to rule out the possibility that any other medical or psychological problem is causing this.

You may be asked to fill out a questionnaire so you don't have to discuss details face-to-face, or your doctor may ask you some very specific questions. You'll probably be embarrassed; most men would rather be almost anywhere else, discussing almost any other topic, than in a doctor's office talking about ED. But you shouldn't be embarrassed. This is private, sensitive, confidential information. Everything you discuss in the doctor's office will remain there. Remember: This certainly won't be the first time your doctor has heard about such difficulties, and it won't be the last. There are millions of other men in the United States alone with this same trouble. And finally, remind yourself that having this discussion is the first step toward solving the problem.

Do you have nighttime erections? Probably one of the first questions your doctor will ask is whether you ever wake up at night with an erection. Most men have several erections while they're asleep; these are usually associated with dreaming, and they happen during a particular phase of sleep called REM, the abbreviation for rapid eye movement sleep. (Because men tend to wake up in the morning with these erections, they often connect them with having a full bladder; this is just coincidence.) The idea behind this question is to make sure there's no mental or emotional problem causing the ED. In other words, if a man can't produce an erection during sexual activity but has several a night while he sleeps, this is a clue that the nature of the problem is not physiological, but psychological. This type of erection problem is called psychogenic, as we discussed above, and it's often treated successfully with counseling. After a radical prostatectomy, things are different. Many men who are potent do not report having nocturnal erections, and some men who are not potent do have them. How can this be? We don't know yet. However, we do know that the stimuli following surgery are different, and most men who are not potent but have nocturnal erections will eventually be able to have intercourse.

How are your arteries? Your doctor will also ask whether you have a history of cardiovascular disease. Men who have had a heart attack; who have coronary artery disease, hypertension, obesity, or elevated blood lipids; or who smoke have a greater chance of having vascular problems. Aside from the obvious health risks, smoking causes arteries to contract and impairs the endothelium (cells lining the penis). *Smoking is an easily reversible cause of ED*; if you quit smoking, you could greatly improve your ability to have an erection. Exercising more than five hours a week has been shown to improve erections. Because exercise helps the vascular system, it also improves the response to sildenafil (Viagra), (tadalafil) Cialis, and other erection-helping drugs mentioned later in this chapter. One of the first steps in erection is for the arteries to dilate; they fill up the penis with blood. If they're contracted, they won't be able to dilate very well. The arteries in the penis are somewhat smaller in diameter than the coronary arteries in the heart; in fact, we now know that when younger men (whether or not they have been treated for prostate cancer) have problems with ED, it may be an early warning sign of coronary artery disease. If you have heart disease, hypertension, atherosclerosis (hardening of the arteries), or high cholesterol (which can contribute to heart disease), it is very likely that the arteries in the penis are already narrowed.

Other Causes of ED

Neurological diseases—diabetes, for example—can cause ED. Also, certain drugs may contribute to sexual problems, and combined with prostate treatment, they may result in ED. Cimetidine (Tagamet), for example, is a drug used to treat ulcers, but it's also an antiandrogen; it blocks the action of testosterone. Other medications that can cause ED include drugs that treat high blood pressure, such as beta-blockers and thiazides; medications that treat depression, such as selective serotonin reuptake inhibitors and tricyclic antidepressants; antipsychotic drugs; sedatives; drugs that treat anxiety; and drugs of abuse, such as opiates. (And don't forget alcohol and cigarettes—they're drugs, too.) Basically, it's a good idea if you're on any medication—even herbal or dietary supplements—to check with your doctor to make sure the side effects don't include ED. Switching from one drug to another may make a big difference.

Diagnostic Tests

Your doctor may want you to undergo further evaluation. If your doctor suspects a problem with penile blood flow, you may need to undergo a duplex Doppler ultrasound of the penis. This test uses high-resolution ultrasound to evaluate the arteries' blood supply to the penis and to test for venous leak. In the duplex Doppler ultrasound, medication that causes the smooth muscle to relax is injected through a small needle directly into the penis; the idea here is to see whether an erection can be produced. If this shot doesn't cause an erection, this is a good hint that there's a vascular problem—trouble with arterial blood flow or venous leak. Sometimes during this test a man develops an erection but gradually loses it; this usually signifies that there's a problem with the veins—they're not shutting off the blood supply, so the blood is escaping from the penis, and thus the erection is failing. Note: Surprisingly, psychological factors can prevent the penis from becoming erect in spite of this powerful pharmacological stimulation. This shows the true influence of mind over matter, and here again, counseling may provide significant help.

Recovery of Potency After Radical Prostatectomy

You've had a radical prostatectomy, and one or both bundles were preserved, which means that the potential for erection is there. So what's the problem? Why isn't it happening?

The first bit of advice your doctor will probably give you here is, "Be patient. Erections return gradually." Maybe better advice is, "Be very patient. It can take up to four years for some men to experience full recovery of potency. Your body has been through a trauma; it needs time to recover." This doesn't mean you should give up on sexual relations until the day you wake up with a full erection or until four years go by—whichever happens first. By no means. Also, know that the erection you have two months after surgery is not the same one you'll have two years from now. *Most patients experience an improvement in their erections over time; the quality improves month by month.*

Before surgery, men became sexually aroused, had an erection, and then pursued sexual activity. But after radical prostatectomy, the stimuli that cause an erection are different; visual and mental stimulation are not nearly as important as tactile sensation—what the penis can feel directly. Usually, shortly after surgery, the only way a man can achieve an erection is with direct sexual stimulation.

PEYRONIE'S DISEASE AND RADICAL PROSTATECTOMY: IS THERE A LINK?

Peyronie's disease is a fairly uncommon disorder of the connective tissue within the penis that can cause curvature during erection. It is estimated to affect nearly four hundred of every thousand men between the ages of forty and seventy, but the true numbers are probably higher; there may be many cases we don't hear about due to patient embarrassment and limited reporting of this disorder by physicians. However, as more men are being treated successfully for ED, we are seeing more men with Peyronie's disease. Johns Hopkins urologists have spotted what they believe may be a small yet significant trend: Peyronie's disease seems to be more common in men who have had a radical prostatectomy. Is this just coincidence? The age group is roughly the same. Or does the procedure itself—or a man's recovery from it—somehow contribute to development of the disease?

A former Johns Hopkins urologist, Jonathan Jarow, has described Peyronie's disease as being like "arthritis of the penis." He says, "When you get scar tissue deposited in the connective tissue of your joints, you get arthritis. It's a similar problem in the penis." Peyronie's disease causes a telltale bend, or curvature, in the penis (which appears only during erection). It may also manifest itself as palpable or painful lumps, or plaques—which may be terrifying for a man to discover. (The plaque is found on the side of the penis where the curvature is directed.) "Many men worry that they have penile cancer," says Jarow, "but we can tell just by examining them exactly what it is." He reassures his patients that although the disorder may be annoying, it is not life-threatening: "Men aren't going to live any longer or shorter because of it."

Although nobody knows exactly what causes Peyronie's disease, scientists suspect it has several causes. In some men, it is most likely related to a series of minor injuries—or, as Jarow explains, "wear and tear"—that result in a low-level autoimmune response.

"Peyronie's disease is a wound-healing disorder," says Johns Hopkins urologist Trinity J. Bivalacqua, who specializes in the treatment of erectile disorders. "Following microtrauma associated with sexual intercourse or injury to the penis, abnormal inflammatory cells called cytokines are released. This is what causes the scar tissue to build up and the Peyronie's plaque to form." Most men, he adds, recover completely from microvascular trauma to the penis. But for whatever reason, men who develop Peyronie's disease don't. Bivalacqua believes the microtraumas may happen because of repetitive buckling, which happens when a man is attempting sexual relations with an incomplete erection.

Peyronie's disease is more common among men who have ED. "But again," notes Jarow, "it's not clear whether it's caused by some of the treatments, such as vacuum erection devices or injection therapy, or whether it's due to having erection problems to begin with."

In some men, there may be an inherited component to Peyronie's disease, as there is with other connective tissue or wound-healing disorders that result in a buildup of dense scar tissue. "If we can understand the mechanism behind Peyronie's disease, we may be able to prevent it," says Jarow.

Why do men who undergo a radical prostatectomy seem slightly more prone to developing Peyronie's disease or, if they already have it, to having their symptoms get worse? Besides the fact that prostate cancer and Peyronie's disease tend to develop in men at about the same age, we don't know yet. However, there is evidence that a man's risk of Peyronie's disease increases to 15 percent (from an average risk of less than 4 percent) within three years of a radical prostatectomy. Further research is necessary to determine exactly why this happens but there appears to be one lead: it is more common in men in whom the nerves were not spared.

The good news is that Peyronie's disease does not progress forever. "About 12 to 20 percent of men will have complete resolution of their penile curvature, and in more than 90 percent of men, the pain goes away," says Jarow. "For most men, it eventually stabilizes. The lump becomes less prominent, and the curvature lessens. In just about everybody, the disease process, the deposition of scar tissue, stops with time."

If a man's problem is penile curvature—if the penis is bent so he cannot engage in sexual activity or it's uncomfortable to his partner—then an outpatient surgical procedure to straighten the penis can be performed, notes Jarow. "However, if he has significant curvature that prevents sexual relations and severe ED, then the treatment of choice would be placement of a penile prosthesis combined with penile straightening," also an outpatient procedure. If a man simply has erection problems but no serious curvature, he is "treated like anyone else with an erection problem, starting with pills, then shots and vacuum erection device, and, if necessary, a penile prosthesis." (All of these are discussed in this chapter.)

This changes the sequence of events. Before surgery, visual or psychogenic stimuli would bring on an erection, which led to interest in sexual activity. Men need sexual stimulation to produce an erection sufficient for intercourse. *Over time, psychogenic erections almost always return.* For now, you will need to be proactive. In other words, you and your partner need to bypass the brain as an instigator or even a middleman and speak directly to the penis. Thus, don't be afraid to experiment with sexual activity.

If you have a partial erection, go ahead and attempt intercourse—vaginal stimulation is the best stimulation to improve your erection. So don't wait until you have the perfect erection. If you do, you could be waiting a long time and missing out on this important aspect of your life. Use whatever erection you have to attempt vaginal penetration; you will probably find that the erection soon becomes much firmer. The use of lubricants such as Astroglide (available on Amazon and at most drugstores) also will help tremendously. Remember, you can have an orgasm even without an erection (and don't be surprised if it is dry).

Early on, however, erections are often not sufficient for traditional vaginal penetration. One common reason for this is the venous leakage described above. Even though the arteries are doing their job and filling the penis with blood, producing a partial erection, the veins aren't keeping the blood trapped inside the penis. To improve this situation, many men find that if they attempt sexual activity standing up, they are able to achieve a much firmer erection. (The escaping blood has to travel all the way back up to the heart, and this takes longer if a man is standing up than if he's lying down.) Sexual activity can continue either while a man remains standing or while he's kneeling. Also, it may help to attempt entry from behind; the vagina opens more easily if a woman is bending forward.

Another way to combat venous leakage is for men to place a soft tourniquet at the base of the penis *before they begin foreplay or sexual stimulation.* The purpose of the tourniquet is to keep blood in the penis once the stimulation causes the arteries to dilate and penile blood flow to increase. The tourniquet doesn't impede blood flow into the penis; it just keeps it from going back out. You can achieve the same effect with a rubber band, a ponytail holder, an O-ring that you can buy in a hardware store, or—if you're brave enough to venture into a novelty store—a device called an erection ring.

To Sum Up

The return of sexual potency is different in every man. Recovery is faster for men younger than age sixty-five. In men who were experiencing some ED before surgery, recovery will take longer, and despite having one or both nerve bundles spared, the recovery of spontaneous erections is less likely. For some men, it can take as long as four years for full potency to return. For others, intercourse is possible just a few weeks after surgery. In any case, you don't have to wait for the penis to become erect on its own.

Again, almost all men who can't obtain an erection after radical prostatectomy still have normal penile sensation and are able to achieve a normal orgasm. *Even if you are not having erections—and even if you need some extra help—your recovery of sexual function is almost certain.* Take heart. As for the extra help you may need, there are five basic approaches, discussed below.

Loss of Potency After Radiation Therapy

Radiation's effect on potency is much more gradual than surgery's immediate impact. Sexual function may be fine immediately after radiation therapy. However, ED may develop gradually over the next one or two years. Radiation-induced ED affects between 10 percent and 70 percent of men; the range is broad because it depends on many things, including the definition of erectile function and the presence of other conditions known to affect erections—hypertension, diabetes, obesity, smoking, and sleep apnea, for example. Other factors are the type of radiation delivery and amount of radiation given, the use of hormonal therapy, and even the length of follow-up of a particular study. The slow, late progression of ED has been blamed on radiation damage to the arteries that provide blood to the penis. However, there is some recent evidence that radiation also may damage the neurovascular bundles, especially after brachytherapy; radiation also may cause venous leakage.

Also, not all men respond to medications such as sildenafil (Viagra), tadalafil (Cialis), avanafil (Stendra), and vardenafil (Levitra) after radiation for prostate cancer. A man's age, the dose of radiation, and whether he had hormonal therapy—and for how long—all play a role in determining how effective these pills can be in radiation-induced ED. In an effort to protect these delicate nerves and reduce the chances of ED, radiation oncologists are developing new ways to estimate the amount of radiation delivered to this area and, if possible, protect the neurovascular bundles with "nerve-sparing" techniques.

Solutions to the Problem of ED

Before we go any further, let's just say right here that some men have very little sexual activity before treatment for prostate cancer and frankly aren't that interested afterward. That's very common, particularly in older men, and there is absolutely nothing wrong with a man who is not concerned about having an erection.

However, many men who were very sexually active before treatment want this part of their lives to continue. What's next? The first thing that needs to happen is that you need to involve your partner. The worst thing you can do—take it from a doctor who has seen the unnecessarily devastating effect ED can have on patients' relationships—is to clam up; wrap yourself up in shame, self-pity, failure, anger, or any other negative emotion you can think of; retreat to a distant corner of the bed; sulk; agonize; and not talk to your partner about this. Your partner should understand what's going on and should be part of the solution.

Second, as mentioned above, experiment early (as soon as four weeks after surgery, sooner after radiation treatment). Anything you can do to bring new blood into the penis will speed up your recovery of spontaneous erections. Many men don't understand this. They don't want to use a crutch because they think it will slow down the body's own efforts to recover potency. This is hogwash. Think of it, if you will, as recovering from any other injury—a broken leg, for example. At first, crutches are necessary. Two of them. Then, as you get stronger, maybe you taper down to one crutch, then a cane. Then you walk, run, and join a marathon, if you wish. The same is true for sexual activity. Experiment early—with a tourniquet, O-ring, or elastic band, if necessary—and if you need more help, we suggest the following crutches, in this order:

- ED drugs—these are called phosphodiesterase type 5 (PDE5) inhibitors, and include sildenafil (Viagra), tadalafil (Cialis), avanafil (Stendra), and vardenafil (Levitra)
- Intraurethral therapy (MUSE)
- Vacuum erection devices
- Penile injection therapy: PGE1, papaverine, phentolamine
- Inflatable penile prostheses (penile implants)

We suggest you begin with a pharmacological approach—ED drugs, intraurethral therapy, or self-administered penile injection—because these truly bring new blood flow into the penis and are most likely to jump-start the spontaneous recovery of erections. Some men worry that if they start using some of these approaches, they will always need them—they'll become dependent on them, and spontaneous sexual activity will never return. *This couldn't be further from the truth. These approaches will actually speed up recovery by bringing blood flow to the penis.* Again, think of them as a crutch. Once spontaneous activity begins to recover, you can throw them away.

ED Drugs

PDE5 inhibitors, including sildenafil (Viagra), tadalafil (Cialis), avanafil (Stendra), and vardenafil (Levitra), are a remarkable breakthrough. Note: Although they are similar, these drugs are not identical, and one of them may turn out to be more effective for you than another. They work very well in many men after radiation therapy and in men after radical prostatectomy, too—but *only if the neurovascular bundles have been spared.* Investigators who report that ED drugs aren't terribly effective after radical prostatectomy are probably working with men who did not undergo an effective nerve-sparing operation.

ED drugs have been called wonder drugs. What does this mean? Will they put a spring in your step, revitalize your relationship, pay your bills, and generally solve all your problems? No. Are they instant erection pills? No. Contrary to the plots of some recent TV sitcoms, and despite many a comedian's monologue, taking one of these drugs is not followed by a hearty *"boing!"* Instead, to understand what happens, we need to take a brief look at the biochemistry of erection.

Several years ago, researchers discovered that the chemical messenger, or neurotransmitter, nitric oxide plays a crucial role in erection. We discussed this briefly above, but here are some of the nitty-gritty details. When a man is sexually stimulated, tiny nerve endings in the penis and the vascular endothelium (cells in the lining of blood vessels) release nitric oxide, which causes the smooth muscle tissue in the penis to relax and the blood vessels to dilate. If an erection, like every chemical process in the body, is a domino effect, or cascade of events, then nitric oxide is roughly step one. For the next link in the chain, nitric oxide activates another chemical switch, called cyclic GMP—known in scientific terms as the second messenger; this is the active agent within the blood vessels and smooth muscles that causes the dilation and relaxation. Here we might consider cyclic GMP to be the gasoline running the engine. How much cyclic GMP you have determines how strong your erection is and how long it lasts. Obviously, erections aren't meant to last forever, so there is also an off switch—another chemical, an enzyme called phosphodiesterase. Cyclic GMP is active in many organs of the body, and the off switch phosphodiesterase comes in many forms, each specifically targeted to various tissues. In the penis, the particular type of phosphodiesterase that's active is called type 5. ED drugs act by blocking the action of phosphodiesterase type 5 (which is why you may also see them referred to as PDE5 inhibitors). In this way, they amplify the action of whatever cyclic GMP is present.

Side Effects

Most ED drugs have little effect on other tissues in the body—except for Viagra, which can temporarily cause minor vision disturbances (a blue color is seen by 3 percent of men who take it). This is because

Viagra also affects phosphodiesterase type 6, which is in the cones of the retina. This side effect is temporary and does not cause any permanent damage.

The major problem with these drugs affects men who are taking a form of nitrate—nitroglycerin, for instance—for heart disease. *Men on nitroglycerin or similar medications should never take these drugs. Both ED drugs and nitroglycerin lower your blood pressure, and when taken together, they can lower it to a dangerous level. Also, men who are on an alpha blocker for the treatment of hypertension or men who have symptoms of BPH after radiation therapy should talk to their doctor about taking an ED drug, because these agents also lower blood pressure. The same goes for other drugs used to treat high blood pressure. Patients on these drugs should have stable blood pressure, and ED drugs should be initiated at the lowest dose.*

Otherwise, the list of side effects for these drugs is relatively modest. Most common are headaches (in 16 percent), flushing (in 10 percent), and an upset stomach (in 7 percent). Men also may experience muscle aches, back pain, and a runny nose. (Flushing is more common with Viagra, Stendra, and Levitra; muscle aches and back pain are primarily associated with Cialis and can be severe.)

How well do ED drugs work after radical prostatectomy? At Johns Hopkins, of men who are unable to have intercourse more than one year after an operation in which both neurovascular bundles were spared, 80 percent are able to have successful intercourse after treatment with an ED drug. But again, not only are these not instant erection pills, they may not even work very well in the first few months or even the first year after surgery. We think this is because the nerves are temporarily paralyzed. However, as these nerves recover, ED drugs work better and better. Thus, if you take an ED drug six weeks after surgery and it doesn't work, you should try again *multiple times a month until it does.* Note: If you have undergone surgery, PDE5 inhibitors will only work if you underwent a nerve-sparing radical prostatectomy.

Also, be sure you're taking it right. All these drugs begin to work within about twenty minutes. But if you take an ED drug with food, especially fatty food, this can delay stomach emptying, so the drug just trickles in small amounts into the small intestine and never reaches the high blood levels necessary to facilitate an erection. This problem is most evident with Viagra, less so with Levitra and Stendra, and not a problem with Cialis. The reason for this relates to each drug's length of action. The effect of Cialis can be felt for as long as thirty-six hours; thus, it lingers in the bloodstream for a long time. Levitra can last as long as eight hours. The most fleeting drug here is Viagra, which can last four hours, at most. Thus, for Viagra to work, it needs to reach a high level in the blood fairly quickly, and if there's fatty food in the stomach (or a big meal of any kind or one rich in dairy products), this just won't happen. If you're going to take Viagra on a full stomach, you might as well not take it at all; it's a waste. Viagra works best on an empty stomach. Then, it takes about an hour to reach its peak strength in the blood. At this point, a man needs to have sexual stimulation. (Remember, immediately after surgery, just thinking about sex isn't going to be enough. Sexual stimulation needs to be tactile.) Soaking in hot water increases blood flow in the pelvis; this might be a good way to spend the hour between the time you take Viagra and attempt intercourse. (This has also been reported to improve the effectiveness of MUSE—see below.) Remember, Viagra does not create an erection; it only facilitates one.

What Dose Should I Take, and When Should I Begin Taking It After Surgery?

As long as you have no contraindication (medical reason not to use a drug such as treatment with nitrates or an alpha blocker, discussed above), it makes sense to start out with the maximum dose. For Viagra, that's 100 milligrams; for Stendra, 200 milligrams; and for Levitra and Cialis, it's 20 milligrams. If the drug works at that dose but there are side effects, you can always try taking less. The most cost effective way to do this is to get a pill cutter (available at drugstores and at many online health stores) and just split the pills in half. The next question is, how often should you take it? Some doctors believe that you should take one of these every night or every other night for the first year after surgery. However, multiple randomized trials showed that the recovery of sexual function one year after surgery was the same in men who took a pill every night, men who took it only when they wanted to have sexual activity, and men who were on a placebo for the first nine months. Thus, in my opinion, it's up to you. I encourage patients who want to resume sexual activity soon after surgery to take these drugs only when they want to have intercourse. For patients in whom this is less important, or men who, because of expense or side effects do not want to take them, I feel that they are not compromising their long-term chances of recovering potency by waiting. However, there are many experts who disagree. They point out that there are many men who would benefit from aggressive rehabilitation using oral or injectable drugs more often. Certainly, if that is your wish, then you should try it.

Who Should Not Take ED Drugs?

If you have any history of cardiovascular disease, retinitis pigmentosa, or significant liver or kidney disease, talk to your internist or cardiologist before you take ED drugs. Despite the fact that they're mainly targeted at the penis, ED drugs are not safe for men with certain medical conditions.

Do not take Viagra, Cialis, Stendra, or Levitra if:

- You are taking any form of nitrate, such as nitroglycerin; or
- You have had an irregular heartbeat or heart attack in the last six months; or
- You have low blood pressure (lower than 90/50 mm Hg); or
- You have high blood pressure (greater than 170/110 mm Hg); or
- You have congestive heart failure or chest pain; or
- You have retinitis pigmentosa.

ED drugs are broken down by an enzyme in the liver. If you have severe liver dysfunction, the action of these drugs may be prolonged. Also, the breakdown of ED drugs can be delayed significantly by eating grapefruit or drinking grapefruit juice (or mixed juices containing grapefruit juice); and by taking drugs such as cimetidine (Tagamet), ketoconazole (Nizoral), erythromycin, or protease inhibitors such as ritonavir (Norvir) for the treatment of

HIV. If you fall into one of these categories, you must discuss the risks of taking an ED drug with your internist first.

Some men who have used ED drugs to have intercourse have had heart attacks and died. This is probably not a direct effect of the drug but was related to the exercise associated with intercourse. Many men who have heart disease do not exercise or don't exercise regularly. These are the weekend warriors who have heart attacks after exertion they're not accustomed to—playing pickup basketball, perhaps, or shoveling snow or moving heavy furniture. If these men have ED, they may rarely experience intercourse and the sexual excitement that goes with it. However, if ED drugs make them able to have intercourse and this causes them to exercise to a point where they shouldn't, this is probably the reason for the heart attacks. The safest bet for you is to talk to your doctor first. If you can't exercise or you have any other limitations on your physical activity, do not take an ED drug.

Which ED Drug Works Best?

There have been no good comparisons of all drugs done in a single study. It's safe to say that all of them are effective and that one drug may work better for one man and another for a different man. Indeed, it may be that there are genetic and physical variations that influence the way each man responds to and tolerates these drugs. Which one should you get? The best way to find out is to get samples of all from your urologist. Try each one to see which works best for you—and give each at least four chances. Just because it doesn't work the first time, you may find that in a different setting— possibly with less in your stomach, for instance—one may work better than another. Remember, "If at first you don't succeed, try, try again." There is evidence that it takes *three or four attempts* using the ED drugs before you may see the maximal benefit. We are fortunate to have four effective drugs to choose from.

WILL IT MAKE ME GO BLIND?

In 2005, a scary story made the news—a published study of about thirty men who developed blindness soon after taking sildenafil (Viagra). This frightened many men (and activated several personal-injury law firms, who advertised class-action lawsuits against Pfizer, the maker of Viagra, on the Internet). But this blindness occurred in thirty men out of about *twenty million* who had taken the drug. The study's investigators identified that this problem occurred *only* in men who had nonarteritic anterior ischemic optic neuropathy (NAION), which is the most common acute optic nerve disease in adults over age fifty. Its typical victims are people with other health complications—such as diabetes, hypertension, coronary artery disease, or hyperlipidemia—and people who smoke. These are the same risk factors for the development of ED.

If you are a smoker or if you have one of these conditions and are worried that you might be at risk for NAION, you should go to an ophthalmologist and be examined for the anatomical abnormality that leads to this problem; it's called low cup-to-disc ratio, or crowded disc. It is not known for certain whether taking Viagra absolutely caused the blindness in these thirty men or whether they would have developed it eventually because they had this abnormality and were at high risk. But if you turn out to have this predisposing factor, which may affect one or both eyes, you should seek your ophthalmologist's advice before you take an ED drug.

How Long Will I Have to Stay on an ED Drug?

In a study of men after radical prostatectomy who were taking Viagra, at three years, 71 percent were still responding to the drug. Of the remaining patients, half of the men stopped taking it because of the return of normal erections, and the other half stopped because the drug didn't seem to help anymore. These results suggest that the vast majority of men with erectile dysfunction after radical prostatectomy who initially respond to ED drugs continue to do so at three years and are satisfied with the effect. Again, the younger man who had no trouble with erections and who had both nerve bundles spared is going to do better than the man who is twenty years older who had one nerve bundle spared and who was having some ED before surgery—but if these drugs don't work for you, don't lose heart. Keep reading.

What Does the Future Hold for ED Treatment?

We've talked about why injury to the nerves that control erection can cause ED. A number of experimental studies currently under way are aimed at preserving these nerves. In animals, several studies have shown that growth factors and stem cells may enhance the recovery of nerve function more rapidly. There is also some exciting evidence that gene transfer may one day be used to transfer growth factors or even genes responsible for nerve function directly into the penis and boost nerve stimulation.

New methods of application are also being studied. Urologists at Johns Hopkins are investigating medications used to treat hypertension or anemia as potential drugs to improve penile blood flow and nerve function after radical prostatectomy. Clinical trials are under way.

Intraurethral Therapy

Another type of pharmacologic treatment is the use of agents that can be placed directly into the urethra. One of these is called MUSE (medicated urethral system for erection), a tiny suppository that contains a vasodilator called prostaglandin E1 (Alprostadil). The best thing about MUSE is that it's easy to administer. First, urinate (to empty and moisten the urethra). Then, place a suppository into the end of the urethra while you are standing. Then, massage the penis for fifteen minutes while the drug is absorbed; it may help to use a tourniquet at the base of the penis as well. MUSE works in about 40 percent of patients. However—and this is a big "however"—MUSE probably won't be ideal for many men after radical prostatectomy. For some reason, prostaglandin E1 often causes severe pain or burning in the penis in men who have undergone a radical prostatectomy. But men who have ED for other reasons (including ED after radiation therapy) do not experience such pain as often, and for these men, it can be a valuable resource. That said, a survey taken by the American Urological Association showed that MUSE is at the very bottom of the list of ED therapies: PDE5 inhibitors are number one, then the vacuum erection device, then injection therapy.

Penile Injection Therapy

Intracavernosal injection (ICI) therapy is one of the best ways to bring new blood flow into the penis and encourage the recovery of sexual function. If PDE5 inhibitors are not working for you, then ICI is the logical next step, because it is the most natural of all ED pharmacotherapies. Also, men who are motivated can start it as early as six weeks after surgery. Ideally, you won't need this forever—consider it a crutch or a jump-start, as described above, until your body recovers enough to handle erection on its own.

How does it work? The keys to a normal erection are for the arteries to open and fill the penis with blood and then for the veins to close so the blood can't escape the penis. The smooth muscle tissue also needs to relax. Several drugs can produce erections by making these events happen; some of these are in a class of drugs called alpha-blockers, which are used to treat some forms of hypertension and also to treat benign prostatic hyperplasia (BPH). The other medications are direct vasodilators; they cause the penile arteries to dilate, which opens up the erectile tissue, making a wider channel for blood to go through. They also cause the smooth muscle tissue to relax and the veins to close. The main advantage here is that these drugs produce an absolutely normal erection using a man's natural erectile machinery. These drugs—papaverine (Pavabid), phentolamine (Regitine), and prostaglandin E1 (Alprostadil, the same medication in MUSE)—can be administered in combination to cause an erection.

It usually takes less than ten minutes for one of these drugs to work, and the erection can last as long as a couple of hours. It will be important for your doctor to determine the lowest possible dose you need to achieve an erection; this will help reduce the risk of side effects. Other ways to help lessen side effects include limiting injections to no more than once a day and using an insulin syringe (which has a smaller needle than many syringes) to minimize pain and bleeding from the injection site. Also, you should compress the site where the needle went in for about two minutes after the injection; this also helps reduce bleeding and tissue damage.

Again, a common side effect for men after radical prostatectomy is that prostaglandin E1 treatment is often very painful. These men should ask their physician to prescribe a different blend of injection, called Bi-mix or Tri-Mix, which contains papaverine, phentolamine, and smaller amounts of prostaglandin E1. This may reduce the pain considerably.

Penile injection is not for everybody. These erection-producing agents may not help men with vascular problems. However, they do work in patients. Because of the nature of this therapy—giving the penis a shot—it obviously is not ideal for men who can't see well, men with poor hand-eye coordination, or men who are very overweight. However, a man's partner can learn how to inject the drugs into the penis. Also, because many erection-producing drugs reduce blood pressure, this therapy can cause problems for some men with heart disease.

One side effect is that if the injection is too strong, it can produce a prolonged erection (this is called priapism) that may require medical therapy to be relieved. Some doctors ask patients who opt for penile injections to sign a consent form because of some other side effects—some of them long term—associated with the injections. These can include tiny blood clots, burning pain after injection, damage to the urethra, or minor infection. But the worst is that in some men, over time, painless, fibrous knots of tissue build up in the corpora cavernosa, which can cause the penis to become curved. (This condition, also called Peyronie's disease, is discussed in this chapter.) Doctors aren't entirely sure why this happens; the medications themselves may cause fibrosis, or it may be related to the frequency of injection, the strength or dosage of the drug used, and the amount of bleeding resulting from the shots. Some doctors believe compressing the site at the time of injection may be critical to minimizing this risk; also, keeping the dosage to a minimum or using a blend of several drugs may help.

Vacuum Erection Devices

The idea here is to create suction using an airtight tube that is placed temporarily around the penis. An attached pump withdraws air, creating reduced atmospheric pressure—a vacuum—around the penis, causing it to become engorged with blood. The penis becomes erect. Then a constricting ring, like a rubber band around the neck of a balloon, keeps the blood trapped in the penis so the erection can be sustained. (This imitates the clamping action of the veins in normal erection.) It usually takes about five minutes to produce the erection, and it generally lasts for about half an hour. (The erection probably shouldn't last much longer than that; leaving the constricting band on too long can cause distention or swelling due to fluid retention in the penis.)

This erection is not quite the same as a normal erection—it begins only above the constricting band. But it is sufficient for successful intercourse. However, the penis is usually cold and sometimes numb, and from the man's standpoint, the erection is often less than desirable because the rigidity is poor. Also, because this approach does not bring new blood flow into the penis, it may not do much to facilitate the recovery process. Vacuum devices have few complications; these can include trouble with ejaculation, pain in the penis, and tiny, pinpoint-sized bruises. (Men taking aspirin or other blood-thinning medications may be more likely to experience such complications.) Some men are highly satisfied with the result of vacuum devices; the majority are not. However, there is some evidence that, if used early on as part of your recovery, they will prevent mild penile length loss following surgery.

Penile Prostheses (Implants)

Penile implants, or prostheses, are available in several varieties; the simplest are malleable, and the more sophisticated ones are inflatable or mechanical. The implants are not a new idea, but they have improved considerably since they were first introduced more than fifty years ago. The malleable prostheses, for example, were exactly the same size all the time—whether or not the penis was in the erect position—which, as you can imagine, often proved awkward in social settings. Earlier models of the inflatable prostheses that did allow for a nonerect size sometimes failed to work and needed to be replaced.

If these relatively clumsy but functional early designs were the prosthetic equivalent of the typewriter, then the latest models are more like a smart phone—sleek, sophisticated, and user-friendly. They are more reliable and designed to look more natural in the nonerect phase. *And they can restore sexual function entirely to normal.*

Most prostheses are implanted into the penis through an incision in the scrotum. A three-piece penile prosthesis is an inflatable implant available in a variety of models and sizes for a custom fit. Each consists of a reservoir implanted above the bladder, a pump placed in the scrotum, and a pair of cylinders implanted in the penis. The entire device is totally concealed in the body. The man is able to inflate the prosthesis by using a pump that is placed in the scrotum. Fluid is pumped into the penis to create an erection and is held there by a valve. Afterward, when the man is finished with intercourse, the valve is released, and the fluid returns to the reservoir. Most men report that it feels like a normal erection, expands the girth of the penis, and provides the rigidity necessary for intercourse. Sensation is completely normal. Note: Contrary to what many men believe, these implants do not make the penis longer; in fact the biggest complaint following implantation is less penile length.

Penile prostheses used to be offered routinely to most men with ED. Now, with oral medications and other good treatments available, many urologists have come to regard penile prostheses as a last resort because they do involve surgery—and thus they carry the risk of complications. These can include infection, scarring, damage within the corpora cavernosa, or a problem with any part of the prosthesis. However, these side effects are relatively rare. *Most men who have penile prostheses are satisfied with the result and have a normal sex life.*

Testosterone Replacement After Radical Prostatectomy or Radiation Therapy

Low testosterone, or hypogonadism, occurs in older men; it can also occur after a man has a radical prostatectomy. Restoring testosterone levels to the normal physiological range with testosterone replacement therapy can improve a man's mood, energy level, and sexual function. However, the relationship between testosterone and promotion of prostate cancer has led most urologists to hesitate before replacing testosterone, because of the fear that this may cause prostate cancer progression or put men at risk of developing distant metastatic disease.

Good news: To date, there is no direct evidence that restoring testosterone levels to the normal range increases the recurrence of prostate cancer in men who have undergone a radical prostatectomy and have an undetectable PSA level. Consequently, for patients who clearly have low testosterone levels (less than 200 ng/100 ml) and who are not at a high risk of having their cancer return, I advise topical (not injectable) replacement with careful monitoring of testosterone levels to make certain they remain in the physiologic range.

Prostate cancer is tough on everybody. Wives and partners feel the stress of prostate cancer and treatment, too. You're all sharing the burden of this disease. Your priorities change, your focus shifts, and your usual best lifeline—each other—may temporarily flag from the physical and emotional stress. The worst thing you can do during this recovery process is try to go it alone. The best thing you can do is talk about it with each other, your doctor, other patients and their partners, a counselor, or a member of the clergy. And go back and read this chapter over again, as many times as you need to, because it is full of hope. Be patient. You *will* get your life back.

12

HORMONAL THERAPY/ ANDROGEN DEPRIVATION THERAPY (ADT)

This chapter was written with expert opinion from Michael A. Carducci, M.D.

THE SHORT STORY:
The Highly Abridged Version of This Chapter

Do you need hormonal therapy? Doctors use hormonal therapy to treat prostate cancer in four specific clinical situations:

- In men with localized disease as a first line of treatment. We strongly discourage the use of hormonal therapy in this case. There are two effective ways to cure cancer that is confined to the prostate, both discussed earlier in this book: surgery and radiation therapy. Hormonal therapy does not cure prostate cancer, and *should not be used as a primary treatment.*
- In men with locally advanced disease, in combination with radiation therapy for a finite period.
- In men who have a rising PSA level after primary treatment with surgery or radiation.
- In men with metastatic disease.

In this chapter, we will help you understand how hormonal therapy works, what it can and can't do, its side effects, and when you should consider starting it.

HORMONAL THERAPY/ANDROGEN DEPRIVATION THERAPY (ADT)

The mainstay for the management of advanced disease is hormonal therapy, also called androgen deprivation therapy (ADT)—shutting down the hormones that feed the prostate and nourish the cancer. Unfortunately, some prostate cancer cells aren't affected by hormonal therapy at all. These are called hormone-resistant (or androgen-independent) cells.

When a man with metastatic disease starts ADT, the early results are successful and highly encouraging: the tumor shrinks, prostate-specific antigen (PSA) levels drop in the blood, and the patient feels better. This remission may last for many years, but it is only a partial victory; only the hormone-dependent cancer cells have been affected, and the drop in PSA level may be misleading. Here, when PSA falls, it signals that the cancer is responding to treatment—which is good—but it is not a guarantee that the cancer is completely gone. The cancer cells that have nothing to do with hormones are unaffected by ADT.

There are several forms of ADT, which can be used individually or in combination. They are all designed to accomplish the same goal: to lower testosterone levels in the blood or block the effects of testosterone at the target organ. The most direct and least expensive way to control testosterone is to surgically remove a man's testicles; this is called an orchiectomy, or surgical castration. The same effect can be accomplished medically, with drugs called LHRH (luteinizing hormone-releasing hormone) agonists, LHRH antagonists, or antiandrogens. For obvious reasons, this is the more popular approach. Recent studies indicate that some men with metastatic disease benefit from the combination of ADT plus abiraterone (Zytiga) or chemotherapy.

WHEN SHOULD YOU BEGIN ADT?

If you have metastases to bone, bone pain, or a large mass of cancer that is obstructing your kidneys or bladder, you need to start ADT *right now*. In this situation, it is the right course of action—one that can make a huge difference in your quality of life and can protect your body from the ravages of cancer.

But what if you have no cancer in your bones and no sign that anything is wrong except a rising PSA level after surgery or radiation, or the presence of cancer in your lymph nodes, and you feel fine? Many doctors would advise you to start hormonal therapy as soon as possible. Others—and I'm in this group—believe that in most cases there is no evidence that starting hormonal therapy immediately, as opposed to later, will prolong life. Hormonal therapy does two things. It stops cells from making PSA, and it shrinks the hormone-sensitive cell population; a man's PSA falls, and it takes longer for his bone scan to become positive for metastases. But it doesn't stop the clock; the hormone-insensitive cells keep right on growing silently, and you may need additional treatments to help keep them in check.

Revolution in Treating Advanced Prostate Cancer

The mainstay for the management of advanced disease today is hormonal therapy. (Note: Androgens are male hormones, and many doctors use these two words interchangeably. This may be confusing; hormonal therapy is also called hormone or androgen deprivation therapy [ADT], or hormonal or androgen ablation.) But before we begin to talk about it, let us add that all of us who treat prostate cancer hope that this will not be the case forever—or even for very many more years. Obviously, the best thing would be to prevent prostate cancer from ever developing. We're not there yet. The next best thing would be to catch it in every man while it's still confined to the prostate, and to cure it with surgery or radiation. And the next best thing after that would be to find a way to stop the cancer, to starve whatever feeds it, to keep it from spreading—or, if it has spread, to kill it where it lies. One thought is that we might control prostate cancer as we do diabetes and heart disease—with some form of daily medication to keep it in check. Another thought is that we might be able to treat it for a time with a medical version of the weed killer Roundup—kill the cancer by preventing it from getting nourishment—and then not even need to use further medication. (We will talk about some promising drugs that work along both of these lines, along with many others, in the next chapter.) Still another avenue of much hope is that new drugs will be able to overcome the cancer-caused stupor of the body's immune system, and will unleash its formidable power to fight off cancer. With these scenarios, men would not need long-term hormonal therapy. And doctors would rejoice right alongside their patients.

Nobody likes hormonal therapy. But we prescribe it because it works. For some men, it can work for many years—even decades. Hormonal therapy means shutting down the hormones that feed the prostate and sustain the cancer.

Why does it work? Prostate cells need male hormones to grow and develop—think of a houseplant that flourishes because it receives a steady supply of fertilizer. If the supply of hormones is shut off, the normal prostate shrinks but does not disappear. If a houseplant doesn't get fertilizer, it doesn't die, either. It might struggle along on nothing but sunlight and water, but it still hangs in there. Normal prostate cells can survive without hormones, and so can cancerous prostate cells. Not having the hormones is a setback—one from which it can take years for prostate cancer to recover—but it's not a lethal blow. In fact, some prostate cancer cells aren't affected by hormonal therapy at all.

Why doesn't ADT serve as a knockout punch for prostate cancer? Because prostate cancer is *heterogeneous*, which means it's a cellular melting pot. It's a bunch of different cell types mixed together. When all of these cells are confined within the prostate, the fact that they're not all alike is not much of an issue. No matter how many different kinds of cells there may be, if they're all in the prostate, they're all equally dead when the prostate is surgically removed or effectively irradiated. But when some cancer cells have escaped to distant sites, this diversity becomes a major challenge. A drug or hormone treatment that targets only one kind of cell won't have any effect against another variety; the one-size-fits-all approach doesn't work here. Plus, some of these cells have learned to be resistant—to grow in the absence of male hormones. These are called androgen-independent or androgen-insensitive cells. Cancer that seems to defy hormonal therapy is called castrate- (or castration-)resistant prostate cancer (CRPC) or hormone-refractory disease.

When a man with metastatic disease starts ADT, the early results are successful and highly encouraging: the tumor shrinks, the PSA level drops in the blood, and the patient feels better. But this is only a partial victory, because *only the hormone-dependent cancer cells have been affected*, so the drop in PSA may be misleading. Guess what controls the production of PSA? Hormones. When male hormones are shut off, the PSA-making process may indeed stop, but this doesn't necessarily mean that the cancer cells are dead or that they've stopped growing. In animal models, scientists have shown that cancer cells can continue to grow even when PSA is no longer made. One process has little to do with another; in fact, the nastiest, most malignant cells don't make much PSA anyway. So when the PSA level falls, it signals that the cancer is responding to treatment—which is good—but it is not a guarantee that the cancer is completely gone.

The cancer cells that have nothing to do with hormones just go on about their merry, proliferative business, oblivious to the hormonal war being fought just cells away. Say you had a weed problem in your garden, and instead of spraying Roundup, you sprayed Raid. What effect would this have on the weeds? Not a lot.

Scientists believe that these androgen-independent cells probably inhabit the prostate for years; they don't suddenly appear one day after the cancer is diagnosed. Ultimately, the androgen-independent cells manage to dominate through different means. One of these is called *genetic drift*. In this case, each time the cancer cells reproduce, or divide, they accumulate more mutations and become increasingly malignant. In the process, cells that used to depend on hormones manage to wean themselves; they learn to survive without them. Another mechanism is called *clonal selection*. Here the most malignant cells (which originally may have been in the minority) grow faster than the better-differentiated, more sedate cells. Over time, they overtake these more normal cells. This may actually be aided, inadvertently, by ADT: the androgen-dependent cells shrink back, and the androgen-independent cells take their place.

Androgen Deprivation Therapy (ADT)

Specific Ways to Control Hormones

Doctors have long known that hormones play a major role in the life of the prostate. In 1786, a British surgeon named John Hunter became the first to demonstrate in animals that a radical operation—castration—caused the sex accessory tissues, including the prostate, to shrink. But it wasn't until the 1930s that anyone discovered *why* this happened. At the University of Chicago, Charles Huggins discovered that removing the testes shut down production of testosterone. And when shots of testosterone were injected into castrated animals, shrunken sex accessory tissues were restored to normal size and function. This Nobel Prize–winning research resulted in another valuable finding—that castration also could shrink prostate cancer.

Huggins was able to achieve the same effect chemically; he found he could shut down testosterone with doses of female hormones called estrogens. Estrogens blocked a signal transmitted in the brain by the pituitary gland called *luteinizing hormone (LH)*, which stimulates testosterone. The oral estrogen, called diethylstilbestrol (DES), produces what's known as chemical castration; it lowers testosterone levels, just as removal of the testicles does.

For now, hormonal therapy, or ADT, means one of two main choices: surgical castration, a one-shot treatment; or chemical castration, a lifetime of medication. Loss of sexual function is likely with almost every kind of hormonal therapy; 90 percent of men on hormonal therapy lose sexual drive and the ability to have an erection.

What's the best method of stopping these male hormones? Think of a car going through a series of checkpoints—points A, B, C, and D—to cross over a border into another country. You want to stop this car from reaching the other side. At what point do you stop it? Do you set up a roadblock at point A, the first stop? Or do you wall off the border at point D, so the car can never cross over? Or do you divert the car at some point along the way? The androgens that affect the prostate reach their destination through a multistep process that begins in the brain. Medical roadblocks are now available to stop or detour this process at point A (the brain), point D (the prostate), or several spots in between.

How ADT Works

Each therapy targets a different link in the chain of hormonal interactions that affect the prostate. Some of them work better than others, and some are more expensive. The chain of hormonal actions is long and complicated; put down on paper, it's a confusing jumble of letters that looks like alphabet soup. And if you're like most men, just thinking about this muddle will make your eyes glaze over. But, stripped down to its essential steps, this code is not so tough to crack—you can do it! (And you need to master this information so you can not only understand what your doctor's talking about, but help choose the treatment option that's best for you. See fig. 12.1.)

To understand this hormonal chain, let's start at the beginning—the brain, where the hypothalamus makes, among other things, a substance called luteinizing hormone–releasing hormone (LHRH), which acts as a chemical signal. It's dispatched in pulses, like Morse code or flashes of light, to the nearby pituitary gland. Its message? "Make LH and FSH."

Luteinizing hormone (LH) and follicle-stimulating hormone (FSH) are other chemical signals, and they bring us to the testicles, or testes, where LH motivates certain cells (called testicular Leydig cells) to make testosterone. (FSH has its major effect on sperm production.)

And testosterone brings us to the prostate. Testosterone circulates in the blood and enters the prostate by diffusion, like water through a tea bag. Soon it undergoes a metamorphosis: testosterone is transformed by an enzyme called 5-alpha reductase into a hormone called dihydrotestosterone (DHT)—which is more than twice as powerful as testosterone. Several studies have shown that the prostate contains less 5-alpha reductase when it is cancerous; therefore, DHT is not believed to be as important in prostate cancer as it is in the normal prostate or in benign enlargement of the prostate (BPH). Both testosterone and DHT can bind to the same receptor in the prostate cell, like two different keys fitting the same lock. (DHT *really* binds to it with great affinity; testosterone does not cling as strongly to the receptor.) When DHT or testosterone hooks up to the receptor, this complex attaches to DNA, which then activates certain genes.

Testosterone in the blood circulates back to point A, the hypothalamus, which acts as a thermostat. It measures the level of testosterone and decides whether to boost or cut back on its LHRH production, and the cycle begins all over again; scientists call this a feedback loop.

Meanwhile, the adrenal glands, which sit on top of the kidneys, also make weak male hormones called adrenal androgens, including androstenedione, dehydroepiandrosterone (DHEA), and dehydroepiandrosterone sulfate (DHEAS), plus small amounts of testosterone. These are minor players, believed to make up only 5 percent or less of the total androgen stimulation to the prostate. Their total effect on the prostate has been a controversial issue (see below).

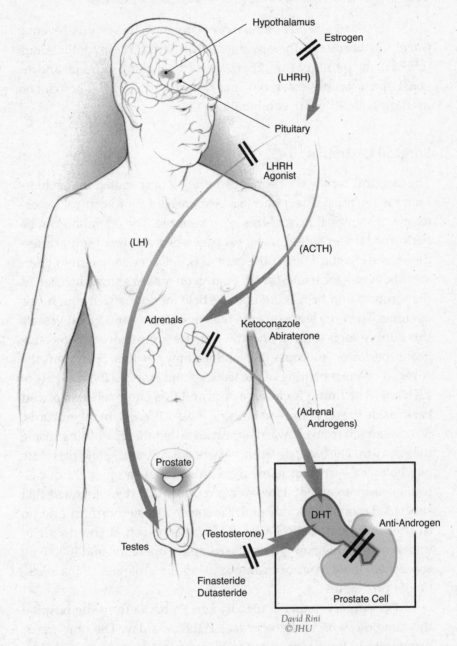

FIGURE 12.1 Where Men Make Hormones and Where Hormonal Therapies Actually Work

There are drugs that block either the effect of testosterone and other androgens (anti-androgens, dutasteride, and finasteride) or the production of testosterone itself (LHRH agonists, estrogens, abiraterone, and ketoconazole).

So there are several potential checkpoints in this chain of events. Currently, hormonal therapy agents can target the hypothalamus (LHRH), the pituitary (LH, FSH), the adrenal gland (adrenal androgens), the testes (testosterone), and the prostate (DHT). They can be used individually or in combination.

Surgical Castration

The surgical removal of a man's testicles (also called an orchiectomy) is the most direct and least expensive way to control testosterone. As surgical procedures go, it's simple. The operation can be performed under spinal anesthesia (for a description of spinal anesthesia, see chapter 8) or, if the patient is not strong enough to tolerate this, even a local anesthetic. A surgeon makes a small incision in the scrotum and brings out each testicle individually through this opening. Then the surgeon cuts the vas deferens and blood vessels that supply each testicle, and the testicles are removed. Some surgeons perform "subcapsular" orchiectomy. In this operation, the surgeon opens the lining of the testicles and empties the contents of each one. The lining is closed again, and this empty shell is placed back inside the scrotum—so nothing looks different; in other words, no one can tell from outward appearance that there's nothing inside the scrotum. The basic differences here are cosmetic—and therefore psychological—and for some men, this makes the thought of castration easier to accept. However, a recent study demonstrated that subcapsular orchiectomy's ability to lower testosterone is inferior to treatment with an LHRH agonist. For this reason, if you decide to undergo an orchiectomy, have the complete operation and if you are concerned about your appearance ask your urologist to place testicular prostheses.

After surgery, patients usually can go home from the hospital the same day—or, at the very latest, the next day. The only major complication to worry about with surgical castration is bleeding. However, this shouldn't be a problem if the surgeon makes a point of checking that all bleeding is stopped before the scrotum is closed and that a compression dressing is left in place to control the smaller, harder-to-see blood vessels.

Castration works fast; it reduces the body's amount of testosterone by 95 percent almost immediately and permanently. Within about three hours of surgery, testosterone levels begin to plummet to a level called the *castrate range*. This is considered the gold standard, an important point of comparison in monitoring the success of hormonal therapy, as certain drugs are judged by their ability to reduce testosterone to this range.

Some doctors used to believe that several months after castration, the body began producing more testosterone at other sites—and that this was the reason prostate cancer continued to grow. This is not true. There is no delayed increase in testosterone and, anyway, that's not why prostate tumors keep growing. They continue to spread because of the cancer cells that are *not* affected by hormones.

What happens to the prostate tumor? It begins to shrink, and men with symptoms of obstruction or pain caused by the cancer begin to feel better right away.

Castration's advantages are that it is effective almost immediately and its results are permanent—there's no need to take daily medication. And, because it is a one-shot treatment, it's relatively inexpensive.

Specific Side Effects

Its disadvantages are certainly psychological (this can vary, depending on a man's age and stage of illness) and cosmetic. Testicular implants—which make the scrotum appear normal—are available for some men. However, castration is irreversible, and for many men this is too final a treatment. (For a discussion of the general side effects of hormonal therapy, see below.)

Medical Castration

Medical castration can be accomplished in three ways: by shutting down the hypothalamic-pituitary connection (see page 389), by directly blocking the ability of the testicles to make testosterone, or by blocking the effects of testosterone at the target organ—the prostate (see fig. 12.1).

Drugs That Shut Down the Hypothalamic-Pituitary Connection

Estrogens

Many men, for many reasons, don't want to undergo surgical castration, so they opt for drugs that accomplish the same result. DES, the main oral estrogen, targets a different checkpoint—the hypothalamus. It works by blocking the release of LHRH. In turn, the pituitary stops making LH, and this virtually shuts down the Leydig cells, the testicles' testosterone-making factories. So testosterone drops to the castrate range.

The effect is not as speedy as with surgical castration; it generally takes ten to fourteen days for testosterone to fall to the castrate range. And it's not permanent—in most cases, the testicles start making testosterone again soon after a man stops taking DES.

We talk about DES here because it's the most widely used oral estrogen, and it's the gold standard of estrogen therapy (but no longer the mainstay of ADT) for prostate cancer. Other compounds, such as conjugated estrogens (Premarin) and ethinyl estradiol (both used for estrogen replacement by women during menopause) have been used, although they are not considered as effective as DES. A drug called polyestradiol phosphate (Estradurin), used mainly in Europe, is injected once a month and may be easier to tolerate for men with gastrointestinal problems. Another drug, called chlorotrianisene (Tace), is a synthetic estrogen that lowers testosterone but doesn't completely shut down its production; it also permits the body to make a little bit of LH. Because its estrogenic activity is weak, it requires large doses to be effective. For this and other reasons, we no longer use Tace as a treatment for prostate cancer.

Twenty-five years ago, oral estrogens—easy to administer and much cheaper than other forms of treatment—were the foundation of medical treatment for advanced prostate cancer. They aren't today, mainly because of their major, potentially fatal side effect—they raise your risk of having a heart attack or developing a blood clot. European physicians use Estradurin in hopes of lowering these risks. Some physicians believe that the clotting complications of oral estrogens happen because the hormones are absorbed by the intestine and metabolized in the liver. This can be avoided when the injectable form of the drug is used, because the body processes it differently. However, the efficacy and safety of Estradurin compared with DES were never well established, and the drug was never widely used. Even efforts to make estrogen easier to tolerate—delivering it in a skin patch, for instance, to minimize nausea and vomiting—have not proven worthwhile (see below).

Other Specific Side Effects

Estrogens cause painful enlargement of the breasts, a condition called gynecomastia. This problem can be minimized, however, with one to three low-dose treatments of radiation given directly to the breast *before estrogens are started*. Edema (water retention, which causes swelling in the ankles and legs) is also common and may complicate problems in men with heart disease and high blood pressure; however, this swelling can be reduced significantly with diuretics. Some physicians also recommend that their patients on DES take an aspirin every day to help them avoid other cardiovascular side effects, such as thrombophlebitis (blood clots in the legs), and to lower the risk of this clot migrating to the lungs (this is called a pulmonary embolism) or heart. Because of the risk of cardiovascular problems, men with a history of heart disease or thrombophlebitis should not use estrogens as their main form of treatment. Also, older men (over age seventy-five) do not tolerate them well. (For a discussion of the general side effects of ADT, see below.) Estrogens can also cause thinning of the skin and the loss of body hair, including facial hair.

LHRH Agonists

Like oral estrogens, LHRH agonists shut down the production of LH and FSH. Here's how they work: LHRH is a small protein, built of ten blocks of amino acid. A synthetic substance called an LHRH analog, or agonist, made by changing one of the ten blocks, works by blocking LH (the hormone that tells the testicles to make testosterone). The hypothalamus acts like a lighthouse, sending out LHRH in signal pulses—like Morse code in flashes of light—to the pituitary gland. LHRH *agonists* work by providing prolonged signals—by turning on the light and keeping it on instead of just sending flashes. So these drugs trick the pituitary; because the pituitary receives no flashes, or pulses, it thinks no signal is being sent, and it doesn't make LH. In turn, the testicles do not produce testosterone.

These drugs don't work right away. In fact, for about a week after a man begins taking an LHRH agonist, his testosterone level kicks into overdrive. This is called a flare, and it happens because the constant LHRH signal initially stimulates LH production. But after about ten days, testosterone falls into the castrate range. For the first few weeks, doctors often prescribe an antiandrogen, bicalutamide (Casodex), to block this surge.

A new class of compounds known as LHRH antagonists do not produce this brief testosterone flare and cause a faster reduction in testosterone than the LHRH agonists. (However, if an antiandrogen is given along with an LHRH agonist, the net effect is the same.) Two such agents, abarelix (Plenaxis) and degarelix (Firmagon), have been approved by the FDA. These agents are best suited for the man who needs treatment as soon as possible—to treat spinal cord compression, for example. Otherwise, given the requirement for monthly injections, most patients are eventually switched over to LHRH agonists. Some investigators claim that the antagonists are more effective in suppressing testosterone consistently to a low level, and that they have fewer cardiovascular side effects. Although these observations have yet to be confirmed in clinical trials, men who have heart disease may prefer treatment with an LHRH antagonist.

The most commonly prescribed LHRH agonists are leuprolide (Lupron, Eligard), goserelin (Zoladex), and triptorelin (Trelstar). In large studies, researchers have found that these LHRH agonists are equivalent to treatment with DES or surgical castration in their ability to lengthen the time until the cancer progresses and to prolong survival.

To Sum Up

LHRH agonists are basically equivalent to DES and to surgical castration in testosterone-lowering and life span–lengthening results. Their chief advantages are that they negate the need for surgery and don't carry the risk of cardiovascular complications that can accompany estrogen treatment. Also, they don't cause breast swelling as often as treatment with estrogens.

Specific Side Effects

LHRH analogs require an injection. Long-acting agents need to be injected either monthly or every three or four months, and new pumps have been developed that dispense medication for a whole year. However, they must be implanted, and this requires a small incision to be made, under local anesthesia. Other disadvantages include the tremendous expense—LHRH agonists cost thousands of dollars a year. (For a discussion of the general side effects of ADT, see below.)

Drugs That Block the Effects of Hormones at the Prostate

Antiandrogens

These drugs don't care how much LHRH, LH, testosterone, or DHT you make; it doesn't matter to them. (Actually, antiandrogens cause testosterone levels to go *up* because of an increase in LH.) All they do is make sure testosterone and DHT don't reach their targets—the receptors. In other words, antiandrogens act as dummy keys in the "locks," or receptors. When testosterone and DHT reach the receptors, there's already a key sitting in the lock, so they can't enter the lock and activate the receptors. Therefore, the tumor doesn't get the hormones it needs to nourish its androgen-dependent cells.

Bicalutamide (Casodex), flutamide (Eulexin), and nilutamide (Nilandron) are the most widely used antiandrogens. Casodex and Nilandron are given once a day, while Eulexin requires two tablets, three times a day. Because of this (and also because it has more side effects, including diarrhea and liver abnormalities), Eulexin is rarely used today. In Europe, cyproterone acetate (Androcur, Procur) is also common. (This drug, however, acts like estrogen, and rather than stimulating testosterone, it actually suppresses the hypothalamic-pituitary connection, so it lowers LH, thus reducing testosterone.) The newest agent in this class is enzalutamide (Xtandi). It is normally reserved for the treatment of men with castrate- (or castration-)resistant prostate cancer (CRPC; see chapter 13).

Originally, antiandrogens were used for specific reasons in combination with other treatments. For example, their most common use, even today, is to block the surge, or flare, of testosterone that occurs during the first week or ten days after treatment with an LHRH agonist. (To stop this surge, antiandrogens are usually given for the first month of treatment with an LHRH agonist.) Antiandrogens also have been given to men who needed more urgent treatment—men who came to the doctor with severe bone pain, for example, or who had large, local cancers that were obstructing urinary flow. Treatment with an antiandrogen immediately blocks the effect of testosterone and brings relief to men who are awaiting either surgical castration or for an LHRH agonist to achieve its full effect. They also have been administered chronically in combination with castration or an LHRH agonist—a form of treatment called combined androgen blockade (see below).

More recently, however, doctors have become interested in using antiandrogens, especially bicalutamide, as monotherapy—that is, as a single agent, without any other form of treatment. The main goal here is to attempt to preserve sexual function. When bicalutamide is given in doses of 50 milligrams, three times a day, sexual interest is maintained in many men; however, beyond one year, only about 20 percent of men remain potent. This 150 milligram daily dose of bicalutamide has been used in men with various stages of prostate cancer. For men with metastatic disease, it is less effective than an LHRH agonist and should not be used as a substitute. In men who don't have metastatic disease, there is a major red flag. Although bicalutamide at this dose was never approved for use in the United States, it was in other countries. However, in England and Canada, the license for this use was withdrawn. This was based on the findings of a study in which men with localized disease were randomly assigned either to receive a placebo or to receive 150 milligrams of bicalutamide a day. More men in the bicalutamide group died—25 percent versus 20 percent of the men taking the placebo. The reason for this is unclear, but (as we will discuss later) this study's results are similar to the long-term findings of the Medical Research Council study. The newest agents in this class are enzalutamide (Xtandi) and apalutamide (Erleada). They are normally reserved for the treatment of men with castrate- (or castration-)resistant prostate cancer (CRPC; see chapter 13).

Thus, men with metastatic disease should not be treated with antiandrogen monotherapy. However, for men who start taking antiandrogens when they have locally advanced disease, the survival rate appears to be about the same. Thus, there is great interest in using these drugs in men with advanced cancer that has not yet metastasized to bone. Note: As we will discuss later in this chapter, no form of early hormonal therapy really prevents prostate cancer from progressing. The only thing it delays is your knowledge of this progression.

Specific Side Effects

In addition to allowing men to maintain sexual interest, antiandrogens appear to have a lower risk of osteoporosis than surgical castration or treatment with LHRH agonists, most likely because testosterone levels are maintained. Both bicalutamide and flutamide cause breast enlargement in about 75 percent of the men who take them. If you are advised to take one of these drugs as monotherapy, insists on breast radiation *before* beginning the agent; if not you will likely develop breast enlargement that will not reverse if the drug is discontinued. Flutamide's major side effect is diarrhea. Also, it can cause significant liver damage in some men; therefore, it's a good idea for men taking flutamide to have their liver function checked after the first few months of treatment.

Conclusion

The fact that men can retain sexual interest makes antiandrogens the focus of intense research—specifically, scientists are investigating combining these drugs with others in hopes of improving quality of life in men undergoing hormonal therapy. However, the use of high-dose antiandrogens as the only form of hormonal therapy for prostate cancer has not yet been approved in the United States. We need to understand the reason for the higher risk of death in men who receive 150 milligrams a day of bicalutamide before patients can safely consider this option.

5-Alpha Reductase Inhibitors

In prostate cells, testosterone is converted by the enzyme, 5-alpha reductase, into a more potent hormone, DHT. Five-alpha reductase inhibitors—drugs such as finasteride (Proscar) and dutasteride (Avodart)—block this enzyme. Their big advantage is that they preserve potency, because testosterone levels in the blood remain unchanged.

These drugs work well in shrinking BPH, in which DHT plays a major role. But in prostate cancer, testosterone is more of a villain than DHT, and finasteride and dutasteride do little to stop it. So by themselves, 5-alpha reductase inhibitors are not enough. Some scientists are investigating whether these drugs may prove more effective when combined with an antiandrogen.

Drugs That Inhibit the Production of Testosterone

One of the first drugs in this class, ketoconazole (Nizoral), got its start as an antifungal agent. Then doctors noticed that men taking it developed breast enlargement—clearly, more than fungal problems were being treated here! Doctors learned that ketoconazole blocks the production of testosterone by the testicles as well as androgens by the adrenal glands. It works quickly; taking 400 milligrams of ketoconazole every eight hours reduces testosterone to the castrate range within twenty-four hours. Because ketoconazole also blocks the production of steroid hormones made by the adrenal glands, low doses of prednisone are administered with it. Another drug in this group, aminoglutethimide (Cytadren), has a similar effect. Neither drug is used very commonly today. Before antiandrogens were available, these drugs were the only way to suppress testosterone quickly. When antiandrogens were approved, these drugs became more or less obsolete for this purpose. However, they are effective in many men who develop CRPC. The newest agent in this class, abiraterone (Zytiga), has been shown to prolong life in these men (see chapter 13) and in men to whom it is administered with ADT (see below). This agent must be administered in combination with prednisone or prednisolone to provide a certain level of background steroids needed by the body on a daily basis.

Combined Androgen Blockade

This idea is not new. Investigators have been pursuing this concept since the 1930s, when scientists first began to understand the ramifications of shutting down every single hormone that could possibly affect the prostate. Some approaches have been more drastic than others—surgical removal of the adrenal glands or the pituitary, for instance.

The theory here is that even low levels of testosterone and DHT—engendered by the adrenal androgens—can stimulate cancer in the prostate, and they must be stopped. This can be accomplished by combining whatever achieves a castrate level of testosterone—surgical castration, estrogens, or an LHRH agonist—with an antiandrogen.

Combined androgen blockade became a hot topic in the medical community in the 1980s, due largely to the work of one scientist. This scientist reported that combining an LHRH agonist with an antiandrogen was far more successful than using either approach alone. But there are a few things you should know about this research: one is that *no other scientist has ever reproduced this man's original spectacular results.* In his study, 97 percent of men with advanced cancers who were treated with an LHRH agonist plus flutamide were still alive eighteen months later. The sad truth is that in nearly every other doctor's experience, *during that era* only half of patients diagnosed with metastatic prostate cancer were alive two or three years later. Most studies since then have shown either no difference in survival or an overall survival time lengthened by only a few months with this approach. The idea that combined therapy can somehow stretch out the time that hormones work—lengthening by several months the time to progression of cancer—just hasn't borne fruit. These findings confirm those of another study of men on the combined treatment. In a huge analysis of about five thousand prostate cancer patients in Europe and the United States, doctors studied overall survival and found, at five years after treatment, *virtually no difference* between the men on combined androgen blockade and the men who underwent castration or took LHRH agonists alone.

It is important to note that after a certain point, some patients actually benefit from *stopping* antiandrogens. For example, if a man taking an antiandrogen in combined therapy begins to relapse—if his prostate cancer begins growing again and his PSA level goes up—one step his doctors should take right away is to *stop* the antiandrogen. In 20 to 25 percent of these men, PSA levels drop when the antiandrogen is stopped (see chapter 13).

Paradoxically, antiandrogens can make some patients who initially were helped by them worse. Exactly why this happens is not clear. In certain prostate cancers, over time, the androgen receptors (the parts of the cell responsive to hormones) undergo a mutation—and all of a sudden, the antiandrogen *stimulates* the cancer. Remember, antiandrogens normally act like a dummy key in the "lock" (the receptor) whose purpose is to block testosterone and DHT from activating the receptor. With this mutation, however, the antiandrogen key actually works—it turns in the lock and activates the receptor. Because of this odd twist, some doctors have questioned the long-term value of taking these drugs and believe they should be used only for a month by men taking LHRH agonists.

Another Approach to Combined Androgen Blockade—Adding Abiraterone to ADT: Hopeful Results from the LATITUDE and STAMPEDE Studies

In June 2017, two studies were reported in the *New England Journal of Medicine* that may change the standard of care for men with newly diagnosed metastatic prostate cancer. In these two large-scale international studies, men with metastatic disease were randomly assigned to receive either ADT alone or ADT plus the combination of abiraterone plus prednisone (or prednisolone). In both trials, the overall survival of patients with metastatic disease who received the combination of drugs was prolonged by 38 percent. In the STAMPEDE trial, half the patients had nonmetastatic advanced high-risk disease and received radiation therapy to the prostate in addition to the randomized drugs. In these patients, although there was no difference in overall survival at the time the trial was analyzed (fifty-four months), there was an 80 percent reduction in the clinical progression of cancer in patients receiving abiraterone plus prednisolone. The implication of these findings will be discussed below.

General Side Effects of Androgen Deprivation

Testosterone is the hormone that makes men feel "manly." When it is missing, some of the characteristics associated with being male, including sexual desire and potency, go away. Side effects of castration—surgical or medical—can include a loss of muscle mass (because male hormones are involved in making men muscular) and osteoporosis ("thinning" of the bones), which eventually can lead to fractures (one study has found that the long-term bone loss is worse for men who undergo surgical castration than medical castration). The loss of bone density—because testosterone helps strengthen bones—may be as much as 7 to 10 percent in the first year; men who smoke may be more susceptible. Men can help prevent this bone loss by taking vitamin D supplements (400 IU daily) and boosting their calcium intake to 1,200 milligrams a day. There is strong evidence that drugs called bisphosphonates help increase bone density. Studies have shown that the drug alendronate (Fosamax), taken by women during menopause to treat osteoporosis and osteopenia (decreased bone mass), can help maintain bone mass during hormonal therapy. A newer and stronger drug in this class called zoledronic acid (Zometa) has been shown to do this even more effectively. Zometa—which is thought to be twenty times stronger than Fosamax and also stronger than another bisphosphonate called pamidronate (Aredia)—also seems to help prevent bone pain and other bone complications of hormonal therapy. It is given intravenously for fifteen minutes, every three months. (Note: Specific risks are discussed with each form of hormonal therapy.)

Protect Your Bones

If you are starting or already receiving hormonal therapy, you should be evaluated for osteoporosis. Your risk is higher if osteoporosis runs in your family. You may also be at higher risk if you have a low body weight, if you have already broken one or more bones, if you drink a lot of alcohol, if you smoke, if you have low levels of vitamin D in your blood, or if you have taken prednisone or other steroids. (Note: If you smoke or consume excessive alcohol, here's an excellent reason to stop. Do it for your bones.) Even if you aren't at particularly high risk for osteoporosis, you should start taking calcium and vitamin D supplements. Do you need bisphosphonates? Not particularly, according to a review article written by scientists at the National Institutes of Health, published in the *Journal of the*

American Medical Association, unless you have osteoporosis (or are at high risk for it) or if your cancer has spread to bone and has become resistant to hormonal therapy. In this instance, bisphosphonates and other new compounds like denosumab (Prolia, Xgeva) have been shown to protect your bones (see chapter 13).

Hot Flashes

Another major side effect is hot flashes, similar to the hot flashes experienced by women during menopause—a sudden rush of warmth in the face, neck, upper chest, and back lasting from a few seconds to an hour. Although they aren't harmful to a man's health, they can be bothersome. They probably occur because the change in hormones affects the hypothalamus, the brain's thermostat for regulating body temperature. The brain's response to changes in the hypothalamus makes the body feel out of kilter. The blast of heat happens because blood vessels underneath the skin are dilating; this causes sweating, which helps bring the body back to normal temperature.

Hot flashes are unpredictable; no one knows what sets them off or what makes them go away. Some men don't have any; other men are plagued by them. There is some evidence that outside triggers such as being near radiant heaters, eating hot food, drinking alcohol, or taking certain medications can bring them on. Hot flashes can be treated with progestational drugs such as medroxyprogesterone (Provera) and megestrol acetate (Megace). It is possible that one shot can put an end to, or severely diminish, hot flashes for six months or more. For some men with an active public life and speaking engagements, taking a single oral dose of Megace before an engagement may be effective in preventing the embarrassment of hot flashes. Mario Eisenberger, a medical oncologist at Johns Hopkins, cautions, "I only suggest this approach on rare occasions, and try to avoid treating hot flashes, because megestrol acetate is very similar to the androgens that we are trying to suppress—and because of this, PSA levels have been reported to rise in men who take it." If you decide to have this treatment for hot flashes, you need to have your PSA level monitored closely. In some men, treatment with an antidepressant called venlafaxine (Effexor) has proven effective in treating hot flashes.

EXERCISE AND ADT

Metabolic syndrome" includes an unholy cluster of bad things that can lead to a heart attack or stroke. Elevated blood pressure; unhealthy levels of blood sugar, cholesterol, and triglycerides; and abdominal fat–a big jelly doughnut of visceral fat, also known as "heart attack fat," right around your belly, a cardiac spare tire. A big gut equals a bigger risk for diabetes, heart attack, and stroke. *All of this is magnified with ADT.*

If you are on ADT–especially if you already have some of these risk factors–you need to fight what ADT is doing to the rest of your body, even as it saves you from dying from prostate cancer. You need to get mad at it. Work hard to take back your life–work doubly hard, because not only will ADT try to turn you into a tub of butter, but you might get mildly depressed. Your brain will tell you that you're too tired to exercise. It's deceiving you. Exercise anyway.

Here's what you're up against: *Normally, if a man wants to lose a pound, he needs to burn 3,500 calories. A man on ADT who wants to lose that same pound needs to burn 4,500 calories.* He's slogging upstream with ankle weights. His metabolism is slower, his sugar metabolism is messed up, his blood pressure may be higher, and, for many reasons, he may not feel very good.

You need to be aware of this, because it might not be on your doctor's radar. Just as important, enlist your family and friends, not only to help push you to exercise and eat right–cut way down on the carbs and sugar, especially–but to tell you if you seem depressed, because depression might sneak up on you.

All these things can be fought. However, if you just go back to the urologist or oncologist for a five-minute appointment and another Lupron shot, you are probably not getting the monitoring you need. Depression may not show up in a brief doctor's visit. Even if the scale shows that you've put on weight, your doctor might say, "Well, that's common with ADT."

Yes, and it's also bad, and it's something you can help prevent, with exercise–cardio (walking, swimming, riding a bike, aerobics, jogging, etc.) plus weights for strength. These can be light weights; you don't need to turn into Arnold Schwarzenegger. You just need to keep your muscles working. Exercise will help with depression, with the cardiac risks, and with the risk to your brain.

The metabolic syndrome that ADT causes may be a major reason–nobody knows for certain yet–why some men who are on ADT have cognitive impairment. Exercising and watching your diet will keep you healthier.

TABLE 12.1

TYPES OF HORMONAL THERAPY AND SIDE EFFECTS

Treatments That Suppress Testosterone	All Side Effects
Bilateral orchiectomy (surgical castration)	Chronic fatigue
LHRH analogs (medical castration)	Osteopenia/osteoporosis
LHRH antagonists (medical castration)	Weight gain
Estrogens	Decreased muscle mass; higher body fat
High-dose ketoconazole	
Abiraterone	Anemia
	Hot flashes
	Decrease in body hair
	Decreased libido and impotence
	Metabolic problems (glucose intolerance, lipid abnormalities)
	Breast enlargement
	Depression; reduction in cognitive function

Other Changes

Other general risks of hormonal therapy include anemia (because male hormones act on the bone marrow to encourage the formation of red blood cells in men) and decreased mental acuity. According to results of an Australian study published in the *British Journal of Urology International*, the loss of male hormones can mean temporary changes in verbal fluency, visual recognition, and visual memory. There are conflicting reports in the literature as to whether it increases the risk of Alzheimer's disease—because there are questions we can't answer yet. For example: If a man shows signs of cognitive impairment, would he have gotten it anyway? Did he start ADT with some risk factors already on board? Or, when he got on ADT, did he stop exercising and gain weight, or experience depression—and was one of those factors the tipping point? That said, in older men, testosterone levels are strongly linked to cognitive function—particularly verbal memory (being able to name the months of the year backward, for instance) and mental control (for example, the ability to recall a name and address after a ten-minute delay).

Although most men undergoing ADT experience loss of sexual desire and the ability to have an erection, impotence is not an absolute certainty; 10 percent of men do remain potent. However, they are rare exceptions to the rule. Impotence here, unlike impotence in other situations, means not only the loss of erections but also the absence of desire, and for this reason drugs like Viagra are ineffective. Indeed, this is the one form of impotence for which there is no effective treatment. It's not a case of "the spirit is willing, but the flesh is weak"; instead, the spirit is not stirred. Some men also experience tenderness, pain, or swelling of the breasts (gynecomastia). This is not common after castration or treatment with an LHRH agonist, but it occurs in 50 to 70 percent of men treated with antiandrogens alone, and in all men on estrogens. It can be prevented by treatment with low-dose radiation to the breasts *before* treatment begins or by treatment with an antiestrogen, which adds further to the cost of an already expensive regimen.

Finally, many men on hormonal therapy report that they don't feel "normal." They may feel irritable and less aggressive. Subtle changes in physical appearance—differences in skin tone and hair growth—also are common. However, contrary to popular belief, there is no change in the pitch of the voice; nor, unfortunately, do balding men regrow a full head of hair.

If you don't fight it with diet and exercise (see page 403), ADT can raise your weight, increase your cholesterol and triglycerides, decrease your muscle mass, and cause you to have more body fat. All these factors can make you more prone to diabetes, heart disease, and stroke.

The American Heart Association, American Cancer Society, and American Urological Association have developed a joint statement advising men who are going on ADT. Diabetes can develop or get worse for men on hormonal therapy, they caution, and men on this treatment have a higher risk of death from heart disease or stroke. They recommend that men on this therapy be followed by a primary care physician, and that they have regular checkups to monitor their weight and blood pressure and blood tests to check glucose control and lipid levels.

Beginning ADT, then, is not a measure to be taken lightly; it is life-changing, and there needs to be a very good reason for it. It is very important for you to know that you're not alone, that many men undergoing this same treatment are experiencing the same feelings. Ask your doctor about a local support group. (For more information, see Where to Get Help on page 503.)

When Should You Begin ADT?
Some Factors to Consider

If you have metastases to bone, bone pain, or a large mass of cancer that is obstructing your kidneys or bladder, you need to start ADT now. In this situation, ADT is the right course of action—one that can make a huge, vital difference in your quality of life and can protect your body from the ravages of cancer. And in this setting, it has been shown to prolong life. A 2007 study of six thousand Medicare patients with metastatic prostate cancer showed that 25 percent of them never received hormonal therapy. The survival of these men was shortened by at least one year (their average survival was two years instead of three).

Then there is the group of men who *should not* be treated with ADT: older men with a limited life span who are diagnosed with *localized* prostate cancer. Many well-meaning physicians, believing that they should be doing something for these men, place them on ADT. This is wrong. In a recent study in the *Journal of the American Medical Association*, investigators looked at 67,000 Medicare patients with localized prostate cancer. They compared the survival at ten years in 25,000 men who received ADT *as their primary treatment* to 42,000 men who did not. There was no difference in their overall survival or their risk of dying from cancer—just an unnecessary difference in their quality of life and side effects. The authors concluded that ADT should only be used in this patient group to relieve symptoms caused if the cancer progresses.

But what should you do if you have a rising PSA level after surgery or radiation, or the presence of cancer in your lymph nodes, and you feel fine? Although many doctors would advise you to start ADT as soon as possible, others—and I'm in this group—believe there is no evidence that starting ADT now, as opposed to later, will prolong life. There is no evidence that ADT cures prostate cancer, nor that it has any effect on the androgen-insensitive cell population, which, for so many men, is the factor that eventually determines life and death. Instead, I believe there is way too much evidence that starting ADT early will only add side effects—that it will actually take life out of the years a man has to live, without adding any years to that life.

If a man adopts this philosophy and decides to wait until he needs ADT, he must be followed very closely and treated at the earliest sign of progression. This means he should go back to the doctor at least every six months. At each visit, he should be questioned closely about any signs or symptoms that could be bone pain, undergo a physical exam to check for any increase in the size of a local tumor, have a bone scan every six or twelve months or any time a new pain develops, and have blood tests—a PSA test and a serum creatinine test to measure kidney function. (An elevated creatinine level in the blood may signal that the cancer has silently obstructed the kidneys.) Other blood chemistries such as alkaline phosphatase should be measured at least once a year.

Not all doctors feel this way. Some will say, "Start hormones right now. Time's a-wasting, and if you start hormones today, you can delay the progression of the androgen-insensitive cell population and add years to your life." Others say, "Let's use hormones intermittently. We'll start and stop them, maintain the quality of life, and have the best of both worlds." And there's a new group using what's called "step-up" treatment, in which men start with innocuous therapies that have little effect and hardly any side effects and then increase the intensity of treatment (and the potential for side effects) as the cancer progresses. We will discuss all these approaches in detail.

Does Early Treatment Prolong Life?

The real issue in debating when to start ADT does not relate to symptoms and quality of life, because if you choose to delay it and are followed carefully, you will be started on active ADT at the earliest signs of progression (such as a positive bone scan), before you have any symptoms. This also delays the adverse side effects from hormones as long as possible. Instead, the simple question is: Does *early* ADT prolong life? The best evidence to date is based on

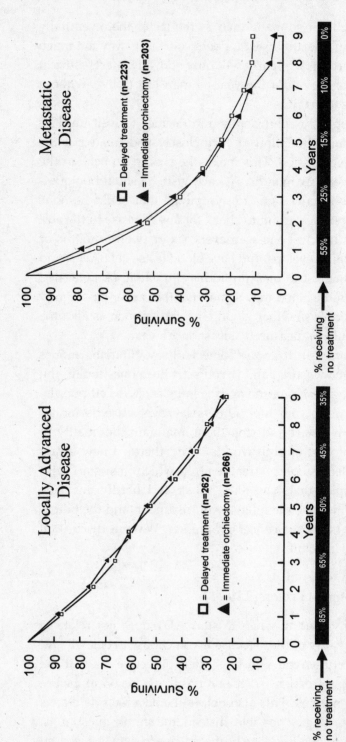

FIGURE 12.2 Does Early ADT Prolong Life?

These two graphs show the results from the Veterans Administration Cooperative Urologic Research Study 1 of 954 men with prostate cancer. The men were randomly assigned either to immediate surgical castration or were given placebo therapy and followed closely until their cancer progressed, at which point they underwent definitive ADT. The percentage of men left untreated is shown in the dark band below the x-axis. With follow-up intervals up to nine years, there is no difference in survival in the men who received early versus later treatment. This study must be addressed by anyone who tries to argue that early ADT prolongs life—because if it does, then what's wrong with this carefully executed, long-term study of almost one thousand men? Modified from Blackard, C.E., D.P. Byar, W.P. Jordan, Urology, 1972, 1: 553–560; reproduced with permission.

a study done by the Veterans Administration Cooperative Urological Research Group (see fig. 12.2). When prostate cancer began to progress in the men on the placebos—this eventually happened to 65 percent of the men with locally advanced disease and all of the men with metastases to distant sites—they began hormonal therapy, too. The study, though not originally intended for this purpose, turned into a comparison of early hormonal therapy versus delayed treatment. *There was no difference in survival between the men who started hormonal therapy late and the men who had been on it all along.* This study took place fifty years ago, but its results are rock solid and still hold up today—because, unfortunately, hormonal therapy still doesn't cure; at best, it palliates cancer, often for many years.

What about the studies that *do* show a benefit to early ADT? To answer this question, the American Society of Clinical Oncology analyzed all the randomized trials that evaluated early versus late ADT in men with metastatic or progressive prostate cancer, including men with positive lymph nodes. They concluded that early ADT results in a moderate decrease (17 percent) in the relative risk of dying from prostate cancer, a moderate increase (15 percent) in the risk of dying from other causes, and no overall survival advantage. What does this mean? If early ADT produces a 17 percent reduction in deaths from prostate cancer, doesn't that make it a worthwhile approach? No. The reduction in death from cancer is an artifact, because men taking ADT are more likely to die from other causes—thus they don't live long enough to die from their cancer!

None of these randomized trials of delayed treatment included men with a rising PSA following surgery or radiation. However, a very large observational study followed two thousand men who, based on their doctor's advice, received either ADT initiated within three months of their first PSA elevation or after they showed signs of disease progression. At ten years, their overall survival and risk of cancer death was identical.

Big Difference

ADT by itself is one thing. But a temporary course of ADT in conjunction with radiation therapy is something else altogether. In chapter 9, we reported that men with intermediate and high-risk disease benefit from hormonal therapy when combined with radiation therapy. Why is this? *Because ADT makes the radiation work better.* There's a big difference between going on ADT for the rest of your life and taking it for a limited time in conjunction with radiation therapy. If your doctor is talking to you about early ADT, you need to know exactly what's being proposed.

But doesn't receiving early ADT delay the progression of cancer? The answer is yes and no. Remember, ADT delays your *knowledge* of progression, but it doesn't stop the clock. Another way to look at it is "pay me now or pay me later." Eventually, the result is the same. ADT does two things: it stops cells from making PSA and shrinks the hormone-sensitive cell population. Say a man begins ADT when his PSA is elevated but his bone scan is negative. His PSA level will drop dramatically, and he may feel that his cancer is gone. But it's not; it has just slipped below the radar. Those hormone-insensitive cells continue to grow silently. There is a euphemism for this, called a "delay in progression." What it really is, unfortunately, is a *silent* progression. Over time (and this may take years), these hormone-insensitive cells will reappear on the medical radar. The PSA level will begin to rise again, the bone scan will become positive, and the tumor will begin to attack bone, producing the signs and symptoms of advanced, hormone-refractory disease.

Actually, this delay is just a time shift. Say the man waited to start ADT until his bone scan was positive. Right away, his tumor would shrink, his PSA level would fall, and he would experience a remission of indefinite duration—until, just as in the first scenario, his hormone-insensitive cells reached a critical mass. Eventually—whether he started ADT early or late—the result would be the same and the survival would be identical. If the man had begun ADT early, his cancer would have progressed, but he wouldn't have been aware of it. The trade-off is that he would have endured the side effects of ADT for a much longer time. If he had begun ADT later, he would have had fewer side effects. What about peace of mind? Well, in both cases, the cancer is growing. The man who begins treatment early has a false peace of mind based on the idea that what he can't see won't hurt him. Unfortunately, as we've discussed at length, hormones are not the long-term answer to controlling prostate cancer.

The best hope is in the nonhormonal approaches we're going to discuss in chapter 13.

Is this absolutely the final answer? There are always two words that we should never use in medicine—*always* and *never*. This is because any analysis like the one above looks at patients as a homogeneous group, without the ability to distinguish the many factors that could influence their outcome. A long-term study from Europe randomly assigned men without metastases either to immediate ADT or delayed treatment. After following these men for an average median of thirteen years, investigators found no difference in the two groups in terms of overall mortality or risk of dying from prostate cancer. However, when they drilled down into the data, they discovered that deaths were higher in the men who had the most aggressive disease (those who died from cancer within the first five years) who received delayed treatment. So if we apply these results to men with a rising PSA after surgery: men with a Gleason score between 8 and 10 (Grade Group 4 or 5) in their radical prostatectomy specimen, whose PSA recurrence is within three years, and in whom their PSA doubles faster than every three months (see chapter 10), may fall into this same category. These men should strongly consider starting ADT early.

What I Believe

So far, there has been no convincing scientific evidence to prove that in most men, early ADT prolongs life. In chapter 10, we talked about the Johns Hopkins study that followed men who had an elevated PSA level after radical prostatectomy. We found that, on average, it took *eight years* for these men to develop metastases in the bones. We also developed a means of predicting when metastases may show up, using the Gleason score on the radical prostatectomy specimen (whether it was more or less than 8), the time after radical prostatectomy when the PSA level first increased (whether it was more or less than two years), and how long it took for the PSA level to double (whether it was more or less than ten months). Using this information, a man can quickly determine his risk of developing metastatic disease. In one of the most common scenarios, a man with

Gleason 7 disease who developed a PSA level elevation more than two years after surgery who had a PSA doubling time longer than ten months had an 82 percent likelihood of being metastasis-free at seven years. On the other hand, if the PSA had gone up within the first two years and the PSA doubling time was less than ten months, then the likelihood of freedom from metastatic disease at seven years would be only 15 percent. This information can tell men how long it will be before they actually need ADT—*if they ever do.* Why should they subject themselves to these serious side effects if they don't have to, and if there is no convincing scientific reason to do so?

Whether a man is treated with ADT immediately, as soon as the diagnosis of advanced disease is made, or his doctor waits until the man has signs of progression and *then* begins treatment, I believe—and study after study proves—that *survival is exactly the same, with the possible exception of the patients mentioned above who are at the highest risk for early death from cancer.* There is no compelling evidence that any kind of hormonal therapy works better earlier than later, when a man begins experiencing symptoms such as urinary obstruction or has a positive bone scan. It is highly unlikely that a man who is symptom-free (also called asymptomatic) is going to feel any better once he has been deprived of his normal hormones. Again, the cancer cells that ultimately prove fatal in prostate cancer are the hormone-insensitive cells. They keep right on growing. To these cells, whether ADT comes earlier or later *does not matter.*

For an asymptomatic man, early ADT means going from feeling fine and normal to experiencing hot flashes; loss of desire and the ability to have an erection; weight gain; changes in muscle mass, skin, and hair growth; subtle changes in personality; and most of all, an increase in the risks of developing diabetes and dying of heart disease. Worse, the long-term effects of ADT can include osteoporosis and cognitive impairment. What's the point of going through this early when, ultimately, you could achieve exactly the same benefit if you wait to start it until there is evidence of disease progression?

The idea of early ADT appeals to many men because it's "doing something rather than nothing." Many doctors, too, promote a proactive approach, telling their patients that this will delay progression of the disease. Actually, it takes a lot of time for a doctor to convince a man *not* to start early ADT—and unfortunately, many doctors don't have very much time to spend with their patients. *If you want to attack the cancer aggressively, don't pin all your hopes on hormones.* Instead, read the next chapter on nonhormonal approaches and consider enrolling yourself in a clinical trial—there are many— aimed at killing the cancer cells that hormonal therapy can't touch.

Intermittent Hormonal Therapy (Intermittent Androgen Deprivation)

In searching for some kind of compromise between early and late ADT, many doctors have embraced the idea of the happy medium— intermittent androgen deprivation (IAD).

Basically, it works like this: Men start ADT early—after an elevated PSA score following a radical prostatectomy, for example— before signs or symptoms of advanced cancer begin. Then, when their PSA levels drop, they stop taking them and get a little "vacation" from treatment. The men are monitored closely, and at the first sign that the tumor is growing, they start taking the hormones again.

The major benefits of all this, advocates say, include better quality of life—recovery of sexual function and a greater sense of well-being during the downtime between treatments. Advocates of this approach believe prostate cancer can be cycled, like a rubber band that stretches and then—*boing!*—snaps back to a smaller state, then stretches again. In this way, they believe they can stave off the emergence of the androgen-insensitive cells that ultimately prove fatal in men with metastatic prostate cancer. And this was its major selling point—that patients would live longer and have a better quality of life.

Here we have another entry in the "sounds good but really isn't that great" category. In a large randomized trial in Canada, investigators compared continuous versus intermittent androgen deprivation in men who had a rising PSA after treatment with radiation therapy. They found no difference in survival at ten years of follow-up, and no delay in the development of androgen independence (when hormonal therapy stops working). Also, in men who were potent when IAD began, only 29 percent had recovery of potency.

Moreover, it seems that IAD may have a hidden complication: cardiovascular disease. In a reanalysis of a randomized trial of IAD compared to continuous treatment, investigators found that older men assigned to intermittent ADT had no apparent reduction in bone, endocrine, or cognitive events, but they had an increased incidence of cardiovascular events. The later finding is not that surprising considering that cardiovascular events are most common in the first six months of hormonal therapy and men on intermittent treatment start and stop it multiple times—so it's always new, and their bodies are always adjusting to it. This should give men pause—especially those with a history of heart disease—if intermittent therapy is recommended. It should also encourage them to ask their doctor why they need any treatment now other than observation.

So if intermittent treatment provides no survival benefit over continuous treatment, and if delayed treatment is the same as continuous treatment, why shouldn't most men with a rising PSA and no symptoms after surgery or radiation just be followed closely and receive hormonal therapy when there is a sign of clinical progression—such as urinary difficulty or a positive bone scan? This is certainly the best way to avoid the complications of hormonal therapy. Note: *Men with metastatic disease should not be on IAD* (see below).

Step-Up Hormonal Therapy

This is a gradual approach to hormonal therapy, and it has great appeal to many men with micrometastases, who have no signs or symptoms of cancer progression but want to "do something" now. The idea here is to start modulating the male hormones with agents that have the fewest side effects and then to escalate as needed, if the disease progresses. For example, as we discussed, prostate cancers don't make a lot of DHT; thus, we would not expect a drug that blocks the production of DHT (a 5-alpha reductase inhibitor) to be very effective in controlling prostate cancer. And it isn't. But hey! It doesn't have many side effects! And so men on step-up hormonal therapy start with the most benign option, a 5-alpha reductase inhibitor. If the PSA level continues to rise, or starts rising again, they move to the next level: an antiandrogen as monotherapy (discussed on page 395). If that begins to lose its effectiveness, they then add a different 5-alpha reductase inhibitor. If that doesn't work, they then add an LHRH agonist.

Although there is no scientific evidence to tell us whether this step-up therapy—in effect, a candy-coated approach to hormonal therapy—is any more or less effective than any other form of treatment, it's safe to say that it's probably a lot more expensive. But it's attractive, too. Many men feel better when their PSA level falls, especially when the treatment has few side effects. It's hard to convince these men that there is no evidence that this works—nor that any form of hormonal therapy is better than delaying treatment until there are signs of cancer progression, as discussed above.

If this is what you want to do, you should do it. However, there are two drawbacks, besides the expense. One is that the men who choose step-up hormonal therapy are also excellent candidates for a trial of one of the new nonhormonal therapies (see chapter 13)—and in the long run, these have a much better chance of killing the prostate cancer cells that don't give a hoot how much, or how little, male hormone you have. It will be hard for medical science to make progress in finding ways to kill these androgen-insensitive cancer cells if the patients who could benefit most from these trials are taking hormones that make them feel better psychologically but ultimately may not control their cancer. Two, remember the silent progression of cancer discussed above? This happens with step-up therapy, too. You may not feel it, but the cancer is still there, growing stealthily, and *when it breaks out from below the medical radar, it can burst back into your life with a vengeance, and suddenly, you have castrate-resistant disease!* Thus, you should ask yourself whether the good feeling you have now, that sense of doing something positive to fight the cancer, is enough to outweigh any second-guessing you may have later for not enrolling in a trial of a drug that would have fought the androgen-insensitive cancer cells when they were more vulnerable.

Treatment of Metastatic Disease

Metastasis is the spread of cancer cells beyond the primary organ. Although this definition includes invasion of the pelvic lymph nodes, when we talk about metastatic disease in prostate cancer, we are basically referring to *distant metastases*, most commonly to bone. Less often, it can refer to metastases to the lung and liver, and very rarely to the brain, adrenal glands, and other sites. For a long time, all men with metastatic disease were lumped together and all treated the same—with hormonal therapy.

Recently, however, things have changed dramatically. Thanks to a major randomized trial called CHAARTED (Androgen Ablation Therapy With or Without Chemotherapy in Treating Patients With Metastatic Prostate Cancer), we now realize that some men who have high-volume metastatic disease do much better if they undergo chemotherapy with docetaxel when they start ADT; they have a dramatic improvement in survival. We also know, because we have learned more about the biology of the disease, that some men who have only a few tiny metastases are candidates for targeted radiation to these sites.

Today, then, we separate men who are first diagnosed with metastatic prostate cancer into three categories, each with different recommendations for treatment. However, in this section we will be referring only to *men who developed metastatic disease while not receiving hormonal therapy.* If you are on ADT (continuous, intermittent, or step-up) and you develop metastases, you are considered to have CRPC and your treatment is entirely different (see chapter 13).

Oligometastatic Disease

In the spectrum of cancer from localized to advanced metastatic disease, this is a kind of midpoint. There are bits of cancer that have spread, or metastasized, beyond the prostate—but not that many, and not at very many locations in the body. *Cancer in this state is still vulnerable, and still responds to treatment.* As Johns Hopkins radiation oncologist Phuoc Tran (see chapter 9) says: "Local radiation treatment to the primary tumor for oligometastatic sarcomas and colorectal cancers combined with radiation to isolated metastases plus chemotherapy, can result in long-term, disease-free survival in between 25 and 40 percent of patients. *Our own clinical experience suggests an oligometastatic state exists in a subset of prostate cancer patients* who benefit from local radiation treatment to the prostate and to all sites of macroscopic (visible) metastatic disease." This refers to men who have three or fewer metastases to bone—a group who in the past had an average survival of about seven years when treated with hormonal therapy alone, compared to a three-year survival with a higher tumor burden.

If you are in this category, you should seek out a center where stereotactic ablative radiation (SABR) is under investigation. This is highly focused, localized, high-dose radiation delivered in a hypofractionated course—in several large doses, spread out over several days. Tran feels that it's ideally suited for treatment of oligometastatic disease, and has shown "high local control rates with minimal toxicity," he says.

Low-Volume Metastatic Disease

These men have no metastases to organs like the liver or lungs, nor metastases to bone beyond the pelvis or spine. In the CHAARTED trial, these patients had the best survival with or without chemotherapy, with more than 50 percent still alive beyond five years. Men in this category should be treated with one of the standard options discussed earlier: either an LHRH agonist with seven days of an antiandrogen to block the brief increase in testosterone, or an LHRH antagonist. They should not receive treatment with high-dose antiandrogens alone as monotherapy (such as 150 mg bicalutamide per day), because this has been shown to be inferior to an LHRH agonist or antagonist. Also, *men with metastatic disease should not receive IAD.* A randomized trial published in the *New England Journal of Medicine* demonstrated that 10 percent more men in the intermittent arm died from prostate cancer, and erectile function was only improved for the first three months.

What else should you do? It is always wise to get a second opinion and consultation with a medical oncologist regarding the advisability of adding chemotherapy or abiraterone (see below). In chapter 6, we discussed the rationale for eliminating the primary lesion in men with high-risk disease. Because of the potential for prolonging life, there are new clinical trials evaluating radical prostatectomy or definitive radiation therapy to the prostate in patients who have limited metastatic disease who have not previously had surgery or radiation therapy.

High-Volume Metastatic Disease

These men have metastases to the liver or lung and/or four or more bone metastases, with at least one metastasis beyond the pelvis or spine. In the CHAARTED trial, men with high-volume disease who started chemotherapy and ADT at the same time experienced a seventeen-month improvement in their average survival. A similar benefit from chemotherapy was demonstrated in STAMPEDE, another randomized trial.

What About the Addition of Abiraterone to ADT?

As mentioned earlier, in June 2017, two studies demonstrated that adding abiraterone plus prednisone (or prednisolone) to traditional ADT prolonged overall survival by 38 percent in men with metastatic disease. This significant improvement in survival is comparable to the effect observed with docetaxel in the CHAARTED trial. It also raises the question as to which form of treatment should be considered the standard of care. Abiraterone is an oral drug that is well tolerated. However, it is also very expensive—$9,000 a month—and requires long-term use. Note: It is expected to be available in a much cheaper generic form soon. Docetaxel (Taxotere) is chemotherapy. It is an intravenous drug that is covered by insurance and after six cycles of treatment, it's over. However, it is associated with more side effects, and is not the best option for some men who are frail or who have other health problems. The bottom line: These developments are very new and there are many unknowns that are yet to be resolved. For this reason, it is imperative that all men with metastatic, or advanced, disease consult an experienced medical oncologist for help.

How Long Do Hormones Work?

This varies from man to man. The numbers have improved considerably and are getting better all the time, particularly with the development of new strategies for attacking hormone-resistant cancer (see chapter 13). Just to give you an example, in 1980, only 10 percent of men with metastatic disease who were treated with hormonal therapy lived one year; 50 percent died within three years; and only 10 percent lived longer than 10 years. Pretty grim—but remember, in 1980 70 percent of men were diagnosed with high-volume metastatic disease. Today, 70 percent of men are diagnosed with low-volume disease. Also, today the outlook is much better because men are being diagnosed earlier, more men have undergone treatment to the primary tumor with surgery or radiation therapy, and there is now effective chemotherapy. There are some exceptional responders to hormonal therapy who have lived many years on ADT, with no apparent change in their cancer.

Still, men want to know how long they are going to live. In the past, I have always told my patients that if they found a doctor who gave them a solid answer to that question, they should not believe anything else he or she said. But some progress is being made. A scientist from the Cleveland Clinic, Nima Sharifi, has discovered an inherited mutation in an enzyme (3beta-hydroxysteroid dehydrogenase, or HSD3B1) that enhances the accumulation of DHT

LOSS OF SEXUAL FUNCTION: WHAT'S REALLY IMPORTANT HERE?

Loss of sexual function is a thought that makes most men shudder. This loss of identity can be even worse when combined with the fear and uncertainty that are part of having cancer. This is a scary time, but you are not alone. It might help to talk to your doctor or family, or to men and their partners who are going through this, too (see the Where to Get Help section on page 503).

For many men with prostate cancer, when it comes down to choosing between sexual potency and holding off cancer, the sex life takes a backseat to survival. If ADT can truly mean the difference between life and death and you're preoccupied with sexual potency, you're missing the bigger point. (On the other hand, *if you have no signs or symptoms of advanced cancer, this is one of the best reasons to delay ADT until you do—and remember, it may be a long time.* The long-term benefits are the same, but the difference in quality of life can be tremendous.) But if you have cancer in the bones or other symptoms of advanced disease, starting ADT now can prolong your life, ease your pain, and make you feel better in countless ways.

One of the greatest challenges with any illness is to find a way past the physical limitations imposed on your body. Even if your sex life has moved to the back burner, you can still be intimate. In fact, intimacy—physical and mental closeness and sharing—is more important now than ever. It's easy, and very tempting, to let yourself become angry at what you *can't* do, and many people fall into this trap as they struggle to come to terms with a serious illness. This kind of frustration ultimately boils down to a control issue—it's human nature; we want to be in charge of our lives. But most of us, throughout our lives, have the point made—repeatedly—that there's remarkably little over which we have direct control. We are at the mercy of—well, God, if you believe in God; infinite other factors if you don't.

One of the most difficult pieces of advice doctors can give to patients—but one of the best things we can do for them—is to tell them to take the hard road: Make it your daily mission to avoid bitterness, which is not only unproductive and time-wasting, it consumes your vital energy and strength like the plague. Don't just ignore negativity; go a step further and substitute positive thoughts and actions in its place. A rabbi once told his congregation, "We all have the same amount of time—today." With this in mind, treasure every extra, precious moment you get to spend with your loved ones. Now is the perfect time to do some things you've always wanted to do—take that trip you've always dreamed of, for instance. Take your partner out dancing. Learn to sail. Teach your grandchild how to fish. Investigate your family tree, and look up long-lost relatives. Realize that there is so much more to living than sexual potency.

Finally, remember that *it's tough on your partner, too.* Of all the things nobody wants to talk about, the impact of sexual dysfunction on the partner is right up there. Karen Boyle, a urologist formerly at Johns Hopkins and an expert in the management of sexual dysfunction, says many women in this situation describe feeling a surreal sense of loss—that there's a "stranger in my bed." For couples who have shared an active, loving relationship, the loss of intimacy can present a great hardship for the patient's partner. For example, all of a sudden, a woman's husband of thirty years isn't interested, but more devastating than any of the physical aspects is that he doesn't seem to care. He has changed. As delighted and grateful as she is that her husband is feeling better, she is also conflicted; she is in mourning—grieving over this change in her best friend. *But this can be worked on*, says Boyle. The challenge is getting the man first to recognize the problem, to realize and understand the feelings of the woman he loves and perceive the changes in himself, and then to agree to participate in a treatment plan geared not to optimizing sexual intercourse but to optimizing sexual intimacy. Erections are not a requirement. Instead, the ultimate goal is for a dedicated, committed man to understand the needs of his partner.

in tumor cells. Individuals who inherit both copies of this mutation, which represents approximately 10 percent of men, experience a shorter duration of response and decreased survival following treatment with hormonal therapy, and should look for a clinical trial or consult with a genetic counselor who may be able to recommend a nonhormonal strategy. This test is currently available at NeoGenomics.

ADT: Conclusions and a Look into the Future

ADT doesn't work forever—but this is not to say that it does not work. *It does work. It does prolong life, and it does ease many symptoms of advanced prostate cancer.* The message here is this: there's no evidence that giving a man *early* ADT—intermittent or continual—or giving more ADT than is necessary works any better than giving adequate ADT *if and when the patient needs it.* Many men are told that early ADT will delay the progression of the disease. Unfortunately, as we have discussed, this is not true. The only thing delayed is your *knowledge* of the progression.

If it were simply a matter of controlling the hormone-responsive cells, we'd have it made. We are very good at that. But it isn't; it's the tricky hormone-insensitive cells—those are the ones we must learn to kill or at least disable. So what we need, and are working hard to find, is a better way to target this group of cells. Many exciting new approaches for doing exactly this are being developed and tested. We will discuss them in the next chapter.

SHOULD YOU BE IN A STUDY?

It depends on the study and the medical institution that's conducting it. Make sure, before you enroll, that you know exactly what's being tested, how the study works—whether some patients (and perhaps yourself) will be receiving placebo treatment, for example—and whether there are any potential side effects. Generally, there are many advantages to participating in a study. Medical studies are strictly controlled, with well-defined rules (participants can stop being in the study whenever they want) and review boards that include doctors, nurses, lawyers, scientists, clergy members, and laypeople. Often, people who take part in medical studies are followed more closely, and thus probably receive better medical care, than the general public—and usually at little or no cost. (Sometimes, if a medication proves helpful, participants are even given a free supply as a reward for their help.)

Participating in a study often means gaining access to new drugs that aren't yet available to others; you may get first crack at a new breakthrough. And many people who volunteer for a medical study say that they feel they are doing something important—that their contribution will advance medical science and ultimately help other people.

"If they're motivated and feel well, patients should always explore this option," says Johns Hopkins oncologist Mario Eisenberger. "They shouldn't give up. For many patients, being in a study gives them a new outlook and new hope."

If You're on ADT, How Often Should You See the Doctor?

If you're on ADT—no matter what kind, and even if you feel perfectly fine—you should be followed closely. For most men, this means seeing a doctor every three to six months. At every visit, you should have:

- A careful history taken, to help your doctor spot subtle symptoms—such as back pain or other bone pain, difficulty with urination, or blood in the urine—that may suggest progression of cancer; and

- A physical exam—to feel for any lumps or changes in the prostate or the prostatic bed; and
- Certain laboratory tests. This is mainly blood work, including a PSA test, a serum creatinine test, which monitors kidney function (an elevated creatinine level in the blood may signal that the cancer has been silently obstructing your kidneys).

Also, as we discussed above, men who are on ADT have a higher risk of developing diabetes (or having their diabetes get worse), cardiovascular problems, osteoporosis, depression, and cognitive impairment. You need to see your primary care physician regularly to monitor your weight and blood pressure, and have regular blood work to check your glucose control and lipid levels.

Your PSA should fall to close to the undetectable range and remain that way. If your PSA stays at a very low level, you don't need any imaging studies, such as a bone scan or CT scan, unless your doctor detects something during a physical examination or you develop new symptoms. In fact, if a man is having a great response to ADT, a bone scan may look worse, because the bone, freed of cancer, is actually healing—and this new bone growth can make the bone scan light up like a Christmas tree. If, after a long period of remaining stable, your PSA level starts to go up, this usually means that the tumor is growing more actively. It usually takes a few months after this first elevation in PSA level before there are any signs or symptoms of progression or before a CT scan or bone scan may pick up new signs of cancer. However, if you started hormonal therapy before your scans showed any evidence of cancer, it may take a long time until your scans become positive, sometimes a year or even longer.

If Your PSA Level Begins to Rise Now, What Should You Do?

First, let's make sure that the laboratory test is correct. Just about every doctor who treats men with prostate cancer can tell you that labs sometimes make mistakes. Have the test repeated to confirm the reading. If the PSA level still comes back elevated, the next step is for you and your doctor to make sure that you're receiving the maximum benefit from hormonal therapy—that it's doing the job it's supposed to do, and that it's not making things worse.

If you have been castrated, make sure that all the tissue was taken out. This is easier than it sounds; all you need is a blood test to measure your testosterone level. Similarly, if you are taking estrogens or an LHRH agonist, make sure you're getting the recommended dosage and getting your shots regularly (if you're not, the levels of hormones may be fluctuating). Again, a blood test can confirm whether your testosterone level is at the crucial castrate range. In either case, if there's too much testosterone in the blood, this is probably the problem, and it can be fixed. Ideally your plasma testosterone should be less than 20 ng/100 ml.

If your testosterone is in the castrate range and you're not on an antiandrogen, you should try taking one to see whether this makes your PSA level fall. Some men are helped by this. If, however, you already are taking an antiandrogen in addition to castration, estrogens, or an LHRH agonist, try stopping it (see above). In some men, going back and forth—stopping an antiandrogen, starting another one, stopping that one, restarting another one—causes repeated declines in PSA and stretches out the time that hormonal therapy can control cancer. For example, if you are taking bicalutamide (Casodex) and your PSA level begins to go up, you can try stopping it and waiting for about six weeks to see if your PSA level goes down. If it doesn't, or if it does and then rises again, you can try another antiandrogen and repeat the same sequence. Some men—especially those who respond to this sequence—will respond to other hormonal approaches, such as estrogens or phytoestrogens.

If it becomes clear that your PSA is no longer being controlled, it is time to act. You need to see a medical oncologist, someone who is an expert in all of the new drugs and approaches we're going to talk about in chapter 13. If your urologist doesn't suggest it, bring this up and say you would like to see someone who has expertise in the latest breakthroughs in the medical management of advanced prostate cancer.

13

HELP IF HORMONAL THERAPY/ ADT STOPS WORKING

Mindfulness Meditation

Faith, Prayer, and Spirituality

Can Changing Your Diet Affect
Your Cancer?

**Note for Partners and
Caregivers—Take Care of
Your Own Health, Too**

This chapter was written with expert opinion from Michael A. Carducci, M.D.

THE SHORT STORY:
The Highly Abridged Version of This Chapter

What should you do if hormonal therapy is no longer working? Take heart: This is the area of prostate cancer research and treatment where we are seeing the greatest momentum and the most exciting advances. Breakthroughs in basic science mean that entirely new drugs and agents—which work in very specific and different ways, allowing for a multipronged attack on cancer—are coming through the clinical-testing pipeline and are now available to men with varying stages of prostate cancer. The time it takes to move an idea from the laboratory to the patient's bedside has sped up. In clinical trials of new drugs, some men with advanced, widely metastatic prostate cancer have gone into remission—something we have never seen before. There is not one treatment that works for every man, but there are drugs that work very well in some men, other drugs that work very well in other men, and many more in the pipeline. There is hope.

It's a far cry from the old chemotherapy drugs with their buckshot approach of killing everything in range—good and bad—and causing terrible side effects while having a limited effect on prostate cancer. These new, precision treatments are tightly focused, and they work like high-powered rifles. They're specifically designed to target the biological mechanisms involved in cancer progression and metastasis, and we have grouped them based on their target and mode of attack. There are new chemotherapy agents, additional drugs that target the androgen receptor, a vaccine to boost the immune system, immunotherapy drugs, drugs that target cancer as it tries to reach the bones, and other emerging targets including blocking DNA repair by cancer cells. We are also figuring out the smartest ways to use all these new drugs. For example, vaccines or newer immunotherapies may be more likely to work when the tumor burden is very low, and combining therapies may to lead to enhanced cell killing.

We are at the dawn of an entirely new era of cancer-fighting.

A word for caregivers: Take care of yourself, too. You need your strength, emotional as well as physical, now more than ever.

Do You Have Castrate-Resistant Prostate Cancer (CRPC)?

As we discussed in chapter 12, the standard first approach for advanced or metastatic prostate cancer is androgen deprivation therapy (ADT). In some men, this can hold cancer at bay for many years; in other men, it doesn't work for very long. When ADT is no longer working—when your PSA starts to go up, or your bone scan or CT scan shows new signs of disease—we call this castrate- (or castration)-resistant prostate cancer (CRPC). What we're dealing with—like sea creatures that somehow manage to survive the darkness and great pressure at the ocean's depths—are wily cancer cells that have figured out not only how to stay alive despite very low levels of testosterone, but how to grow and spread, rewiring themselves to use alternative pathways. The cancer adapts and evolves.

How do you know if you have CRPC? When you start ADT, your PSA falls. It reaches its lowest level around nine months to a year later, and it can stay there for many years. Eventually, however, it is likely to start rising. In some men, the change in PSA is very gradual; even though this indicates early castrate resistance, your doctor may choose to watch your PSA number for many months— or even for years—if your rise is particularly slow.

If your rate of rise is substantial, it is reasonable to get another blood test to confirm that the PSA changes are real, and to check your testosterone level to make sure it is in the castrate range (20 to 50 ng per 100ml). If you are on an LHRH agonist/antagonist, make sure you're getting the recommended dosage and getting your shots regularly (if you're not, the levels of hormones may be fluctuating). If the blood test indicates that there's too much testosterone in your blood, this is probably the problem, and it can be fixed.

If your testosterone is in the castrate range and you're not on an antiandrogen, you should try taking one to see whether this makes your PSA level fall. Some men are helped by this. If, however, you're already taking an antiandrogen in addition to ADT, try stopping it. *In some men, stopping an antiandrogen is treatment in itself; PSA can decline in up to 30 percent of men who attempt this approach.* Switching to another antiandrogen is also an option: this can cause repeated declines in PSA and stretch out the time that ADT can control cancer. For example, if you are taking bicalutamide (Casodex) and your PSA level begins to go up, you can try stopping it and waiting for about six weeks to see if your PSA level goes down. If it doesn't, or if it does and then rises again, you can try another antiandrogen such as nilutamide (Nilandron) and repeat the same sequence. Some men—especially those who respond to this sequence—will respond to other hormonal approaches, such as estrogens or phytoestrogens. Recent data suggest the more potent antiandrogen, enzalutamide (Xtandi), should be tried as the first antiandrogen. However, it is hard to tell whether the benefit of enzalutamide is clinically meaningful, given its cost and side effect profile as compared to bicalutamide—which is cheaper and has few bothersome side effects.

If your testosterone is low and your PSA is steadily rising, you should get new scans to see what's happening—to determine the amount of cancer and see if new sites have appeared. If there is no evidence of tumor on these scans, your diagnosis is *nonmetastatic CRPC,* and your long-term prognosis is more favorable than that of men with positive scans, or *metastatic CRPC.* If metastases are present, don't lose hope: there are now a number of approved life-prolonging agents, which we will be discussing in this chapter.

If you have CRPC, you need to have a medical oncologist who is an expert on all of the new drugs and approaches as part of your team. If you can, find a Center of Excellence in prostate cancer research and treatment. If your urologist doesn't suggest this, bring it up and say you would like to see someone who has expertise in the latest breakthroughs in the medical management of advanced prostate cancer. This is important: many of these drugs are very new, and not all doctors are up to date on the newest advances.

It is also important to know the rate of increase in your

PSA—whether it is doubling in less than three months, the extent and location of any metastatic cancer, and whether you have any physical symptoms near where the cancer is located. Physical symptoms like bone pain or changes in kidney function prompt more urgent approaches—changing drug therapy, perhaps, or delivering radiation to painful sites. Your urologist may need to do a procedure to relieve obstruction of your kidneys as a result of large lymph nodes or worsening of your cancer related to the prostate itself, if it is still in place.

If you don't have other symptoms, or if scans show that progression is slow, there is more breathing room—less urgency to change therapy, and time for more detailed discussion of your next steps, including participation in a clinical trial.

A Transformation in Thinking

For more than two decades, in this book and in earlier books, we have been telling the story of prostate cancer—and we've needed to keep retelling it because the story is constantly changing. It used to be that the only way to treat advanced prostate cancer was with ADT, because chemotherapy wasn't very good at treating this particular form of cancer. Now the question is, which of the new therapies should we use, and when? The realm of chemotherapy has exploded with new breakthroughs from basic science and our better understanding of biology—of prostate cancer, of the cells and pathways that support and encourage metastasis, and even of the body's own weapons for fighting off cancer. Novel drugs and agents that work in very specific and different ways have proven to be life-prolonging, and more are coming down the clinical-testing pipeline. This is allowing for a multipronged attack. The timetable for moving an idea from the laboratory to the patient has sped up, as well. Even more good news: Many of the latest drugs have fewer or more tolerable side effects because their methods of action are so tightly focused.

Scientific thinking about cancer has undergone a transformation. We have moved from the general idea that cancer represents an uncontrolled growth of cells to the realization that cancer develops and progresses through a series of distinct events. There are steps within steps that define how cancer cells grow, spread, and cause particular symptoms, such as bone pain. Each of these steps is a potential target of attack. So if you think of advanced prostate cancer as a freight train—like the one careening out of control in the movie *Unstoppable*—maybe we don't have to stop the entire train. Maybe just putting the brakes on a few cars, or disrupting the track, or taking the fuel out of its engine will be enough to change the course of this disease.

Before we get to these new types of drugs, it is important that you know something else about progress. It can happen in another way, too, and it's not through dogged scientific investigation, but through serendipity. *The world of advanced disease can change on a dime.* Never forget this. Many doctors—including myself—have seen it happen. As a young doctor, I served for two years at the San Diego Naval Medical Center, caring for young men dying of metastatic testicular cancer. The picture was grim; in those days, chemotherapy cured only 10 percent of these men. And then came a miracle: a drug called cisplatin (Platinol) was discovered. A scientist noticed that bacteria did not grow around the platinum electrode on a battery and wondered whether platinum might have an effect on cancer. He developed a derivative of platinum and tried it on a number of mice that had tumors. It didn't work. But somebody noticed something unusual about the mice in this study—they had shrunken testicles—and asked another question: Could this compound have any effect on testicular cancer? Bingo. All of a sudden, 70 percent of men with this terrible cancer were being cured. Young men weren't dying of testicular cancer as often anymore.

Men with prostate cancer should understand this story well. There is hope that through serendipity, a similar discovery will be made. It could happen tomorrow. It might be happening already, if one or more of the tactics we're about to discuss proves as successful as scientists expect.

We write this with the great hope and expectation that there will be new treatments that will work like high-powered rifles with only one target in their sights—prostate cancer cells. They will be specifically designed to target the biological mechanisms involved in cancer progression and metastasis. What follows is a rundown of where we stand today and what the future may hold.

Cancer Biology and Targets for Treatment

Take a look at the diagram in Figure 13.1. It's like a little solar system, with cancer cells in the center. Orbiting around it are different types of normal cells, all of which play a role in the development and survival of prostate cancer. Multiple factors and cells come into play in the development and survival of prostate cancer cells. From a tactical standpoint, this is good—the more potential targets, the better. Scientists have been learning much over the last few decades about these cells and how they interact with each other and with prostate cancer. Their discoveries have led to the development of agents

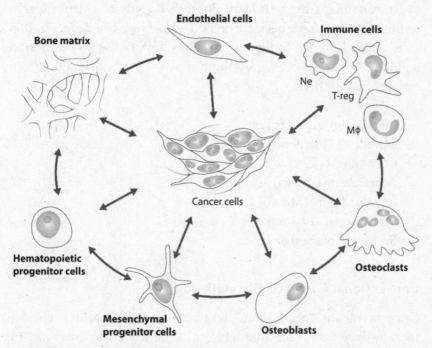

FIGURE 13.1   The Supporting Cast: Cells Prostate Cancer Needs

Cancer cells would wither and die if they didn't get a lot of support from other cells. Wouldn't that be great? This diagram shows five major targets of treatment: the cancer cells themselves; the bone, which includes cells called osteoclasts, osteoblasts, and bone matrix cells; immune cells; endothelial cells; and stem cells (also called progenitor cells). This figure was adapted with permission from an original designed by Kenneth J. Pienta, M.D., medical oncologist and director of the Research Laboratories at the Brady Urological Institute at Johns Hopkins.

designed not only to kill cancer cells but also to prevent cancer from progressing and to strengthen the immune system. The investigational and already-approved agents we'll be discussing next involve these key players. Because the situation is so dynamic—literally, changing every few months—it is important that you have an experienced medical oncologist who can walk you through the options available to you, including these and other drugs being tested in clinical trials.

Target: Prostate Cancer Cells

Something happens to normal cells to make them become cancer cells: their growth goes out of control. Also, they don't die; the normal mechanisms for cell death no longer apply to them. Clearly, certain switches have been turned off somehow. The agents in this section are designed to flip the switches back to the on position to regulate the cancer cells' growth, to slow their rate of cell division, and also to kill them.

Life-Prolonging Drugs:
Docetaxel (Taxotere)
Cabazitaxel (Jevtana)
Abiraterone (Zytiga)
Enzalutamide (Xtandi)
Sipuleucel-T (Provenge)
Radium-223 (Xofigo)

Conventional Cytotoxic Chemotherapy

Cytotoxic means "cell-killing," and conventional cytotoxic chemotherapy drugs are drugs that actually kill cancer cells. They work by affecting the vital mechanisms of a growing cell at different points in its life cycle, hindering its ability to divide and multiply, and ultimately causing it to die. Because these drugs work best on rapidly dividing cells, they can affect normal cells, including hair follicles and cells in the bone marrow that make blood cells, along with the cancer cells.

More than a decade ago, there was a breakthrough in chemotherapy: a drug called docetaxel (Taxotere), which works by interrupting an important process in cell division. Johns Hopkins oncologist Mario Eisenberger, with colleagues from twenty-four countries, conducted a study of 1,006 men with CRPC. This study compared two different schedules of Taxotere (one group received the drug every three weeks and the other received it weekly) versus treatment with a drug called mitoxantrone (Novantrone)—which, when given with prednisone, had been shown to improve quality of life but not to prolong life. The study showed that the men taking Taxotere every three weeks lived longer and had a better quality of life compared with the men taking Novantrone. Taking Taxotere on the three-week schedule reduced the risk of dying from prostate cancer by 24 percent; the men in this group lived an average of 18.9 months, compared to 16.5 months in the Novantrone group; some men lived even longer.

Data from this study prompted the FDA to approve Taxotere for the treatment of men with CRPC in 2004. This important study not only offered men a new treatment alternative, it confirmed that prostate cancer can be a chemosensitive disease. In other words, Taxotere proved that there are chinks in the armor of even the worst prostate cancer.

Next question: Would it work even better if given earlier? In the CHAARTED study (see page 416), scientists evaluated Taxotere in men with hormone-sensitive metastatic prostate cancer in conjunction with traditional ADT. This approach has been successful in breast cancer, when chemotherapy is given early to patients with the highest risk for recurrence. The CHAARTED study showed an average seventeen-month improvement in survival for men who got both Taxotere and ADT, as compared to men who received ADT alone (and again, some men lived significantly longer). The U.K.-led STAMPEDE study (see page 400) showed similar results for the same comparison of chemo plus ADT versus ADT alone. These findings provide a new standard of care for men presenting with newly diagnosed metastatic prostate cancer. The men who showed the greatest benefit were men with high-volume disease. However, Taxotere is not for everyone, because there are side effects. Very good news comes from the landmark LATITUDE study and from another arm of the STAMPEDE study—both of which found that giving abiraterone (Zytiga) plus prednisone and ADT produced identical results to giving Taxotere and ADT (see chapter 12), with minimal to no side effects.

Other chemotherapy

Eisenberger, his colleague Michael Carducci, and others participated in a trial of a chemotherapy agent called cabazitaxel (Jevtana) that led to its approval by the FDA. In this study of men who were no longer responding to Taxotere, men who received Jevtana had about a two-month improvement in survival over men who took Novantrone—15.1 months versus 12.7 months. Jevtana is administered intravenously once every three weeks at a recommended dose of 25 mg/m^2, although recent studies showed that the lower dose of 20 mg/m^2 may be as effective with fewer side effects. Jevtana has its own set of side effects. Although it increases survival, it also causes neutropenia, a drop in white blood cells; thus, drugs that increase the white blood count are often given along with it. A small percentage of men receiving Jevtana have a higher likelihood of blood in the urine, caused by bleeding from the bladder. Jevtana extends life after Taxotere. Each life-extending drug is like a puzzle piece. Carducci and other medical oncologists are wondering if, by changing the order in which these pieces are placed, they can extend life even further. "There are even more options and now many more research questions," says Carducci. "What is the right sequence of therapy—even more exciting, can these drugs be combined for a greater cytotoxic effect?" If, for example, abiraterone and ADT extend life, maybe for years, could Taxotere buy more time after that, and then Jevtana after that—or would a triple approach of ADT, abiraterone, and Taxotere really knock cancer out for an indefinite period of time? Expect new studies to be asking these questions soon. Another question: Could these drugs be even more effective combined with something else entirely, such as immunotherapy?

Other cytotoxic chemotherapy drugs have not yet been shown to prolong survival. These include paclitaxel (Taxol), mitoxantrone (Novantrone), vinblastine (Velban), cyclophosphamide (Cytoxan), and 5-fluorouracil (Efudex). These drugs are rarely used these days, and if they are, they are used to treat men whose metastatic CRPC has progressed despite the many agents available to medical oncologists.

In some men, particularly those with neuroendocrine or small cell cancer (discussed below), platinum-based drugs such as cisplatin (Platinol) can be more effective, combined with Taxotere or Jevtana. Men with mutations in DNA repair genes and processes also seem to respond better when platinum is part of the regimen. PARP inhibitors, another class of drugs (discussed below), show great promise in targeting faulty DNA repair genes, as well. *Note: If you have metastatic cancer, it is important to get genetic tumor sequencing from a biopsy of one of the metastatic sites.* This is because cancer can evolve over time. The genetic mutations that show up in a metastatic site may be very different from those evident in the needle biopsy from your initial diagnosis, or from the removed prostate specimen if you had a radical prostatectomy. The new biopsy could direct your treatment toward a PARP inhibitor, platinum-based drug, or other new drug that may prove more effective.

With chemotherapy, there are often side effects, many of which can be overcome. We will discuss these later in the chapter.

Androgen Receptor–Targeting Agents

As we discussed in chapter 12, ADT can be effective for a long time. But in many men, prostate cancer cells eventually find their way around ADT. Remember, when testosterone enters the prostate cell, it is converted to dihydrotestosterone (DHT), which binds to a specific protein called an *androgen receptor* in the nucleus of the cell (see chapter 1). This powerhouse then switches on various genes within the prostate, stimulating growth. When testosterone and DHT levels decline, the cancer cells compensate by making more receptors. They also develop the ability to make their own homebrew—to create androgens internally within the cell. And as we are just now beginning to understand, they switch their power source—think of a diesel engine that can run on used frying oil—to a parallel pathway, the glucocorticoid receptor (see below). Through these sneaky mechanisms, cancer cells begin to grow again and become "castration resistant." Knowledge is power, and understanding what these cells are doing gives us new ways to target these specific mechanisms.

Abiraterone (Zytiga)

Years ago, we had a clue that by blocking all steroid production, we could lower testosterone levels even further than we could with ADT alone. Ketoconazole (Nizoral), a drug used to treat fungal infections of the skin, blocked steroid production and could drop PSA and slow prostate cancer down even in the setting of castrate levels of testosterone. However, it had a number of side effects and also interfered with the metabolism of many drugs used to treat other medical conditions. Worse, studies with Nizoral were never able to show that the drug improved survival.

Then, from the shelves of an old chemical library came abiraterone (Zytiga). Laboratory tests showed that it blocked key enzymes in the steroid hormone production cascade. Abiraterone did not interfere with nearly as many other drugs as Nizoral—and it was highly effective at lowering the precursor steroid molecules necessary for the production of testosterone. Early clinical tests showed dramatic declines in PSA and demonstrated the need to combine abiraterone with a very low dose of prednisone or prednisolone to provide some essential steroids the body must have. For years, however, many scientists were skeptical that abiraterone could improve survival; it was seen as just another hormonal therapy option.

Again, we're dealing with puzzle pieces. Where did abiraterone fit? Abiraterone plus prednisone was compared to prednisone alone in men with metastatic CRPC who had received Taxotere chemotherapy. Abiraterone with prednisone improved survival on average by 4.6 months versus prednisone alone; side effects were minimal and included fatigue, fluid retention, and electrolyte and liver test abnormalities in a small percentage of patients. The FDA approved abiraterone/prednisone based on these findings.

So this was abiraterone/prednisone after Taxotere. But the combination was so well tolerated that it was then studied after ADT—that is, in men who progressed on ADT but had not yet had

Taxotere chemotherapy. This study looked at how well abiraterone/ prednisone delayed time to progression of disease using CT and bone scans to look for evidence of metastasis. Men stayed on treatment even if their PSA was rising, if their scans did not show new areas of spread. Abiraterone/prednisone significantly delayed "radiographic progression" (new sites of cancer that show up on scans) by more than eight months compared to prednisone, and with long-term follow-up also showed an average improvement in overall survival of 4.4 months. This study changed the whole order of when to give chemotherapy; many patients and doctors perceived abiraterone as having fewer side effects than Taxotere, and since both improved survival, abiraterone now is often given before chemotherapy.

Could abiraterone work even better if given even sooner than this? Many new studies have been looking at starting abiraterone at earlier points in the course of prostate cancer: before prostatectomy, along with radiation, and in conjunction with traditional ADT for metastatic disease. In chapter 12, we discussed the exciting findings from the LATITUDE and STAMPEDE studies showing that men who received abiraterone plus an LHRH agonist had a significant lengthening of survival. Given the success of abiraterone, other pharmaceutical companies are developing similar drugs. That's another good sign: you can tell the success of a drug if there are many "copycats."

Enzalutamide (Xtandi)

Right on the heels of abiraterone came enzalutamide (Xtandi). Charles Sawyers at Memorial Sloan Kettering, one of the codevelopers of imatinib mesylate (Gleevec) for chronic leukemia, and Michael E. Jung, at UCLA, sought to design a better antiandrogen based on the crystal structure of the androgen receptor. In clinical testing, enzalutamide proved to be more potent at blocking androgen signaling than bicalutamide (Casodex) and had a greater effect on reducing tumors in animal models of prostate cancer. Enzalutamide also prevented the transport of the androgen/receptor complex into the nucleus where it signals prostate cancer growth. This unique function of enzalutamide set it apart from bicalutamide, nilutamide, and flutamide, the other antiandrogens.

Enzalutamide, like abiraterone, was clinically evaluated in men with metastatic CRPC both before and after Taxotere chemotherapy. Both studies showed that enzalutamide improved overall survival and delayed radiographic progression. The AFFIRM study showed a five-month improvement in survival after chemotherapy in men who took enzalutamide. The PREVAIL study showed an average six-month delay in radiographic progression and an average two-month improvement in overall survival. Enzalutamide is tolerated well by patients, does not require co-treatment with prednisone, and is taken daily as a pill, just like abiraterone. However, it is not ideal for all men; it may increase the risk of cognitive impairment, and it is not to be used in men who have experienced seizures in the past or who have a seizure disorder. Its major side effect is fatigue, but some men experience loss of balance that could lead to a fall, and a few men have liver test abnormalities. Two other head-to-head studies showed that enzalutamide delayed progression of cancer longer than bicalutamide in men with early CRPC.

As with abiraterone, there are copycat drugs for enzalutamide; one of them is called apalutamide (ARN-509). And, as with abiraterone, there are questions about timing: Could it do more if given earlier? Enzalutamide is being studied in men with nonmetastatic CRPC; in conjunction with salvage radiation therapy; with primary radiation and even before radical prostatectomy. In other studies, it is being tested as a potential stimulant for immunotherapy: could enzalutamide somehow prepare the soil, in other words, for immunotherapy to take root and allow the body to wipe out prostate cancer?

Now that both enzalutamide and abiraterone are approved for use before and after Taxotere chemotherapy (and new studies have shown that starting abiraterone at the time of ADT can prolong life significantly—see chapter 12), both agents are being used extensively, and we are learning more about them all the time. *We now know that not only does timing matter, but order matters, too—a lot.* For instance, we know that whichever drug you use first is the one that will have the greatest impact; activity of the second drug, if the first one stops working, is significantly lower. What we don't know is which drug to use first. Both abiraterone and enzalutamide are expensive, and will remain so until generic forms are available or insurance will reliably pay for their use up front. Note: The manufacturers of each agent do offer assistance programs for patients unable to afford the cost of the medications. There is a wide range of costs and copays, depending on a patient's prescription coverage for oral medications. Since these drugs are so expensive, one thing you don't want to do is pay a lot for a drug that is not going to work right now.

AR-V7

Will abiraterone or enzalutamide help you? A new blood test can answer this question. Jun Luo, a scientist in the Brady Urological Institute's Research Labs at Johns Hopkins, discovered a variant of the androgen receptor called AR-V7. This is a mutation of the androgen receptor protein that acts like a permanent "on switch." In men who harbor this mutation, the androgen receptor is active all the time and does not require testosterone or DHT to turn it on. For this reason, patients with CRPC who have a mutated AR-V7 receptor do not respond to either abiraterone or enzalutamide. Luo and Hopkins medical oncologist Emmanuel Antonarakis developed a test that captures prostate cancer cells traveling in the bloodstream and then looks for the AR-V7 molecule. Results so far suggest that if a man does not

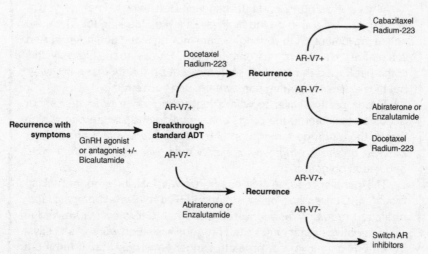

FIGURE 13.2 AR-V7 Results and Sequencing Treatment

have circulating cells to capture, or AR-V7 is not detected, then enzalutamide or abiraterone may keep cancer from progressing for some time. A man who tests positive for AR-V7 is unlikely to respond to either drug and should be considered for chemotherapy. Interestingly, half of men who test positive for AR-V7 don't stay that way forever: during treatment with chemotherapy, they convert to negative and are then candidates for treatment with enzalutamide or abiraterone (see fig. 13.2). These findings need to be confirmed in larger studies and the blood test needs further refinements before it becomes widely available. In the meantime, ask your doctor about sending your blood to Johns Hopkins for this test at the Division of Molecular Pathology.

WHEN PROSTATE CANCER TAKES A BACK ROAD: A NEW IDEA FOR STOPPING RESISTANCE

Suzanne Conzen, M.D., a medical oncologist at the University of Chicago, has been doing research on breast cancer for twenty years. We now know that breast cancer and prostate cancer share many of the same genes and pathways—and the one that Conzen is working on is one that nobody was talking about even two years ago. It is the *glucocorticoid receptor (GR) pathway*, responsible for the primary stress hormone, cortisol.

What's it doing in prostate cancer? Bad things. Imagine you're stuck in terrible traffic on the highway—it's like a parking lot. Then you notice movement off to your right—cars moving along unhindered. And you realize, "Hey, there's a frontage road!" Parallel to the highway, this is the back road the locals take. It may not be the four-lane highway, but those cars are getting somewhere, and you're not.

This is pretty similar to what's happening when prostate cancer becomes resistant to the drugs enzalutamide and abiraterone, which target the androgen receptor (AR). *When prostate cancer gets blocked on the AR highway, it simply cuts over to the frontage road and keeps on going.*

The parallel road, in this case, involves GR. In groundbreaking research, Conzen has been exploring GR's role *in sabotaging antiandrogen drugs.* "We discovered that when GR is overexpressed in triple-negative breast cancer, the prognosis is much worse," she says. When GR gets involved, prostate cancer turns ugly, too. It turns out that AR and GR pathways have an overlapping "cistrome"—a subset of genes controlled by a master switch. When the AR is shut down, GR moves in and occupies some of the exact same places on DNA, switching on and off genes that promote tumor growth.

The implications of this are huge. What Conzen, her co-principal investigator Russell Szmulewitz, M.D., and their colleagues are learning has the potential to transform the care of men with metastatic prostate cancer. Their hypothesis—that blocking GR could *turn back the clock* and force cancer *back onto the main road, making drugs such as enzalutamide work better*—is now being tested in clinical trials for breast cancer as well as prostate cancer. One GR-blocking drug, mifepristone, is already FDA-approved for use in other conditions. Others are in development.

If GR activity is one of the major reasons that treatment for metastatic prostate cancer fails—if, as Conzen suspects, it is causing "even more nastiness and proliferation"—and an effective drug can block that activity, "hopefully there will be significantly longer remissions," she says.

Target: The Immune System

These agents are used to boost the body's own immune response to the cancer. There are two approaches: active immunity and passive immunity.

Active Immunity

Let's switch gears here and talk about another strategy for treating prostate cancer—helping the body become strong enough to help itself. The idea is to even the fight. Imagine any great lopsided battle in history—like the ill-fated charge of the Light Brigade during the Crimean War—and say that you could somehow change the odds. What if those valiant Englishmen had worn bulletproof vests—or, better yet, riot gear and helmets? They would still have been outnumbered, but at least they'd have had a fighting chance.

In about 70 percent of men with prostate cancer, advancing cancer is accompanied by a substantial drop in lymphocytes—blood cells that make antibodies, which help the body's immune system fight off disease. The result is an underpowered immune system.

Think of the scrawny, 97-pound weakling getting sand kicked in his face by the big, mean bully in the old ads for Charles Atlas's body-building isometrics.

More recently, research on the body's immune system and the search for drugs to boost its power have advanced markedly: sipuleucel-T (Provenge) has been approved; PROSTVAC is still under investigation; and a number of monoclonal antibodies and small-molecule inhibitors designed to activate tumor-specific immune pathways are in development.

Sipuleucel-T (Provenge)

This is the first drug designed to use the immune system to treat, rather than prevent, a cancer. The drug started a revolution when it made news for its reported ability to prolong the lives of men with advanced prostate cancer. Provenge is a patient-specific preparation—a vaccine cultured from a man's own blood cells. It is enriched by immune system cells specially engineered to kill cells that make an enzyme called acid phosphatase. The manufacturing is a bit complicated. The first step is to harvest the patient's white blood cells through a process called leukapheresis (done at blood donation centers like the American Red Cross): basically, blood goes out through a needle in one arm, some white blood cells, platelets and red blood cells are taken out, and the rest of the blood is pumped back into the other arm. These are shipped to a central site for processing. The custom-manufactured drug is then shipped back to the treatment site (a clinic or your doctor's office) and given intravenously.

Provenge seems to be well tolerated, with none of the typical side effects associated with chemotherapy. Because of this, and because early testing showed that the drug produced immune responses in most patients, further clinical studies followed, including several randomized, placebo-controlled trials in men with CRPC, to see whether Provenge prolongs life. In two trials, it took slightly longer (11.1 versus 9.7 months) for *cancer to progress* in the men taking Provenge. *Survival* was longer, as well, in men taking Provenge compared to a placebo (23.2 versus 18.9 months). However, Johns Hopkins medical oncologist Mario Eisenberger notes that the key to these early results has much to do with study design. These trials were "originally designed to look at men who had metastatic prostate cancer and who had failed hormonal therapy, to determine whether treatment delayed progression of the disease. Unfortunately, it didn't cause a delay. There was *no significant difference in the time it took cancer to progress*—which means that the primary endpoint was negative."

Scientists were puzzled that although there was no effect on the disease and its clinical symptoms, men who had randomly been assigned to receive the vaccine lived four months longer than men who got the placebo. It turns out that in all of the men, cancer progressed. But when this happened, the men in the placebo group were treated with the vaccine, and the men who had already taken Provenge received Taxotere. Larger studies were needed to sort out the actual benefit of the vaccine. A larger Phase III study followed, with overall survival as the primary endpoint, in men with CRPC that had spread to the bone. In this trial, the men in the Provenge group lived about 4.1 months longer than the men in the placebo group. Again, the findings were puzzling. *While overall survival was increased, there was no improvement in the progression of metastatic disease or in PSA level.*

Provenge has had a rough road to FDA approval, because these studies generated so many questions. This larger Phase III study of Provenge provided enough data for the FDA to approve its use in men with metastatic CRPC who have minimal symptoms of disease. It is generally offered to men who have *not* had chemotherapy. It is not a drug that makes sense if one's cancer is causing symptoms or getting worse at a quick pace. In many ways, Provenge is an investment, like an interest-bearing savings account. You have to wait some time to see enough interest in your bank account to use for something of real value. If you look at your bank account on a daily basis, you may see no real change in the value of the account. It's only after a long period of time that you can see the interest add up. Provenge is like this: while you're receiving it and for months afterward, you may not see any real advantage to receiving it. And the additional time it can provide overall is hard to measure and hard to prove. For these reasons, if you need treatment to feel better now or slow your cancer down now, Provenge may not be the right option.

When it was first approved, Provenge was not widely available. But the manufacturer has increased its production so that Provenge is an option for many men with early progressive disease. The drug's high cost has also been an issue; however, since it is administered in clinic or infusion center, insurance generally covers its cost and administration.

But physician-scientist Charles Drake, formerly of Johns Hopkins and now at NewYork-Presbyterian/Columbia University Medical Center, says we should look beyond the statistics that say Provenge can prolong life by a few months: "It might be able to achieve much more than that if given earlier, in men with a lower tumor volume or less aggressive disease. It also might achieve synergy or extra momentum if it's combined with other treatments." In fact, studies are looking at how Provenge can be combined with other approved agents like radium-223 or agents like abiraterone or enzalutamide, or with other immunotherapy. Drake recently completed a trial, published with Emmanuel Antonarakis as first author, in which men with a rapidly rising PSA after surgery or radiation were randomly assigned to get either a year of ADT with Provenge starting about a month later, or Provenge first followed by a year of ADT. "Men got a better immune response when they got the vaccine first, and then the ADT," he says. "Our trial helped us figure out the right order—the vaccine first, and then the ADT—and that you could do it safely."

Other Vaccines

Other vaccines are in the works. One is based on a modified version of listeria (a bad kind of bacteria that, in its unaltered state, can give you food poisoning). Another, called PROSTVAC-VF (also called PSA-TRICOM) uses a modified smallpox virus as its means of entry into the body and targets any cell that makes PSA. The virus is the means of transportation, like a mail truck, and the envelope it delivers can be read only by cells that make PSA. Early testing showed that PROSTVAC is well tolerated and can indeed stimulate the immune system. Some studies have shown that it can cause a drop in PSA levels, but this is not consistent for most patients. Based on a small Phase II study, 125 men were randomly assigned to receive

PROSTVAC. Like Provenge, it had little effect on the time it took cancer to progress in these men and for them to require additional therapy. Yet with longer follow-up, men in the PROSTVAC treated group lived about eight and a half months longer than men in the control group. The median survival for men in the PROSTVAC group was 24.5 months, versus 16 months for the control group.

PROSTVAC is being tested as part of a worldwide clinical study called the PROSPECT trial, involving 1,200 men with metastatic CRPC from about two hundred centers. The study is designed to see whether early treatment with this vaccine improves survival. Investigators are waiting for the results, and if it performs as well as they hope, men could start getting this vaccine in addition to Provenge. As with Provenge, overall survival may be increased even if there is little apparent change in clinical symptoms.

Still another vaccine, called GVAX, is being tested by Drake and Antonarakis in men with high-risk prostate cancer undergoing surgery. In this study, men are getting either a short course of ADT alone, or GVAX vaccination followed by a short course of ADT. The benefit here is that a pathologist can examine the surgically removed prostate to see whether the immune system has been activated—whether there's evidence that the immune cells have begun to attack the cancer.

Passive Immunity

One of the many evil things prostate cancer does to the body is to secrete a substance that puts the immune system's great warriors, white blood cells called killer T cells, to sleep. These cells aren't dead; they're just sawing logs. A T cell can be sitting in a stupor right next to a cancer cell, and the T cell does nothing because the cancer cell is sending a signal saying, "I'm a normal cell; keep sleeping." New drugs called *checkpoint inhibitors* are like the handsome prince in "Sleeping Beauty": they allow the kingdom of T cells to wake up.

Checkpoints are tiny molecules sitting on T cells, and checkpoint inhibitors target these specific molecules. Many of the drugs in this category end in "–mab." They include ipilimumab (Yervoy), nivolumab (Opdivo), pembrolizumab (Keytruda), and a new one called MDX-1106. There are different checkpoints; one of them is called PD-1. New drugs including pembrolizumab and nivolumab target PD-1. Ipilimumab targets another checkpoint called CTLA-4. Potentially, for each checkpoint—and it's still not clear exactly how many there are—there is some way to block it.

Checkpoint inhibitors are saving lives in many forms of cancer, particularly melanoma, lung cancer, kidney cancer, and bladder cancer. Right now, it seems that a minority of men with prostate cancer respond to PD-1 blocking drugs. Only a few men with prostate cancer respond to CTLA-4-blocking ipilimumab. Scientists aren't sure why—but maybe the men who don't respond to one drug will respond to a drug that blocks a different checkpoint. It's worth pursuing: In small studies, a few men with widely metastatic prostate cancer—metastases in the liver and brain, with PSA levels in the thousands—have responded extraordinarily well to checkpoint inhibitors. Scans have showed those metastases melting away and being replaced with normal tissue. PSA levels have plummeted.

Why wouldn't a drug that's having great success in metastatic *lung* cancer help men with metastatic *prostate* cancer? It may have something to do with the number of mutations on the cancer cell, Charles Drake explains. "Some melanomas have over five hundred mutations; squamous cell lung cancer can have two hundred to five hundred mutations, kidney cancer has about seventy. But prostate cancer only has about thirty." Basically, the more mutations a cancer cell has, the more it stands out to the immune system, and the easier it is to recognize as an enemy. Think about any villain from *Batman*—the Joker, with his green hair and white pancake makeup, for instance. But prostate cancers, even the very worst ones, are more like James Bond villains; they don't look that much different from anybody else.

What can make prostate cancer cells more conspicuous? Enzalutamide may somehow stimulate the immune system to recognize prostate cancer. As part of a recent study, Drake and Oregon scientist Julie Graff, the lead investigator, gave four doses of pembrolizumab to ten men who were also taking enzalutamide. Three of these men had exceptionally good responses. Their PSA levels dropped to the undetectable range; two of the men had been on narcotics for pain and were able to stop taking them. One man's liver metastases went away. Their tumors shrank radiographically—meaning they couldn't be seen in imaging. But the other seven men did not have this response. In three men, the disease did not get noticeably better, but it didn't get noticeably worse, either. Four men did not have any evidence of a benefit, and one of these men died of his cancer. It may be that the men who responded had tumors with a lot of easy-to-spot mutations.

These are early days yet for immunotherapy drugs. New ones are being developed that target other immune system cells—macrophages, B cells, dendritic cells, vista cells, and foot soldier cells called "natural killers." Other drugs are being developed to target different checkpoint molecules. Studies are looking at combining new drugs such as ipilimumab with other cancer vaccines—like Provenge, PROSTVAC, or newer experimental DNA vaccines. Clinical trials of checkpoint inhibitors are being offered by many medical oncologists.

Again, timing may be an essential part of the equation. It may be that immunotherapy drugs should be used earlier, when men are without symptoms and the tumor burden is much smaller. Finally, like all forms of treatment, immunotherapy drugs come with a list of potential side effects. Because these drugs activate the immune system, normal tissue can be affected. About one-third of patients have some immune-related side effects. There is a greater chance of an "–itis"—pneumonitis (inflammation of the lungs), colitis (inflammation of the colon), or hepatitis (inflammation of the liver), for example. Patients on these drugs are watched closely for any of these side effects and most resolve either by stopping the drug or by starting steroids that dampen the immune response.

Drugs That Keep Cancer Cells From Doing Basic DNA Maintenance

The drugs we're going to talk about next could be considered *gene-targeted drugs*, and the genes in question are involved in repair work. Cells do routine maintenance all the time; this is usually a good thing. Among the body's army of fix-it specialists are tumor-suppressor proteins such as BRCA1 and BRCA2. When DNA repair genes such as BRCA1 and BRCA1 are mutated, cancer—breast cancer, and prostate cancer, too—can thrive.

The tools these genes use are enzymes called poly ADP-ribose polymerases (PARPs). PARPs help cells repair naturally occurring breaks in DNA. But when a cancer cell needs maintenance, we don't want it to get fixed. *PARP inhibitors* are drugs that block access to PARP and prevent bad genes from repairing themselves—so they die.

Recent studies have shown that about 12 percent of men have inherited, or *germline*, mutations in genes such as BRCA that repair DNA damage. This percentage is higher than anyone suspected, and when we look at genetic mutations in prostate cancer tumor cells—which can happen over time—even more patients, *nearly one-third* of men with prostate cancer, are found to be possible candidates for treatment with PARP inhibitors.

PARP inhibitors are FDA-approved for the treatment of ovarian cancer that has progressed despite chemotherapy, and clinical trials are under way to study how well these drugs work in prostate cancer. These PARP inhibitor studies stem from a high success rate—a tumor response or even remission that lasts for a number of months—in a small study of men with prostate cancer who had a mutated DNA repair gene.

How do you know if you have a bad gene that might be vulnerable to a PARP inhibitor? Genetic sequencing of your cancer, ideally from a metastatic site. This is precision medicine. It means that a drug targeted to the genes involved in your cancer may work very well; it also means that if you do not have one of these particular mutations, you may need a different treatment.

PARP inhibitors tend to end in "–rib." They include olaparib, veliparib, rucaparib, and niraparib. *PARP inhibitors show great promise*, and some men with the "right" mutations—BRCA1/2, particularly—have responded exceptionally well. Again, we're in the early days. Could PARP inhibitors combine well with chemotherapy—particularly with platinum-based chemotherapy? There is reason to believe so. Platinum drugs can cause DNA damage. Add a PARP inhibitor that stops the cancer cells from repairing that damage, and more cancer cells should die. Radiation causes DNA damage, too—and may make a PARP-inhibiting drug even more effective. Combining one or more of these approaches with immunotherapy agents (described on page 445) may also deal cancer a severe blow.

Target: Bone

Approved Agents:
Radium 223 (Xofigo)
Zoledronic acid (Zometa)
Denosumab (Xgeva)
Strontium-89 (Metastron)
Samarium-153 (Quadramet)

Bone is more complicated than you might think; it's made up of the matrix (calcium), which, in turn, is built by hardworking cells called osteoclasts and osteoblasts (described below). Bone is a living structure, and its molecules are constantly changing, or remodeling. All our lives, our bones are continually being reabsorbed and replaced. When prostate cancer invades the bone, it disrupts this process—but also gives us several potential targets for medical attack. The inflammation that is generated when cancer invades the bone and the bone fights back is another target for therapy.

In 90 percent of men who have metastatic prostate cancer, metastasis happens in the bone; often, it happens *only* in the bone. (We talk about stereotactic ablative radiation in oligometastasis in chapter 9). As cancer sets up shop in bone tissue, many changes take place. Two different, similar-sounding cell types play a major role here: the osteo*blasts* and the osteo*clasts*. *Osteoblasts* cause bone to thicken and become denser. In prostate cancer, these cells are in overdrive; bone metastases are very dense, and the bone often becomes hard, like concrete. These are called osteoblastic metastases. *Osteoclasts* constantly remodel bone by dissolving thick areas. In breast cancer—much more so than in prostate cancer—this is the predominant mechanism in metastases to bone. In these metastases, the bone characteristically becomes very thin, brittle, and easily breakable.

The embattled bones in prostate cancer can also be affected by the treatment itself—particularly by hormonal therapy. When the male hormones are suppressed, there is increased osteoclastic activity. This creates an unfortunate situation—although hormonal therapy can kill prostate cancer cells, it can also weaken bones and make them prone to fracture. However, this also creates an opportunity for treatment. Because of the tendency of prostate cancer to spread to bone, *bone-targeted treatment* is an exciting new avenue of research. If prostate cancer likes bone—and bone, in turn, certainly seems to roll out the welcome mat for prostate cancer—how can we fix it so that this environment is no longer so hospitable? Because there are so many mechanisms involved in bone metastases, there are many promising approaches under study. Let's turn our attention to some of these now.

Radiopharmaceuticals (Radionuclides)

These are radioactive particle–containing drugs that are injected into the bloodstream. Like prostate cancer itself, they have a special affinity for bone and head right for the bone matrix.

Beta particle emitters: Radiopharmaceuticals (also called radionuclides) such as strontium-89 (Metastron), samarium-153 (Quadramet), and palladium-103 were originally designed to combat bone pain, especially pain in multiple sites. They emitted low-dose β-(beta) particle radiation, which could kill cancer cells but also cause changes in the normal bone matrix. Although many men achieved pain relief, these agents did not prolong life and had lingering effects on the bone marrow and blood counts. Attempts to use these radiopharmaceuticals earlier—in men with early or limited bone metastases—showed few advantages, and raised concerns about the safety of giving chemotherapy later.

Strontium-89 has a longer half-life, so its effects on the bone and bone marrow are longer-lasting than those of samarium-153. The downside is that strontium-89's side effects can also last longer, making additional therapies difficult. One study, done at MD Anderson Cancer Center, suggested that using strontium-89 in combination with chemotherapy increased survival in men with bone metastases. Interestingly, newer studies suggest that about 40 percent of men with bone metastases treated with samarium-153 alone had significant reductions in their PSA levels, *suggesting that getting rid of whatever cancer lies in the bones means that the lion's share of the cancer has taken a huge hit.*

Alpha particle emitters

In recent years, because of the marrow toxicity concerns and trouble combining these earlier radiopharmaceuticals with chemotherapy, α-(alpha) particle emitters have taken center stage. Because α radiation has a larger particle size than β radiation, it can travel only short distances and has a short half-life. Radium-223 (Xofigo) is like a bull in a small china shop. It charges right to bone from the bloodstream—where, in the narrow confines of the bone matrix, it bounces around like a Ping-Pong ball, killing all prostate cancer in the immediate vicinity. For the most part, however, the bone marrow is spared and the particles exit the body through the digestive tract with very little effective radiation left; diarrhea can occur, but is generally mild.

Xofigo was FDA-approved after it showed a two-and-a-half- to three-month improvement in average survival when given before or after Taxotere chemotherapy. It is indicated for men with bone metastasis and no evidence of spread within the body except possibly for small lymph nodes. Xofigo is given through the vein once a month for six months. It is generally well tolerated, and along with prolonging life, it can relieve pain. It does not seem to affect PSA, however; only about 1 in 10 men experiences a drop in his PSA. For some men, this is discouraging: Xofigo must not be working if the PSA is not dropping, they think. But PSA is not the issue here. In studies, *even if PSA was rising*, bone scans and how the patient felt were better indicators of benefit. Often the scans do not get worse and the patient has less pain! Xofigo requires referral and coordination of care with radiation oncologists or nuclear medicine radiologists.

In new studies, Xofigo is being combined with chemotherapy, immunotherapy, and drugs such as enzalutamide and abiraterone—and once again, investigators are looking at timing. Could giving Xofigo earlier eliminate the cancer cells that may be hiding in the bone or bone marrow *long before bone metastases develop? There is good reason to hope that this will prove to be the case.*

Even more hope is on the horizon in this field of research and treatment: next-generation, genetically engineered radiopharmaceuticals (also called radionuclides) can seek out targets on prostate cancer cells—including prostate-specific membrane anti-gen (PSMA)—for ultra-precise delivery. Preliminary results in the U.S., Europe, and Australia have been dramatic. There is great hope that radiopharmaceuticals will one day be added to the armamen-tarium of treatments that can put men with metastatic cancer into extended remission.

Bisphosphonates

We talked about these drugs in an earlier chapter, in a different context—as a means of strengthening bone to prevent osteoporo-sis in men on hormonal therapy who are at high risk. These drugs work on the osteoclasts. *Zoledronic acid (Zometa)* relieves bone pain, reduces the need for radiation to the bone because of pain, and helps prevent fractures and spinal cord complications. It also reduces the incidence and severity of osteopenia (loss of minerals in the bone). Zometa in general is very safe. It is given intravenously; this takes about 15 minutes and is usually done once a month, but your doc-tor may prefer to do it every few months, or even yearly. You may experience a brief spate of flulike symptoms (aches or muscle pains) that lasts about a day. Zometa can also cause a slight decrease in the red blood cell count and may change kidney function slightly. Note: Rarely (in 1 to 2 percent of users), it can cause osteonecrosis, death of the bone, in the jaw *if dental procedures are done while the patient is taking it.*

If you take this medication, your doctor will need to monitor your blood count. Also, because Zometa is cleared from the body by the kidneys, you will need to have a blood test to make sure your kidneys are working effectively before you take it. All men who get Zometa should also take calcium (1,000 milligrams daily) and vita-min D (400 IU daily).

RANKL Inhibitor

Denosumab (Xgeva) targets bone, but it's not a bisphosphonate. It's a monoclonal antibody, an artificial antibody made in the laboratory to lock onto a single target; in this case, a receptor known as RANKL. When RANKL is blocked, the osteoclasts are not able to destroy or remodel bone. In a clinical trial, Xgeva proved superior to Zometa in delaying and reducing the risk of bone fractures and other bone complications in men with advanced prostate cancer.

The side effects of Xgeva have proven similar to those of Zometa, except that Xgeva does not cause flulike symptoms. The same monitoring and precautions apply. Xgeva is given by subcutaneous (under the skin) injection, not an IV, and kidney function doesn't have to be monitored. Unlike Zometa, which can remain in the bone for longer periods of time, Xgeva may need to be given more often. In clinical trials, like Zometa, Xgeva caused osteonecrosis of the jaw (see above) in some people and slightly increased the risk of infection, but Xgeva was superior to Zometa in protecting the bones from cancer. Xgeva is now approved for men with bone metastases from advanced cancer. Xgeva lowers calcium levels more than Zometa. Therefore, all men who receive it need to have regular blood tests to monitor their calcium levels, and should also take supplemental calcium (1,000 milligrams daily) and vitamin D (400 IU daily).

If You Have Small-Cell Carcinoma

Small-cell carcinoma is different from "regular" prostate cancer in many ways, although at first it looks just the same. Typically, a man who has small-cell carcinoma of the prostate appears to have the usual prostate cancer and may undergo surgery or radiation to cure it. Sometimes, however, the disease returns with a vengeance. Instead of a few stray cells causing a detectable PSA level, small-cell carcinoma bursts back on the scene as a rapidly growing soft tissue mass, often in the prostate bed. Worse, this is often quickly followed by spots of cancer in the lungs, liver, bone, and brain—*and throughout all of this, a man may have only a low PSA level*. The diagnosis of small-cell carcinoma can be confirmed with a biopsy of one of the metastatic sites. *It is crucial to know whether you have this form of prostate cancer, because the same drugs that work on small-cell carcinoma elsewhere in the body work here as well.* Many doctors prescribe combinations of cisplatin (Platinol) or carboplatin (Paraplatin) and etoposide (VePesid), paclitaxel (Taxol), docetaxel (Taxotere), and topotecan (Hycamtin). Radiation can be very effective in targeting isolated metastases as well.

Helping You Feel Better

A very important issue in advanced cancer is the day-to-day business of palliative treatment—easing symptoms and pain and keeping up nutrition in men who don't feel like eating. In this area, thankfully, there *is* much that can be done to make life better. Many men are amazed at how much better they feel when the individual symptoms of advanced prostate cancer are addressed and eased. And the intangible benefits of simply feeling more like your old self again—being able to go back to work, play a round of golf, or attend a family gathering—are priceless.

Help If You're in Pain

"Pain is very closely associated with quality of life," says Mario Eisenberger. "People in pain have a reduced appetite; they lose weight. They're often depressed. Sometimes they're bedridden, the pain is so bad. If we control the pain aggressively, we often see patients getting stronger and eating better. Aggressive pain management is clearly to the patient's benefit."

It's not only beneficial, it's your *right* as a patient not to suffer. Far too many men with advanced prostate cancer endure excruciating pain in the course of their disease. Several studies have shown that an average of 72 percent of men with advanced prostate cancer have pain at one time or another. In one study of 201 men with prostate cancer, 47 percent reported feeling pain that ranged from "moderate to very bad" despite the use of painkillers. This tells us several things. One is that, as diseases go, prostate cancer may be more likely to induce painful symptoms. Its particular patterns of spreading—metastases to bone and particularly to the spine—make it second only to cervical cancer in terms of causing severe pain. But this study also shows us something else. These 201 men were on analgesics—painkillers—yet they still hurt. Some of them even felt miserable pain. Does this mean that painkillers don't work? No. It means the doctors treating these men *weren't giving them enough medication* to make them comfortable or the men refused to take the necessary amount to relieve their pain out of fear of side effects or addiction. Or they weren't getting radiopharmaceuticals or other drugs that could target the cancer in their bones and help ease their pain.

There is no excuse for that. An article by University of Colorado scientists cited some reasons why men with advanced prostate cancer are often undermedicated. One is that many doctors just don't learn enough about pain medication in medical school and in their subsequent professional training; they learn how to save or prolong lives, but not always how to make their patients comfortable. (This situation is getting better as medical schools and continuing education courses are doing a better job of teaching doctors how to manage patients' pain.)

But perhaps a bigger problem—and this also has to do with the way health-care professionals are educated—is the very real fear that patients will get addicted. This is hogwash. The sole purpose of these drugs is to alleviate pain, and frankly, few patients need these medications more desperately than people with cancer—especially men with metastatic prostate cancer whose pain is extreme. And yet every day all over this country, this study showed, some doctors prescribe painkillers at inadequate dosages, some nurses withhold doses of painkillers, and some pharmacists refuse to provide drugs. With all the media attention focused on addiction to and the over-prescribing of narcotics for less serious forms of pain, the unique misery that is cancer pain remains a big problem. Addiction is quite rare in patients with cancer.

In addition, some doctors worry about the side effects of analgesics (see below). They worry about inadvertently precipitating a patient's death—or worse, being an unwitting part in a patient's suicide attempt if he overdoses. Other problems listed in this study come under the category of communication failure. Some guidelines for drug dosages (printed in medical reference books and other sources) are not appropriate for the particular intensity of cancer pain. And sometimes—this is increasingly common—if a patient is being looked after by a group of physicians, there may not be a clear understanding of who's responsible for pain management. The pain may fall through the cracks. If you have advanced cancer, your doctor should ask you at every visit if you have any pain. If you do, say so!

The good news is that with the many life-prolonging thera-pies we have discussed above, and the use of drugs like Zometa or Xgeva to reduce the likelihood of developing pain, pain symptoms are much less common. Maybe, if you are feeling pretty good and going about your daily life, you find it irritating to be asked all the time about pain; maybe it's a reminder that one day you may not be doing so well. The questions about pain are very important. This is a symptom that may have meaning and imply a need for additional tests. It is also something that can, and should, be treated.

You're a Patient: What Can You Do?

If you're suffering progressing pain, talk to your physician. If you're being treated by a group practice, ask that one doctor oversee your pain management. If you're still not satisfied with the care you're getting, look for another doctor—preferably someone who treats many cancer patients and is attuned to their particular, intense pain.

Another option is to contact the National Hospice and Pallia-tive Care Organization, a group whose goal is to "enable patients to carry on an alert, pain-free life and to manage other symptoms," so their days "may be spent with dignity and quality at home or in a homelike setting." (For more on this, see Where to Get Help, page 503.) Most hospice programs—there are hundreds throughout the country—are directed by physicians, and care is administered by a spectrum of health-care professionals, including nurses, psycholo-gists, members of the clergy, and social workers. Care and advice is available twenty-four hours a day, every day, and it is centered on patients and their families.

There are also some regulatory issues, the University of Colo-rado study showed. When potentially addictive narcotics (strong painkillers such as morphine) are involved, so is the government. That's why most of these drugs are called controlled substances. Some governmental red tape can include limits on refills; however, this is not an insurmountable difficulty—it just means patients need to get their doctors to write new prescriptions when their medica-tion runs out. Many states now have tracking systems to tabulate how many narcotic pills have been prescribed to someone, and who has prescribed them. The purpose of this is to prevent multiple doctors from prescribing the same medicines to a patient who might be on the path to addiction—not to keep someone with cancer pain from relief.

But finally, the study showed a variety of reasons why the *patients themselves* didn't ask for adequate pain medication. Some men aren't very good at expressing their symptoms or conveying the depth of their pain, the researchers found. Some men feel it isn't "macho" to admit that their pain is intolerable. If you have a problem with this, it may help to take along a family member or friend who feels no such hesitation when you go to see the doctor. Other men are afraid of becoming addicted—and some of these men aren't helped any when zealous family members urge them to "just say no" to drugs!

Some men believe—especially if they've seen their own fathers or family members go through it—that the pain is just an inevitable part of having the cancer and that nothing can be done to help them. Others worry about the pain yet to come and want to save the "big guns," the strongest medications, until the pain becomes intolerable. (Actually, with heavy-duty painkillers such as morphine, relief always comes when doctors boost the dosage, so there is nothing to be gained by seeing how much pain you can stand.) Some men don't want to be labeled as "bad" patients by complaining about their pain. And finally, the study said, some men—ever the providers—worry that costly pain medication will use up all their family's resources. For these men, methadone may be a good option. At around $30 a month, it's the cheapest narcotic.

The bottom line is that you—or a loved one with prostate cancer—do not need to suffer any level of pain. There is help available. Ask for it.

Drugs for Pain

It makes sense to treat each level and kind of pain differently. At the lowest level is mild pain that responds to aspirin, acetaminophen (Tylenol), or ibuprofen (Advil, Motrin). Next come such opiate drugs as codeine. As far as opiates go, codeine is considered weak. In terms of pain relief, it can't hold a candle to high-powered opiates such as morphine—the highest rung on the pain-relief ladder. However, this milder opiate generally is sufficient to ease moderate pain. The biggest advantage to using strong opiates is "their lack of ceiling effect," as one study puts it. "Increasing the dose always increases the pain relief," although it can also increase the side effects. Opiates can be administered as pills (both long-acting and short-acting formulations), patches placed on the skin, formulations administered as liquids into the vein, under the skin, or absorbed by the inner linings of the mouth. This flexibility in providing opiates for pain allows your doctor to address your pain needs based on how you are feeling.

In addition, other drugs not generally classified as painkillers—particularly corticosteroids—have proved helpful in reducing inflammation and bringing relief from some spinal pain. Corticosteroids given in high doses also work by interfering with the effects of substances made by the body, or maybe by the cancer cells, that mediate pain. Sometimes the body's response to corticosteroids is fast and dramatic; however, nobody can use high doses of steroids for a long time. Side effects include swelling, bleeding, ulcers, and muscle weakness, in addition to mood changes.

If you are elderly, have other health problems, or are taking other medications, certain painkillers may have a greater effect on you than on other men. Be sure to discuss these factors, the side effects of various drugs, and the form in which you should take these drugs—pill, liquid, rectal suppository, skin patch, or shot—with your doctor. If you need additional information, your pharmacist also may be able to provide you with the package insert sheets for various drugs. These generally are impenetrable, written in tiny print, and confusing—they contain more information than most people want to know. They also tend to list every possible side effect, even the unlikely ones. However, some people find this information helpful. For more sources of information, see Where to Get Help, at the end of this book.

Complementary Approaches to Pain Management

Talk to your doctor before you try any treatment, even if it seems "natural." Having said that, many people benefit from nontraditional forms of pain management, including prayer and meditation (discussed below), acupuncture, deep breathing, aromatherapy, relaxation techniques, massage therapy, biofeedback, hypnosis, yoga, music, and even laughter (also called humor therapy). Advocates of these therapies cite many good effects. They can lower blood pressure; reduce stress hormones, which cause the arteries to tighten; slow the heart rate; block or interfere with pain signals; stimulate the immune system; cause the body to release endorphins, its own natural painkillers; and improve blood circulation. Most important, the above therapies are not harmful. And all of these benefits—particularly those to the cardiovascular system—can improve your quality of life.

Drugs for Milder Pain

Listed here are some nonsteroidal anti-inflammatory drugs (NSAIDS) and some of their brand names. (Just because we don't mention the brand name here doesn't mean it isn't a good drug.) Over-the-counter drugs include aspirin, acetaminophen (Tylenol, Datril), naproxen (Aleve), and ibuprofen (Motrin, Advil, Nuprin). Prescription drugs include diflunisal (Dolobid), choline magnesium trisalicylate (Trisilate), salsalate (Disalcid), naproxen (at a higher strength than the over-the-counter version; Aleve, Naprosyn, Anaprox), indomethacin (Indocin), sulindac (Clinoril), and ketorolac (Toradol).

Drugs for Moderate to Severe Pain

Listed here are prescription drugs and some of their brand names. (Again, not all brand names are mentioned here.) They include fentanyl (Duragesic), propoxyphene (Darvon, Darvocet), codeine (Tylenol with codeine), oxycodone (OxyContin, Roxicodone, Tylox, Percocet, Percodan), meperidine (Demerol), methadone (Dolophine), hydromorphone (Dilaudid), and morphine (Roxanol).

Treating Specific Pain

Not too long ago, a widespread treatment called *hemi-body irradiation* was used to ease pain in prostate cancer patients with metastases to bone in several places. Hemi-body irradiation involved wide fields of radiation—large expanses of the body and comparatively high doses of radiation. The problem was that this often wiped out key blood-forming cells in the bone marrow and compromised the body's immune system, resulting in such complications as infection and the need for transfusions. Now, for pain that is concentrated in one area—a portion of the spine, for instance—more specific pain treatment is a far better approach. Some of these are discussed below.

Spot Radiation

This is localized, external-beam radiation treatment targeted at one or several painful bone metastases. It won't prevent new metastases from cropping up in bone, but it generally helps ease pain in the sites it does treat. Spot radiation often results in several months of dramatic relief from pain, and it helps prevent spinal cord compression (see below). In recent studies, 55 percent of patients received complete relief from pain, 33 percent had partial relief, and only 12 percent had little or no response.

Radiopharmaceuticals (Radionuclides)

Radium-223 (Xofigo) or other agents like strontium-89 (Metastron), samarium-153 (Quadramet), discussed above, are radioactive isotopes (also called radionuclides) injected into the body as an outpatient procedure. They are specially tailored to relieve bone pain. Like calcium, they are taken up immediately by bone, as water is absorbed by a sponge—except these compounds tend to zoom right past healthy bone and zero in on metastatic cancer. Relief from pain has been reported in 50 to 80 percent of patients.

Bisphosphonates/RANKL Inhibitor

Drugs in this group (discussed on page 452), particularly zolendronate (Zometa), have shown promise in easing the pain of bone metastases and slowing future development of bone pain. We also discussed another bone-targeting drug, denosumab (Prolia, Xgeva).

Although it's not a bisphosphonate, it has been shown to be superior to Zometa in delaying and reducing the risk of bone fractures and other bone complications in men with advanced prostate cancer.

When Additional Treatment May Be Needed

In addition to causing extreme pain, metastases of cancer to bone can cause two other catastrophic complications—spinal cord compression and pathologic fracture.

Spinal Cord Compression

About a third of men with metastatic prostate cancer are at risk for spinal cord compression. When cancer eats away at the spine, causing part of the spinal column to collapse, it traps and sometimes crushes nearby nerves. If you have severe pain in your back that accompanies leg weakness, loss of sensation (often beginning with numbness or tingling in the toes), trouble walking, constipation, or urinary retention, you may be at risk, *and you need to get an MRI scan right away.* An MRI scan is essential; it gives details of the spinal cord and can show early signs of compression. If spinal cord compression is an immediate danger, the MRI will show the cancer invading the dura, the membrane surrounding the spinal cord; this is called extradural compression. If your hospital doesn't have an MRI machine, it's worth it to make arrangements to travel to another hospital. *This is a very serious problem—a true emergency—and it requires aggressive, immediate treatment!* It is far better to treat potential spinal cord compression early than to try to repair the damage after it happens.

Patients in imminent danger of spinal cord compression should be treated with large doses of corticosteroids, usually a drug called dexamethasone (Decadron), for forty-eight hours. Then, depending on how the patient responds to this, the doctor will make a decision on what to do next—this could mean spot radiation treatment to the spine or surgical decompression, an operation to ease the pressure on the spinal cord.

If you have not yet begun hormonal therapy, now is an excellent time to begin—and fast—with immediate castration or treatment with an antiandrogen (see above). Giving an LHRH agonist alone in this situation is wrong, because it can cause a surge in testosterone that could aggravate the cancer sitting so precariously on the spine. This may be the perfect job for LHRH antagonists (such as degarelix [Firmagon]).

Spinal cord compression is yet another blow in a series of unpleasant complications of prostate cancer, and it has the greatest potential to ruin quality of life—it can lead to paralysis with an accompanying loss of bowel and bladder function. Most significant, it can result in the loss of a patient's independence and sense of dignity.

If you begin to feel any of the warning signs mentioned above, call your doctor immediately; don't wait until your next scheduled appointment! This may mean the difference between remaining able to walk and becoming bedridden.

Pathologic Fracture

When cancer invades bones, they become brittle. Brittle bones break. Therefore, men with metastatic prostate cancer are prone to broken bones (called pathologic fractures). Most susceptible are the bones that bear much of the body's weight, those in the hip and thigh. Sometimes, doctors can take precautions to protect bones at risk—putting pins into the hip to strengthen it, for example. Such steps are a good idea when a bone has a large area of cancer (greater than 3 centimeters in diameter) that takes up at least half of the bone's outer shell.

Other Complications

It may be the cancer, or it may be the drugs you're taking to treat it. In any case, you may experience some of the following symptoms or side effects. Some of the advice here comes from nurse practitioners at Johns Hopkins—Janet Walczak, Vicki Sinibaldi, and Caroline Pratz—who specialize in helping people who are undergoing chemotherapy.

Fatigue

Develop a healthy respect for fatigue. For many people with cancer—any kind of cancer—it's a ubiquitous shadow. Hard to measure and sometimes hard to see (particularly in men who make the extra effort not to show discomfort or admit any perceived weakness), fatigue can have profound effects. Wendy S. Harpham, a physician who has experienced this "on both sides of the stethoscope," in caring for patients and in her own battle as a long-term survivor of non-Hodgkin's lymphoma, coined the term *post-cancer fatigue*. As she observed in the journal *CA: A Cancer Journal for Clinicians*, this fatigue can manifest itself in unexpected ways—difficulty concentrating or learning new information, forgetfulness, irritability or emotional swings, clumsiness, malaise, loss of interest in the world in general, miscommunication, mistakes, or decreased sexual desire. "Unlike the tiredness that healthy people feel, this fatigue is more difficult for patients to ignore, often impairs patients' ability to function well, and is not relieved with one night's rest....The underlying physical problem...is that extra effort is required for even normal activities and social interactions." Because your energy levels may fluctuate from one day to the next or even from hour to hour, this may affect your ability to "pull your weight" at home or work—and this, in turn, may heap guilt or feelings of inadequacy on top of your other burdens. It may inevitably affect family and colleagues as well. "The situation may be compounded," Harpham adds, "if well partners, caregivers, or coworkers run out of steam. No matter how tired healthy people may be, they feel they can't complain or take a rest because [cancer] survivors are always more tired."

If any of this description strikes a familiar chord, talk about it with the people in your life, Harpham advises, so they can understand what's going on. A "tense facial expression or body language may cause bosses, friends, coworkers, and family members to believe that [you're] angry, sad, or upset when, in fact, simple tiredness is the culprit. Children may worry, mistakenly, that their parents are angry with them." Fatigue can fuel anxiety as well and magnify everything. But learning to recognize fatigue for what it is—and taking a few necessary steps to accommodate it instead of becoming frustrated with what you can't do—can help you deal with this problem. For more help, talk to your doctor.

Muscle Loss

Long-term hormonal therapy can cause weakness and loss of muscle mass. Like fatigue, this can also produce anxiety. One of the best ways to fight this is by maintaining as active a lifestyle as you are able. This doesn't mean that you have to be a marathon runner, but it does mean that regular physical activity helps to keep muscles healthy. Coincidentally, it can also help with cancer-related fatigue. Activities such as walking, swimming, or riding a bicycle can be helpful. Every little bit helps—even very small things, like parking farther away from the grocery store so you have to walk a few steps more. Even if you are being treated for more advanced disease and are undergoing chemotherapy, exercise can help counter the effects of the treatments on your muscle mass and strength. Having said that, please know that this is not a guilt trip. Do what you can—but also listen to your body, and only do what is comfortable for you.

Urinary Tract Obstruction

If you're having any of these symptoms—weak urine flow, hesitancy in starting urination, a need to push or strain to get urine to flow, intermittent urine stream (starts and stops several times), difficulty in stopping urination, dribbling after urination, a sense of not being able to empty the bladder completely, or not being able to urinate at all—it's probable that the cancer has become extensive enough to block your urinary tract. Several procedures are available to ease these symptoms, including a TUR or the placement of stents. Contact your urologist if you are experiencing any of these symptoms.

Weight Loss

What's wrong with losing weight, particularly if you've spent the better part of your life trying to do just that? The problem here is that people who have cancer need to eat. Losing weight means losing strength and the body's energy reserve for fighting off illness.

No appetite? Able to eat just a little at a time? The thought of taking vitamins makes you gag? Then eat less, more often—have small, nutritious snacks throughout the day. Make every calorie count. Empty calories in sugared iced tea or soda won't do your body as much good as the calories in juice, for instance; the same goes for the empty calories in a doughnut versus the calories in a muffin or slice of banana bread. Finally, if you just can't force yourself to eat as much food as your body needs, you may want to try a calorie-packed liquid nutrition supplement, such as Ensure, Sustacal, or Boost. Most hospitals have nutritionists available to help you solve dietary problems like these. That's what these people are there for, so let them help!

In severe cases of weight loss, doctors can insert a gastrostomy tube, which bypasses the upper digestive tract and allows patients to get much-needed nutrition in liquid form. This tube provides a painless route for food to get to your stomach. It's comfortable and discreet—hidden by clothes—and can be removed when your appetite comes back and you don't need it anymore. Don't think the tube will be there forever. Fortunately, such measures are rarely needed or used in prostate cancer.

There may be a time that the amount of cancer in your body overwhelms how you feel, and as a result, you are less active. When your activity level is limited, the amount you need to eat is reduced as well. This is normal, common, and expected. Your family can present foods to you, encourage the high-calorie drinks, or take you out to eat. If you are not hungry, then you are not bothered by not eating. There is no dissatisfaction, and in fact, sometimes eating makes you feel worse. Families need to understand this simple message. In most societies, eating is social. We gather to eat for holidays, for celebrations, for promotions, to share our day's activities. Gathering for a meal can continue, but you may not eat all that is offered, nor should you.

Constipation

This is another big problem for many men taking strong painkillers such as morphine, which sedate the digestive tract as they relieve pain. Many doctors prescribe mild laxatives or stool softeners at the same time they prescribe opiate analgesics. If you are taking opiates for pain, you must take at least stool softeners, as these painkillers will definitely constipate you. For most, a stool softener is not enough—a laxative is needed to stimulate the gut to push the stool along. Also, some antinausea medicines can slow your bowels, so you may need to take a stool softener or laxative occasionally to keep things moving. Another option is adding fiber supplements to your diet; these are available in a variety of forms, including mixtures you can add to fruit juice. Avoid fiber supplements if you are not able to take in enough liquid fluids. You don't have to have a bowel movement every day, but you should be having one every two to three days—and when it does happen, it should not be uncomfortable. Exercise can help with this problem, too, and again, make sure you drink plenty of fluids.

Diarrhea

This can be a result of some chemotherapy drugs that affect the cells lining the intestine. Remember some of the immunotherapies can cause diarrhea too—a form of "colitis." Xofigo is known to induce diarrhea in some men as well. Some medications, such as loperamide (Imodium) and atropine and diphenoxylate (Lomotil), can help stop or slow diarrhea, but talk to your doctor before you start taking one of these, particularly if you're receiving immunotherapy. You need to replace the fluids you have lost through diarrhea; drink plenty of liquids, and eat small but frequent meals. If you are able, try to eat bland foods such as toast, rice, and applesauce. Gatorade, other sport drinks, or Pedialyte can help restore electrolytes and help you avoid becoming dehydrated. Dairy products may make diarrhea worse.

Nausea and Vomiting

These are side effects of several chemotherapy drugs, and they're the symptoms many men fear the most. Nausea is horrible. Some people feel it's even worse than vomiting—that feeling of dread, the heaviness that drains the life out of you and makes you flat-out miserable. This also becomes part of a bad cycle—you feel terrible, so you can't eat, and then your body becomes weak, which makes you feel terrible. Managing nausea can be a challenge for doctors, nurses, and patients; it often requires trial and error, patience, and determination. This is because different drugs to treat nausea and vomiting (called antiemetic drugs) work better for different people, and some people require more than one antiemetic drug at the same time. Some good antiemetics include dexamethasone (Decadron), dolasetron (Anzemet), granisetron (Kytril), ondansetron (Zofran), palonosetron (Aloxi), and prochlorperazine (Compazine). It's important to be proactive. Don't wait until you are miserable or vomiting to start the medicine. Take it as directed, and don't try to go without. Once the nausea and vomiting begin, it is harder to get these symptoms under control.

You may feel like giving up, but you have to try, and keep trying, to get liquids and food down. If you don't, you could become dehydrated, and you may wind up in an emergency room or doctor's office, getting intravenous fluids. Some people with nausea look at a whole plate of food or even a full glass of juice and gag. Well, you don't have to eat a whole plateful of food. Just take a few bites now, and a few bites later, and a few more bites in an hour. If the smell of cooking bothers you, eat your food cold or at room temperature. (Speaking of smells, other odors that never bothered you before, such as perfume, air freshener, or pipe tobacco, may suddenly seem unbearable. Don't worry; this will go away when your treatment is over.) Stay away from fried, fatty foods; most of these require a strong stomach on a good day! You may find it's better to eat dry foods, such as cereal, toast, or crackers. Drink cool, clear, unsweetened juices, such as apple juice, or light-colored sodas, such as ginger ale. Although it's important to get plenty of rest, try not to lie flat for at least two hours after you have finished eating. Eat a light meal before treatment. Also, a tip from a gastroenterologist: If you have trouble swallowing pills, talk to your doctor. You're not alone, and there are good ways to get around this. Some people find it easier to put a pill in a spoonful of applesauce and swallow it that way. You may be able to cut your pills, or have a compounding pharmacy make pills that are easier to swallow, or combine several medications into one capsule, or put medicine into a liquid suspension.

Sores in the Mouth

This is another temporary problem caused by some chemotherapy drugs. Sores in the mouth and throat can cause pain and infection. They can also hinder your ability to eat or drink. You must baby your mouth and throat during this time. Use a soft toothbrush; eat soft, soothing foods, such as ice cream, scrambled eggs, pudding, and Jell-O. Sucking on ice chips or Popsicles may be comforting as well. If your lips are dry, use a lip balm. Try gargling with a mixture of water, baking soda, and salt; use alcohol-free mouthwash such as Biotene; Biotene toothpaste is less abrasive. If the over-the-counter products don't give you relief, ask your doctor or nurse about medicated mouthwashes (such as Magic Mouthwash or Gelclair) that may be helpful.

Hair Loss

This is another side effect of some—but not all—chemotherapy drugs, and it can happen to the hair all over your body, not just on your head. This is almost always a temporary problem. When your treatment stops, your hair will come back—and, as a surprise, it may come back with a different color or texture. Some drugs just cause the hair to thin slightly. Use low heat if you blow-dry your hair, and use a sunscreen or wear a hat to protect your scalp.

Loss of Blood Cells and Platelets

Chemotherapy can destroy the cells in your bone marrow—your white blood cells, red blood cells, and platelets—and rarely, radiopharmaceuticals can also lower your blood count. This isn't good, because your white blood cells help your body fight off infection. If your white blood cell count falls too low, you may need antibiotics to prevent an infection. If you develop a fever when your white blood cells are low, you will need to be admitted to the hospital for a brief time, for evaluation and intravenous antibiotics. If your white blood cell count falls too much, your doctor may decide to give you a break in your chemotherapy or even decrease the dosage. There are drugs (Neupogen [filgrastim] and Neulasta [pegfilgrastim]) that can be given to raise your white cells after chemotherapy to reduce your risk of infection. If you have a low white blood cell count, stay away from crowds and especially from people who are sick. This can be hard, but remember, it's just temporary. Do your best not to cut yourself; wear gloves when you're gardening or cleaning. Remember, an open wound is a gateway for infection. If you feel sick or feverish, take your temperature; if it's higher than 100.5 degrees Fahrenheit or if you have chills, a productive cough, redness, or swelling (which could mean an infection), call your doctor or nurse.

If you have a low red blood cell count, you may feel weak, short of breath, tired, or dizzy, or have a fluttery, rapid heart rate. You may need a transfusion to boost your red blood cells quickly. Transfused blood is heavily screened and is extremely safe. If your doctor recommends a blood transfusion, you should get one: you will most likely feel better soon afterward. Drugs that boost the red cell counts after chemotherapy are rarely used these days because of research that suggested these drugs may actually shorten survival.

If you have a low platelet count, you may have trouble with bleeding. Platelets help your blood to clot. If you cut yourself or have a nosebleed, you will need to apply pressure for a longer time to stop the bleeding. If you develop sudden pain in your head, joints, or lower back, or if you experience sudden dizziness, call your doctor immediately; you may be bleeding internally. If your platelet count becomes too low or if you are bleeding with a low platelet count, you may need a platelet transfusion.

Complementary Medicine

In chapter 3, we discussed many dietary approaches to preventing prostate cancer. Although the situation is different, the caveat still applies—even though something is complementary or alternative and you can buy it in a health-food store, it can still hurt you. Remember, you can overdose on anything, if you get too much of it. Anything can be toxic, if taken improperly. Complementary medicine can include lifestyle therapy (some approaches are mentioned above in the section on pain) and dietary changes. At a minimum, these lifestyle approaches (including spirituality and prayer, discussed below) can change the way you perceive your illness. They can help you cope better, and there is a cascade of good events that can come from this—eating better, for one thing, becoming more rested, feeling stronger, and having a greater sense of well-being.

Changing your diet may help slow the course of prostate cancer, but nobody knows for sure yet. There is evidence to support this, which we'll discuss below. On the other hand, as we discussed above, it is dangerous to lose too much weight; this could seriously impede your body's ability to fight cancer. Also, studies suggest that as many as two-thirds of patients who use alternative therapies don't tell their doctors. This is bad; alternative therapies (even natural remedies such as plant extracts or botanicals) can change the effectiveness of other medications and cause side effects. If you choose to augment your diet with any supplements, be sure to tell your doctor.

The Mind-Body Connection

The mind has a tremendous—and largely untapped—ability to influence the body for bad as well as good. Before we go on, let's take a moment to dispel some guilt. There are a lot of books out there—and countless seminars, articles, and self-help pamphlets—selling the idea that with the right attitude, mental state, spiritual serenity, or even diet, you can heal yourself or control your illness. But the flip side of this mind-set is that if your illness progresses, somehow you've messed up, that you're to blame—you haven't eaten enough vegetables, taken the right multivitamins or supplements, or gotten enough rest or exercise, or you just generally allowed negativity to compromise your health. This definitely is not true.

PROSTATE CANCER AND DEPRESSION

There are some of the things you already have to cope with—stress, fear, anger, anxiety, sweating out one PSA test after another, pain, fatigue, uncertainty, and the cancer itself. But at some point, an estimated 1 in 4 cancer patients battles depression as well. Although it's common, this is not a normal part of cancer, and it can be treated. Not treating your depression in a stoic attempt to ride it out or snap out of it can even shorten your life. This is something beyond the normal sadness that accompanies having cancer.

If you have any of these symptoms, see your doctor: sadness that won't go away; sleeping much more or much less than normal;

waking early in the morning, worried, and being unable to go back to sleep; inability to be happy; eating much more or much less than normal; feeling tired all the time; inability to concentrate or make decisions; restlessness; listlessness; not wanting to participate in normal activities; feelings of worthlessness, helplessness, and guilt; thinking often about death or suicide.

The vast majority of people suffering from depression can be treated successfully. Because the problem—believed to stem from a biochemical imbalance or faulty communication in brain cells—differs in everyone, it may take a bit of trial and error for you and your doctor to find the treatment that works best. Be patient, and don't give up. It may also help for you to talk with other men who are going through this. Ask your doctor about support groups in your area. (For more, see Where to Get Help on page 503.)

"The average patient generally does not have a clear grasp of the molecular biology of carcinogenesis," writes physician and cancer survivor Wendy Harpham in *CA: A Cancer Journal for Clinicians*. "Even to those patients who understand that recurrence is due to mutated cells that escaped the earlier round(s) of cancer therapy, the possibility of having accelerated the recurrence can be disturbing. Just as believers in mind-over-matter worry that negative thoughts can cause cancer cells to multiply, those who want to believe that proper actions can control outcome worry...that they've set themselves up for progression of disease." Too often with cancer, Harpham adds, a vicious cycle of fatigue and anxiety can set in, each feeding off the other.

The British evangelist David Watson, who wrote about his own battle with cancer in the book *Fear No Evil*, points out how unproductive such thinking is: "Many times I have talked with those who are seriously ill, and I have found them anxiously wondering what they had done to bring about their condition. They blame themselves; or if they cannot live with that, they project their guilt onto others or God. It's someone's fault! The trouble is that either feelings of guilt, which are often imaginary, or direct accusations, which are often unfair, only encourage the sickness. Both hinder healing."

Above, we mentioned some therapeutic options that generally come under the heading of alternative or complementary medicine (although these practices, many of them traditionally Eastern, are becoming increasingly respected by Western physicians). All of these have been helpful to somebody, and the way they help one person may not be the way they prove beneficial to you. But we know that using your *mind* to lower your blood pressure, to facilitate deep breathing and relaxation, can help your *body* in its battle with cancer. We also know that the "lone wolf" does not do as well as the man who has many connections—who is married; who has good relationships with family and friends; who goes to a temple, church, mosque, or synagogue. Many studies have confirmed the importance of emotional connection—loving support—to good health. As Tedd Mitchell, director of the Cooper Clinic's Wellness Program, observed, "We are made not to live alone, but to interact regularly with others....In my medical practice, it seems that patients with strong family ties cope better with illness."

Mindfulness Meditation

Many studies have shown that mindfulness meditation can make life better for people in pain. How much better? Well, that's hard to quantify. For example, results from a small study done by Leeds Beckett University investigators, published in *Pain Studies and Treatment*, suggest that just ten minutes a day "can improve pain tolerance, pain threshold and decrease anxiety toward pain." But the study's participants were healthy university students, not men with advanced prostate cancer—so, will meditation make your pain better? The answer may come from another study, published in the *Journal of Pain Management*, in which Canadian researchers concluded that "while mindfulness meditation did not significantly reduce the sensory aspects of pain, it may reduce aspects of pain related to tension, fear, and autonomic arousal"—anxiety, emotional distress, and the perception of pain. "It may be that individuals who incorporated mindfulness into their pain management practice became less negatively affected emotionally by their pain." Will it help you? It's easy to find out. Many centers offer meditation classes, and there are thousands of websites with tips on how to get started.

You can do it at home, just sitting in a chair with your eyes closed. Why not give it a shot?

Faith, Prayer, and Spirituality

If you are religious—whatever your religion—you probably feel great comfort in knowing that you're not alone, that God is always with you. You can draw strength from prayer and from the prayers of others, and from seeking peace. You can surrender the burdens of illness, anxiety, fear, fatigue, and uncertainty—trade them all in for a greater serenity about the future.

If you are not religious but thinking about it, now is the perfect time to explore your spirituality. There are excellent reasons to support this decision. Numerous studies have shown that, among other benefits, religious people—those who put their faith in something larger than themselves—live longer, have lower blood pressure, and need fewer pain medications. *But if you are not interested, then you should not feel pressured;* extra pressure is the last thing you need in your life right now. You should be allowed that freedom, and family members and friends should respect your wishes. (However, you still may want to explore one or more of the complementary forms of therapy mentioned above for stress reduction, relief of pain, and an improved sense of well-being.)

So if you pray for God to take away your cancer, will you be healed? Maybe. But many religious leaders say that the better, far more effective, prayer is the "Thy will be done" kind—because you don't know the big plan for your life (if you believe there is one, that is). Nobody does. It may help for you to talk about this with your doctor as well, if you feel comfortable doing so. Ask your doctor if he or she believes in God and in prayer. You can also direct your prayers toward the greater good—to help the doctors taking care of you, the scientists working to find the cure, and all the men with prostate cancer and their families.

Can Changing Your Diet Affect Your Cancer?

In chapter 3, we discussed the strong circumstantial evidence linking the development of prostate cancer to dietary factors. It also appears that diet can influence the development of prostate cancer throughout an adult's lifetime and that something about the Asian diet seems to prevent this progression of cancer.

Based on these facts, many men believe that once they have prostate cancer, they can slow it down or cause it to reverse itself by changing their diet. One of the most intelligent and vocal advocates of this is Michael Milken, who at the age of forty-seven was diagnosed with advanced prostate cancer. His story is well known because he has devoted his life and considerable resources to fighting this disease and finding a cure. In addition to receiving the standard forms of medical therapy for his disease, he also changed his diet; he drastically reduced the amount of fat he ate (to 9 grams a day) and stopped eating desserts and most dairy products. Furthermore, because the Asian diet is rich in soy protein, he made soy a staple of his diet, substituting tofu or tempeh for meat and mixing soy protein isolate powder with water or fruit juice. To make his Spartan diet more palatable, he worked closely with the chef Beth Ginsberg to create tasty meals. (These recipes are in *The Taste for Living Cookbook*, coauthored by Ginsberg and Milken.) The idea of finding a cancer-fighting diet strongly appeals to many men.

In fact, many men with prostate cancer spend a lot of time at the health-food store, loading up on dietary supplements such as saw palmetto and zinc. It is important to talk to your doctor about supplements because as new information is published, recommendations change. In general, high doses of vitamins and minerals do not provide additional protection. It was previously thought that high doses of vitamin E and selenium were protective against cancer; however, new information tells us that higher doses of vitamin E may actually be harmful, and adequate amounts of selenium can be obtained through diet eating vegetables grown in the ground, such as garlic.

Thus, we don't know the verdict on diet and advanced prostate cancer yet. There has been no scientific, objective study to examine this approach. We do know that in breast cancer—a disease that seems to parallel prostate cancer, with its low rates in Asian women and the increase in risk when Asian women migrate to western countries—the consumption of fat, red meat, or fiber after diagnosis has not been found to lengthen or shorten life. As we discussed in chapter 3, prostate cancer is believed to develop because of oxidative damage to DNA. Hit after hit—mainly from eating too many "bad" things or not enough "good" things—causes a series of irreversible mutations in DNA, which in turn lead to cancer.

It is not reasonable to assume that diet can reverse cancer after the fact—that it can "unring the bell." The best example of this is smoking—we know it causes lung cancer, but it's impossible to make lung cancer go away by stopping smoking. There are a number of studies that suggest that soy and rye bran can inhibit the development of tumors. However, in most of these studies, treatment with soy began at the time the tumors were implanted into the animals. Soy and bran contain significant amounts of phytoestrogens, and these plant-derived estrogens can act like other estrogens and suppress testosterone. Also, some of the cancer cell lines used in the studies can respond to estrogen itself. Thus, it's unclear whether these experimental studies accurately predict what will happen to a man with an established cancer who switches to a soy-based diet.

Another important piece of advice about diet is to keep your heart healthy! Prostate cancer is a disease of aging, and with advances in therapy for prostate cancer, men are living longer. Heart disease also increases with age. ADT can cause weight gain (see chapter 12), and it's important to do your best to fight it with exercise and a healthy diet. Excess weight can contribute to high blood pressure, diabetes, and high blood fats like cholesterol. All these medical problems are also associated with higher rates of heart disease. Thus, to live as long as possible with your prostate cancer, you need to keep your heart healthy, and one way to do that is to eat wisely and stay physically active. If you're on ADT, as we discussed in chapter 12, you have to burn off more calories to lose a pound. Thus, it pays to eat smart: Carbs and sugar, although they may be comforting, are not your friends. Lean meat, fish, and chicken are better than fried chicken, hot dogs, and cheeseburgers. This doesn't mean you can't ever eat those foods if you love them; it just means you should aim more toward healthy and less toward "comfort" foods. Eat more fruits and vegetables. Salmon and tuna are rich in "good" fatty acids—and they don't have to be expensive; you can buy them in cans at the grocery store. Blueberries are packed with antioxidants. Nuts are a great source of protein and a better snack choice than chips. Soda just gives you empty calories without anything of benefit—compared to the antioxidants and zero calories in unsweetened tea, for example. Try to make sure that most of what you eat will be helping you stay healthy.

So what's the bottom line? If you want to change your diet to reduce your intake of fat and increase your intake of soy, you should do it. Finally, be careful not to lose too much weight too quickly. A rapid 10 percent drop in weight can compromise your immune system—which may be the major self-defense mechanism that is holding your cancer in check.

Note for Partners and Caregivers–Take Care of Your Own Health, Too

Alice B. Baldwin, whose husband had a successful radical prostatectomy (but who died a few years later of colon cancer), became a reluctant expert on coping with a husband's illness. She has some excellent advice to offer wives and partners on this subject. "You may be tempted to skip meals, to lose sleep, to forgo exercise, to drive in bad weather, and generally to ignore your own health," particularly if your husband or partner is hospitalized.

But neglecting your own health now may mean you won't have enough strength and stamina left over for the longer haul. "Recognizing your needs and fulfilling them as adequately as circumstances permit is your obligation not only to yourself but also to your spouse and to all who love you."

- Eat right, and take a multivitamin. Baldwin learned this the hard way during her husband's recovery from liver surgery. "Because of my concern for his welfare, I skipped meals off and on for a few days. Suddenly, the corridor blurred, and I found myself gripping a water cooler to keep from falling. For a few awful moments, I was afraid I would faint. In a few minutes I felt better, and after eating a light lunch, I was perfectly all right. I realized what a serious mistake I'd made by skipping those meals." If you can't take time for a regular lunch, be prepared with energy-boosting snacks such as boxes of juice, cheese and crackers, raisins, peanuts, and granola bars. Just don't let yourself become run-down.

- Keep track of your weight. "We all react differently to stress, but you should note and quickly correct gains or losses of more than a few pounds."
- Get some exercise. Take a walk once or twice a day. You'll need your own strength and resilience now more than ever.
- Get some sleep. Your odds of sleeping better will improve if you keep up an adequate diet and get some exercise. Recognize that stress interferes with your body's normal patterns, and snooze when you can—even if it's not when you're used to resting. Relaxation techniques—listening to peaceful music, visualizing pleasant scenes, breathing deeply—may help you unwind. If it helps, "remind yourself that you've done the best you could; your spouse and the medical staff have done the best they could; and now the day has ended," says Baldwin, although she admits that some nights she was simply too upset to sleep. "My husband's condition, his doctors' anxieties, my fears of the future all out-weighed my physical and emotional exhaustion. Even as I write this sentence, my stomach muscles tighten, my throat constricts, my palms begin to sweat, and I remember exactly how scared I felt."
- Ask family and friends for help—particularly if you're commuting to the hospital or doctor's office on unfamiliar roads or in heavy traffic. "At the hospital, you will benefit from their hand-holding and emotional support; on the road, they can handle the tricky turns."
- Check your own vital signs daily. Baldwin recommends asking yourself some basic questions every day, including: How do I feel today? Why do I feel that way? Tomorrow, I will take care of my need for (fill in the blank). What concern interfered with my sleep?
- Finally, when the treatment is over and life is getting back to normal, realize that your relationship has altered in subtle but significant ways, Baldwin says. "If we did not actually love one another more than we did before the illness, we now cherished one another more fully. Our children and our relationships with them were similarly changed. Perhaps the experiences we shared accelerated our normal maturation and led us all to appreciate one another more deeply.

"I recognize that I was physically and emotionally drained, and that I lost much of my resilience. Evidently this was obvious to our children, because I detected them going to new lengths to protect and to help me. My gratitude to them was tempered by my concern for them. Discussing this with the youngest, a recent college graduate, I said, 'We do not want our lives to interfere with your life,' and she replied, 'Your lives are part of my life.' "

About the Authors

Patrick C. Walsh, M.D., is the University Distinguished Service Professor Emeritus at the James Buchanan Brady Urological Institute at the Johns Hopkins Hospital and the Johns Hopkins University School of Medicine. He is best known for his pioneering work in the development of "the anatomic approach to radical prostatectomy," which involves nerve-sparing techniques that have reduced the probability of impotence and incontinence, and for his thirty years as the professor and director of the Brady Urological Institute. He also has made major contributions to the basic understanding of benign and malignant neoplasms of the prostate. Along with co-workers, he was the first to describe the 5 alpha-reductase enzyme deficiency, to develop an experimental technique for the induction of benign prostatic hyperplasia (BPH), to demonstrate the influence of reversible androgen deprivation on BPH, and to characterize hereditary prostatic cancer. He is a member of the National Academy of Medicine, formerly named the Institute of Medicine of the National Academy of Sciences. For fifteen years he was on the editorial board of the *New England Journal of Medicine* and for twenty-five years was the editor-in-chief of *Campbell's Textbook of Urology*, which has been renamed *Campbell Walsh* in his honor. In 1996, Dr. Walsh received the Charles F. Kettering Medal from the General Motors Cancer Research Foundation for "the most outstanding recent contributions to the diagnosis and treatment of cancer." Dr. Walsh was honored as the 2007 National Physician of the Year for Clinical Excellence by America's Top Doctors®, and received the 2007 King Faisal International Prize in Medicine for his contributions to prostate cancer. In 2012 he was awarded the Francis Amory Prize by the American Academy of Arts and Sciences. Together with Janet Farrar Worthington, he authored the bestselling books for lay people, *The Prostate: A Guide for Men and the Women Who Love*

Them, and more recently, *Dr. Patrick Walsh's Guide to Surviving Prostate Cancer*, Dr. Walsh has served as the president of both the American Association of Genitourinary Surgeons and the Clinical Society of Genitourinary Surgeons. To learn more about Dr. Walsh and his views on prostate cancer, watch his interview with Charlie Rose: http://urology.jhu.edu/prostate/videoWalsh.php

Janet Farrar Worthington, an award-winning science writer, has written and edited numerous health publications and contributed to several health books. She is the editor of *Discovery*, a research publication for the Patrick C. Walsh Prostate Cancer Research Fund at the Brady Urological Institute of Johns Hopkins and also the editor of *Leap, a magazine for Johns Hopkins Rheumatology*. The former editor of *Hopkins Medical News*, the alumni magazine for the Johns Hopkins School of Medicine, she is the senior writer for the Prostate Cancer Foundation's website. She often writes about prostate cancer for her men's health blog, vitaljake.com. Worthington has written two nonmedical books, *Bumble Creek Farm* and *Where's the Wine?* and also has a nonmedical blog, janetfarrarworthington.com. For six years, she was a national commentator for *Marketplace*, a program on public radio. She lives in Prescott, Arizona.

Glossary: A Guide to Medical Language of the Prostate, from A to Z

Note: Most of the words here are nouns; where we thought it necessary, we indicated otherwise.

abiraterone (Zytiga): a drug that targets the androgen receptor.

ablation: a method of getting rid of something. Cryoablation, for example, is using freezing temperatures to get rid of a prostate tumor. Hormonal ablation is getting rid of the hormones that nourish a prostate tumor.

acid phosphatase: an enzyme that, like PSA, is secreted by the prostate. Elevated acid phosphatase levels can signal that something is wrong with the prostate.

active surveillance: in prostate cancer, this is the process of delaying definitive treatment until it becomes clear, through vigilant monitoring, that the tumor is growing—waiting for evidence that cancer is on the move and then taking action.

acute bacterial prostatitis: a form of prostatitis associated with urinary tract infections, positive cultures that identify bacteria in the prostate, and an abundance of white blood cells in prostatic secretions. Acute bacterial prostatitis comes on suddenly and is accompanied by fever and symptoms that demand prompt treatment.

adjuvant therapy: an additional therapy. This is more than an extra precaution; ideally, it is designed to treat a problem before it starts. In prostate cancer, this means giving additional therapy, such as immediate radiation or chemotherapy, to high-risk patients *before* there is evidence that cancer has returned, with the hope that it won't return.

adrenal androgens: weak male hormones made by the adrenal glands. These include androstenedione, dehydroepiandrosterone (DHEA), and dehydroepiandrosterone sulfate (DHEAS), plus small amounts of testosterone. They are minor players, believed to make up only 5 percent or less of the total androgen stimulation to the prostate. Their total effect on the prostate is a controversial issue.

ADT (androgen-deprivation therapy): hormonal therapy for prostate cancer, either achieved by surgery (castration) or medicine (drugs including estrogens, antiandrogens, and LHRH agonists or antagonists), given as short- or long-term treatment.

age-specific PSA levels: a new way to evaluate PSA tests using a man's age to determine the significance of his PSA reading.

alpha-blockers: a class of drugs, originally designed to treat hypertension, that act on the prostate by relaxing smooth muscle tissue.

analgesics: painkillers.

analog: a synthetic look-alike of a drug or chemical.

anal stricture: tight scar tissue that can interfere with bowel movements.

anastomosis: the site at which two structures are surgically reconnected after an organ has been removed. After radical prostatectomy, this refers to the connection between the reconstructed bladder neck and the urethra.

androgen-dependent, or androgen-sensitive cells: cells in prostate cancer that are nourished by hormones, which can shrink dramatically when the hormones that nourish the prostate are shut off.

androgen-independent, or androgen-insensitive cells: cells in prostate cancer that are not nourished by hormones and therefore don't respond to hormonal therapy.

androgen receptor: a protein that is a target for treatment of advanced prostate cancer; the receptor is like a lock, activated by testosterone and DHT, which act as keys.

androgens: male hormones, such as testosterone.

angiogenesis: the process of forming new blood vessels. Advancing cancer paves the way by making new blood vessels.

angiogenesis inhibitors: drugs that block angiogenesis. The idea is to starve cancer by cutting off its supply lines. Cancer may not die, but it won't get any bigger, either.

antiandrogens: drugs, such as bicalutamide (Casodex), flutamide (Eulexin), and nilutamide (Nilandron), used in hormonal therapy to treat prostate cancer. These drugs block the effects of testosterone and DHT on prostate cancer cells by neutralizing their effect (they prevent testosterone and DHT from binding to the androgen receptor).

antibiotics: drugs that kill bacteria.

anticholinergic drugs: a group of drugs whose side effects include hindering urination. These may help some men with incontinence.

anticoagulants: medications that help prevent the blood from clotting.

antimetastatic drugs: drugs that put roadblocks in the way of cancer's progress, discouraging it from invading other cells or from developing new blood vessels (this process is called angiogenesis).

antimicrobial drugs: bacteria-killing drugs, such as antibiotics.

apalutamide (Erleada): a drug that targets the androgen receptor.

apoptosis: also called programmed cell death; the process by which cells kill themselves.

arterial (adj.): relating to the arteries.

artificial sphincter: an implanted device used to treat incontinence that has persisted for a year or longer and shows no signs of improving on its own.

AR-V7: a mutated androgen receptor that stops drugs such as enzalutamide (Xtandi) and abiraterone (Zytiga) from working.

ASTRO definition: a definition for relapse, or biochemical failure, after radiation therapy (determined by a panel from the American Society for Therapeutic Radiology and Oncology). According to this definition, failure after radiation means three consecutive rises in PSA levels (taken at least three months apart) after it reaches its nadir—the lowest point PSA reaches after treatment. The date of failure is backdated to the midpoint between the nadir and the first rise in PSA. (Many doctors now are using the nadir + 2 definition.)

asymptomatic (adj.): experiencing no symptoms. A man with asymptomatic prostate cancer doesn't notice anything out of the ordinary; he feels fine.

atypical (adj.): a finding on biopsy; this means the cells do not look normal but are not necessarily cancerous.

benign (adj.): harmless; not cancerous; not fatal.

benign prostatic hyperplasia: see *BPH*.

bicalutamide (Casodex): the most common antiandrogen drug, used to treat advanced prostate cancer.

biopsy of the prostate: a means of sampling the prostate by taking cores of tissue with a needle so it can be checked for the presence of cancer.

bisphosphonates: bone-targeting drugs used for several purposes. They strengthen bone to prevent osteoporosis in men on hormonal therapy; they also reduce the likelihood of bone pain, reduce the need for radiation to the bone because of pain, and reduce fractures and spinal cord complications.

bladder: a hollow, muscular reservoir that functions as a holding tank for urine.

bladder neck contracture: a constriction of the bladder neck caused by scar tissue. This can impede urine flow.

bladder spasms: painful, uncontrollable contractions of the bladder.

bladder stones: tiny formations made from crystals of uric acid or calcium that precipitate out of urine.

bloodless field: a surgical term that means controlling bleeding within a patient to give surgeons a better view as they perform an operation.

blood-prostate barrier: a membrane that prevents many substances, including antibiotics, from entering the prostate. This barrier breaks down when a man has bacterial prostatitis, permitting most antibiotics to enter the prostate.

bone scan: also called *radionuclide scintigraphy*; imaging test in which doctors inject into the bloodstream a radioactive tracer, a chemical that's attracted specifically to bone. The bone scan is an excellent means of finding out whether prostate cancer has spread to bone.

bound PSA: PSA molecules in the bloodstream that are chemically tied to proteins. Other PSA molecules are without these chemical ties; these are called free. If a man has a PSA test and most of the PSA is bound, the PSA elevation is probably coming from cancer.

BPH: benign prostatic hyperplasia, or enlargement of the prostate. A benign condition that occurs in most older men when prostate tissue begins to grow around the urethra, gradually compressing it and hindering urine flow.

BPSA: a particular form of free PSA produced by the prostate's transition zone, a thin ring of tissue that surrounds the urethra, in BPH. BPSA is more of a marker for BPH than for cancer.

brachytherapy (interstitial radiotherapy): implanting radioactive "seeds," or minute chunks of radioactive material, into the prostate to kill cancer.

BRCA1 and BRCA2: the best known genes linked to breast and ovarian cancer risk, which have been shown to also increase the risk for prostate and pancreatic cancers.

calculi: see *prostatic calculi*.

capsule of the prostate: the outer wall of the prostate gland.

castrate range: the level to which testosterone drops after orchiectomy. This is an important point of comparison in monitoring hormonal therapy, as certain drugs are judged by their ability to reduce testosterone to this range.

castration: see *orchiectomy*.

catheter: a tube used for drainage or irrigation; most commonly used to drain urine out of the bladder.

cell division: the method through which the body's cells multiply. A single cell divides into two. Then those two cells each divide into two, and so on.

chemical castration: the use of drugs to accomplish the same effect as orchiectomy—that is, to lower the testosterone level to the castrate range.

chemotherapeutic drugs: a class of cell-killing drugs used to treat many forms of cancer.

chronic bacterial prostatitis: a form of prostatitis associated with urinary tract infections, positive cultures that identify bacteria in the prostate, and an abundance of white blood cells in prostatic secretions. This can be a recurring illness, coming back periodically for years after an initial episode of acute bacterial prostatitis.

chronic prostatitis/chronic pelvic pain syndrome (CPPS): the most mysterious category of prostatitis. Nobody knows what causes the symptoms in this group (which used to be named for what it was not, nonbacterial prostatitis), and antibiotics don't help at all. In some men, the prostate may not even be the problem—the pain and other symptoms may be a result of spasms elsewhere in the pelvis, rectum, or lower back. This category has two subgroups— inflammatory and noninflammatory, based on whether any white blood cells (also called inflammatory cells) are found in the prostatic fluid.

clinical stage of prostate cancer: an estimate of the extent of a man's cancer, based on factors such as the digital rectal exam, PSA test, and bone scan. Pathologic stage is much more certain, but this can be determined only when a pathologist examines actual prostate tissue after surgery.

clonal selection: the process whereby the most poorly differentiated, rapidly growing, aggressive cells overtake the slower, well-differentiated cells as a tumor progresses.

complementary medicine: nontraditional medicine. In pain management, for example, this includes herbal remedies, prayer and meditation, acupuncture, deep breathing, aromatherapy, relaxation techniques, massage therapy, biofeedback, hypnosis, yoga, and even laughter (also called humor therapy).

complexed PSA: the PSA bound to a protein called alpha 1-antichymotrypsin (ACT). The complexed PSA assay is a way of looking at the ratio of bound to free PSA.

conformal radiation therapy: a technique for delivering externalbeam radiation that maximizes the dose of radiation to the prostate tumor while keeping the risk of damaging nearby tissue to a minimum.

corpora cavernosa and corpus spongiosum: spongy chambers in the penis that become engorged with blood during an erection.

corticosteroids: powerful drugs that reduce inflammation and, in men with advanced prostate cancer, bring relief from some spinal pain. However, because of their side effects, they are not good for long-term use.

creatinine test: a blood test (also called a serum creatinine test) that checks for impairment of kidney function.

CRPC (castrate- or castration-resistant prostate cancer): cancer that recurs after remission with hormonal therapy (ADT). This is also called hormone-refractory prostate cancer.

cruciferous vegetables: vegetables in the cabbage and turnip family, including broccoli, cauliflower, cabbage, Brussels sprouts, bok choy, and kale. They can help lower the risk of developing cancer.

cryoablation or cryotherapy: using extremely cold liquid nitrogen to freeze the entire prostate, causing cancer cells within the gland to rupture as they begin to thaw.

CT (computed tomography) scan: a circular series of X-ray pictures taken by a machine that goes around the body. A computer puts the pictures together, generating images that, as in an MRI, are like slices of anatomy.

cystometry: a test that measures bladder pressure and function, done by passing a small catheter through the urethra into the bladder. Changes in pressure are monitored as the bladder fills with water.

cystoscope: a tiny, lighted tube that works like a periscope on a submarine. In cystoscopy, it is inserted into the tip of the anesthetized penis and threaded through the urethra into the bladder; this allows the doctor to inspect the bladder, prostate, and urethra for abnormalities.

deep venous thrombosis: condition in which blood clots form in the deep veins of the legs; it is a potential complication of major surgery, such as radical prostatectomy. At best, these clots can be painful. At worst, they can be fatal, if a chunk of a blood clot in the leg breaks free and shoots up to the lungs. These should be treated immediately.

DES: see *estrogens.*

DHT: dihydrotestosterone, the active form of male hormone in the prostate. It is made when testosterone is transformed by an enzyme called 5-alpha reductase.

DIC: disseminated intravascular coagulation, a blood-clotting disorder that develops in some men with advanced prostate cancer.

differentiating agents: drugs that work by slowing down cancer's rate of growth.

differentiation of prostate cancer cells: how cancer cells look under the microscope. Well-differentiated cells have distinct, clearly defined borders and clear centers, and their growth is relatively slow and orderly. Everything about poorly differentiated cells is murkier and not as well defined. As cancer progresses, these poorly differentiated cells seem to melt together and form solid, nasty blobs of malignancy. These are the most aggressive cells in a tumor, and they are given a high grade (8, 9, 10) in the Gleason scoring system. Well-differentiated cells are called low grade (2, 3, 4). Moderately well differentiated cells fall in between (5, 6, 7), and it's hard to predict what these cells will do.

digital rectal exam: a very important part of the physical examination in which a doctor's gloved, lubricated finger is inserted into the rectum to feel for lumps, enlargement, or areas of hardness that might indicate the presence of cancer. It is uncomfortable but not painful, and it's generally brief, lasting less than a minute.

diuretics: drugs that work by altering the way the body metabolizes sodium; this causes the kidneys to absorb less water, so more of it leaves the body in the form of urine. For most people, taking diuretics means urinating more frequently and having a more forceful stream. Taking them can be disastrous for a man with BPH.

diverticula: pockets of the bladder lining that poke out like balloons through the bladder wall. (A single one of these is called a diverticulum.)

DNA: the genetic blueprint; vital information contained in the nucleus of every cell.

docetaxel (Taxotere): a chemotherapy drug that hinders cells' multiplication.

dorsiflexion exercises: pumping the feet up and down to exercise the calf muscles; a good exercise to do immediately after surgery to prevent deep venous thrombosis.

double-blind study: a study in which neither the doctor nor the patient knows who's receiving the placebo or the standard medication versus who's receiving the new medication being tested.

dry ejaculation: also known as retrograde ejaculation. This is a complication of some prostate procedures, including TUR. For most men, this has no effect on the pleasant sensation of orgasm. Dry ejaculation is pretty much what it sounds like: semen is not expelled out the urethra when a man reaches sexual climax. Instead, it goes the other way—back into the bladder. This happens because part of the bladder neck—a muscular valve whose job is to slam shut at the time of ejaculation, forcing semen out the urethra—is often resected along with the prostate tissue. When this area is damaged or missing, there's nothing to prevent semen from heading the wrong way. This also occurs after a radical prostatectomy or radiation therapy, because the prostate and seminal vesicles, which make the fluid, are either removed or dried up.

ED drugs: drugs used to treat erectile dysfunction. These are phosphodiesterase inhibitors, such as sildenafil (Viagra), tadalafil (Cialis), avanafil (Stendra), and vardenafil (Levitra).

edema: swelling caused by fluid retention.

ejaculate (noun): semen, the fluid that exits the body during orgasm, or sexual climax. *Ejaculate* also is a verb.

ejaculation: emission of semen at the climax of sexual intercourse.

enzalutamide (Xtandi): a drug that targets the androgen receptor.

epididymis: the "greenhouse" where sperm mature and are stored until orgasm.

epididymitis: an infection of the epididymis. This may occur after a surgical procedure that damages the ejaculatory ducts, allowing infected urine to back up into the vas deferens.

epidural anesthesia: a local anesthetic administered through a tiny plastic tube, inserted between the vertebrae of the spine, near the small of the back. The epidural anesthetic bathes the area outside the membrane lining the spinal cord, temporarily numbing the nerves in the lower body. Unlike spinal anesthesia, which is delivered in one dose, epidural anesthesia can be given continuously. The area of numbness can be adjusted; so can the degree of pain relief.

epithelial cells: cells in the glandular tissue of the prostate that secrete fluid that becomes part of semen.

erectile dysfunction (ED): the inability to have an erection sufficient for sexual intercourse.

estrogens: female hormones. Estrogens block the release of a signal transmitted by the pituitary gland called luteinizing hormone (LH), which stimulates testosterone. Oral estrogens, taken as hormonal therapy by men with prostate cancer, reduce testosterone to the crucial castrate range. The main oral estrogen used for this is diethylstilbestrol (DES).

excise (verb): to cut out; to remove surgically.

external-beam radiation therapy: a curative treatment for prostate cancer. It involves beaming X-ray energy into a prostate tumor from the outside, a few minutes at a time, over the course of several weeks.

fascia: a thin blanket of connective tissue.

5-alpha reductase: enzymes in the prostate that convert testosterone to DHT.

5-alpha reductase inhibitors: drugs that block the formation of DHT. This causes the prostate to shrink and improves the obstructive symptoms of BPH. These drugs do not affect levels of testosterone, the hormone responsible for a man's libido and sexual function.

fluoroscopy: an imaging technique in which an X-ray image appears live on a screen instead of as a still photograph.

Foley catheter: a catheter inserted into the penis and threaded through the urethra into the bladder, where it's anchored in place with a tiny, inflated balloon. It removes urine from the body; it also can be used for irrigation to prevent blood clots.

following expectantly: see *active surveillance.*

free PSA: also called percent-free PSA; PSA that is not chemically bound to proteins in the bloodstream. If a man has an elevated PSA level and most of the PSA is free, then the elevation is probably due to BPH.

frozen section analysis: freezing, then slicing tissue into very thin sections to be examined under a microscope. In a staging pelvic lymphadenectomy, lymph nodes are removed, then rushed to a pathologist for frozen-section analysis to check for cancer.

FSH: follicle-stimulating hormone, made along with LH by the pituitary gland. FSH has its major effect on sperm production.

gene therapy: one of the most exciting nonhormonal areas of treatment for advanced prostate cancer. Scientists are now able to program the body's DNA like a computer chip, sending it on a selective search-and-destroy mission targeted only at prostate cancer cells. Gene-targeted drugs are aimed at specific mutated genes or processes found in metastatic cancer.

genetic drift: as a cancer progresses and its cells double over and over again, the DNA becomes less stable. The cancer develops new mutations; it becomes more aggressive. As the tumor progresses, well-differentiated cells deteriorate into poorly differentiated cells. This downslide is called genetic drift.

genetic susceptibility: a complex of genetic factors that create a more hospitable atmosphere for cancer.

Gleason Grade Group (GG or GGG): a simplified system of grading prostate cancer, developed by pathologist Jonathan Epstein at Johns Hopkins, that classifies Gleason scores into five groups based on the aggressive potential of the cancer cells.

Gleason score: a way to classify the severity of cancer based on the way it looks under a microscope. Cells that are well differentiated are given a low grade (2, 3, 4); poorly differentiated cells are given a high grade (8, 9, 10). Moderately well differentiated cells fall in the middle. See also *differentiation of prostate cancer cells.*

glutathione S-transferase Π (GSTP): an important enzyme that helps prevent oxidative damage, which can lead to prostate cancer.

grade of prostate cancer: see *Gleason score* and *Gleason Grade Group.*

growth factors: substances that activate processes that promote cell division.

gynecomastia: tenderness, pain, or swelling of the breasts in men. This is a common, easily treatable side effect of some forms of hormonal therapy for prostate cancer.

hedgehog pathway: the path taken by a cancer in metastasis. Blocking this pathway may mean that we can prevent cancer from spreading.

hemi-body irradiation: a once-common form of radiation treatment delivered to ease pain in prostate cancer patients with metastases to bone in several places. It involves irradiating great expanses of the body.

hereditary prostate cancer (HPC): HPC is present in families if there are three first-degree relatives (a father or brothers) who develop prostate cancer; or two first-degree relatives, if both developed it before age fifty-five; or if prostate cancer has occurred in three generations in the family (grandfather, father, son). HPC can be inherited from either side of the family.

heterogeneity: the state of being diverse or varied; not uniform. In prostate cancer and BPH, heterogeneity refers to a "melting pot" of cells, all jockeying for position in one area.

HIFU (high-intensity focused ultrasound): a procedure that treats spots of cancer within the prostate, rather than the entire gland.

high-dose-rate (HDR) brachytherapy: also called temporary brachytherapy; this is usually given along with external-beam radiation. The seeds don't stay in; they're removed at the end of each treatment session.

hormonal therapy (also called ADT, for androgen deprivation therapy): the use of hormones to treat advanced prostate cancer. Hormonal therapy is aimed at shutting down the hormones that nourish the prostate. Some cells in a prostate tumor are responsive to this, but some aren't.

hormone-dependent, hormone-sensitive: see *androgen-dependent, androgen-sensitive* (*cells*).

hormone-independent, hormone-insensitive: see *androgen-independent, androgen-insensitive* (*cells*).

hormone-refractory prostate cancer: metastatic prostate cancer that has returned after months or years of being controlled by hormonal therapy. This is also called castrate-resistant prostate cancer (CRPC).

hot flash: a sudden rush of warmth in the face, neck, upper chest, and back lasting from a few seconds to an hour; a side effect of some hormonal treatments for prostate cancer. Although hot flashes aren't harmful to a man's health, they can be bothersome.

HOXB13: a prostate cancer susceptibility gene; 60 percent of men who inherit a mutated form of this gene are diagnosed with prostate cancer by age eighty.

hyperplasia: an increase in the number of cells.

hypofractionated radiation therapy: higher doses of radiation delivered over a shorter time period—four to five weeks, for instance, instead of eight weeks.

image-guided radiation therapy (IGRT): radiation therapy in which the location of a man's prostate (which is never constant) is checked every day before treatment so that small adjustments in his position can be made, making the radiation as precisely targeted as possible.

imaging (verb): seeing and taking pictures inside the body using various forms of energy, including ultrasound, magnetic resonance (MRI), and X-rays.

immunotherapy: treatment designed to maximize the immune system's ability to fight cancer.

impotence: also called erectile dysfunction (ED); this is the inability to have an erection, which, in most cases, is treatable.

incidental prostate cancer: apparently dormant, small cancer cell clusters that reside in the prostates of millions of men. In some men, this cancer never poses a danger. In others, however, it eventually does.

incontinence: also called urinary incontinence; it is the unintentional leakage of urine. (Another kind of incontinence, bowel or fecal incontinence, means having an unintentional bowel movement.)

infectious prostatitis: a term some doctors use to describe bacterial prostatitis. Bacterial prostatitis is not infectious; men can have a normal sex life without worrying about giving the disease to someone else.

inflammation: the "gasoline" that accelerates the flames of rampant cell growth by injuring cells, damaging DNA, and causing the body to crank out replacement cells that may be faulty; long-term inflammation is linked to many forms of cancer.

insulin-like growth factors: a class of hormones that may influence the development of prostate cancer.

intensity-modulated radiation therapy (IMRT): an approach to external-beam radiation using multiple beamlets to "sculpt" the radiation dose to fit the individual contours of each man's prostate and pelvic region.

intermittent hormonal therapy: also called intermittent androgen suppression; in this plan, men start taking hormones early, before signs or symptoms of advanced cancer begin. Then, when their PSA levels drop, they stop taking them and get a little "vacation" from treatment. The men are monitored closely, and at the first sign that the tumor is growing, they start taking the hormones again.

intra-abdominal (adj.): in the abdomen.

intraurethral (adj.): in the urethra.

intraurethral therapy: a pharmacological treatment for men with ED using agents that can be placed directly into the urethra.

invasive (adj.): involving an incision; the body is physically entered. In minimally invasive surgery, this incision may be a hole as small as a dime, or there may be no incision at all if the body's own passageways—such as the urethra in the TUR procedure—are used. A noninvasive procedure does not invade the body at all; many forms of imaging are noninvasive.

irritative symptoms in BPH: these include frequent urination, especially at night; a strong sense of urgency in urination; inability to postpone urination; and sleep disrupted by the need to urinate.

ISUP (International Society of Urological Pathology). This abbreviation is used sometimes rather than "grade group" to refer to the simplified system developed by pathologist Jonathan Epstein at Johns Hopkins.

IV: the abbreviation for *intravenous*, which means, literally, "through the veins." Medication, fluids, or nutrition supplements can be administered this way.

kidneys: the body's main filters. They cleanse the body of impurities and, at the same time, salvage and recycle useful materials.

laparoscopic pelvic lymphadenectomy: dissection of the lymph nodes as a means of staging prostate cancer. Laparoscopic surgery is minimally invasive; there's a tiny incision, and much of the surgery is conducted through "telescopes."

latent (adj.): dormant; passive.

lateral lobe enlargement: a form of BPH that results when prostate tissue compresses the urethra from the sides.

LH: luteinizing hormone, a chemical signal transmitted by the pituitary. LH motivates the testes to make testosterone.

LHRH: luteinizing hormone–releasing hormone (also called GnRH, for gonadotropin-releasing hormone); a chemical signal made in the brain by the hypothalamus. LHRH tells the pituitary gland to make LH and FSH.

LHRH agonists: synthetic look-alikes of LHRH. These drugs shut down the pituitary's production of the hormone LH.

LHRH antagonists: these drugs work faster than LHRH agonists to lower testosterone without producing the brief testosterone "flare."

libido: sex drive.

localized prostate cancer: cancer that is confined within the prostate and is therefore considered curable.

local recurrence of cancer: when cancer returns to the prostate or nearby tissue after treatment.

lycopene: an antioxidant found in tomatoes, red grapefruits, watermelons, and berries that fights oxidative damage, which may lead to prostate cancer.

metastasis: a chunk of cancer that has broken off from the main tumor and established itself elsewhere. A distant metastasis means this new site of cancer is far from its point of origin. The word *metastases* is plural, and *metastatic* is an adjective that refers to a metastasis.

micrometastases: tiny, invisible (and undetectable) offshoots of prostate cancer.

middle lobe enlargement: a type of BPH in which a lobe of prostate tissue grows inside the bladder. When it reaches a critical size, it can block the opening of the bladder neck like a cork in a bottle. This explains how some men with a small prostate can develop major symptoms of urinary obstruction.

MRI: magnetic resonance imaging; a means of imaging that's painless, noninvasive, and does not use X-rays. It is time-consuming, however, often taking about forty-five minutes. MRI gives a three-dimensional scan of the body, producing images that are like slices of anatomy.

MRI fusion biopsy: an image taken during multiparametric MRI (mpMRI), used during an ultrasound biopsy to provide a 3-D road map to suspicious-looking areas of the prostate that need to be sampled.

Multiparametric MRI (mpMRI): a form of MRI that looks at the prostate in several ways, including with a contrast dye injected in the blood.

nadir + 2 definition: this defines treatment failure after radiation therapy as a PSA level that has risen 2 ng/ml higher than a man's PSA nadir (the lowest level it reached following treatment).

National Comprehensive Cancer Network (NCCN): an alliance of twenty-seven National Cancer Institute–designated comprehensive cancer centers that issues highly respected guidelines for clinical standards of care.

nerve-sparing radical prostatectomy: what some doctors call the anatomical approach to radical retropubic prostatectomy; they're referring to important modifications that reduce blood loss and allow men to remain potent and continent after radical prostatectomy.

neurogenic bladder: trouble in the bladder caused by a neurological problem, such as Parkinson's disease.

neurotransmitters: chemical messengers; signals sent from a transmitter in one nerve cell to a receptor in another.

neurovascular bundles: cordlike structures that run down the sides of the prostate near the rectum. The bundles contain microscopic nerves that are essential for erection; they also contain arteries and veins that help surgeons identify the location of these nerves.

nitric oxide: a substance released by nerve endings during erection, causing the smooth muscle tissue in the penis to relax.

nocturia: frequent urination during the night. A man has nocturia if he has to get up several times a night to go to the bathroom. This is often a symptom of BPH.

nocturnal penile tumescence test: an evaluation to determine whether a man has erections at night while he sleeps.

nonhormonal therapy: exciting new treatments for advanced prostate cancer specifically designed to target the biological mechanisms involved in cancer progression and metastasis.

noninvasive (adj.): not invasive; in other words, there's no incision.

NSAIDs: nonsteroidal anti-inflammatory drugs, which are used to treat mild pain. Available over-the-counter and in prescription form.

nutraceuticals: drugs extracted from specific nutrients.

obstructive symptoms in BPH: these include weak urine flow, hesitancy in starting urination, a need to push or strain to get urine to flow, intermittent urine stream (starts and stops several times), difficulty in stopping urination, dribbling after urination, a sense of not being able to empty the bladder completely, and not being able to urinate at all.

oligometastasis: the presence of a limited number (usually fewer than four) very tiny spots of cancer outside the prostate in a man who has no symptoms of advanced cancer; this can be treated with stereotactic ablative radiotherapy (SABR or SBRT).

omega-3 fatty acids: fatty acids found in fish oils that may be helpful in preventing coronary artery disease and are not linked to the development of prostate cancer.

oncogene: a gene that acts like a stuck accelerator in a car; the "on switch" that keeps cancer cells growing.

orchiectomy: surgical castration. A form of hormonal therapy involving removal of all or part of the testicles. This causes testosterone levels to fall to the castrate range.

orgasm: the climax of sexual intercourse.

overflow incontinence: when urine leaks out because the bladder is too full to hold any more.

oxidative damage: incremental damage caused over many years as free radicals (toxic by-products of everyday metabolism) attack the DNA in cells, causing mutations that lead to cancer.

palliate (verb): to ease or relieve. Palliative treatment makes symptoms, and therefore quality of life, better, even though it may do nothing to cure the underlying cause of these symptoms.

palpable (adj.): tangible. Palpable cancer in the prostate means there's a lump, lesion, or nodule that a doctor's gloved finger can feel during a digital rectal exam.

pathologic fracture: when cancer invades bones, they become brittle. Brittle bones break. Men with metastatic prostate cancer are prone to getting broken bones, called pathologic fractures. Most susceptible are the bones that bear much of the body's weight—those in the hip and thigh.

pathologic stage of prostate cancer: the definitive extent of a man's prostate cancer. (The possibilities include organ-confined cancer, capsular penetration, positive surgical margins, invasion of the seminal vesicles, and/or involvement of the pelvic lymph nodes.) This is determined after prostate surgery, when a pathologist examines the actual prostate specimen and dissected tissue from the nearby lymph nodes instead of merely making guesses about how far the cancer has spread based on test results and a few cells from biopsies.

pathologist: a doctor who studies cells, tissue, and organs and makes determinations about them, answering such questions as "Is there cancer here?" and "Was all the cancer removed?"

PCA3: a test performed on urine that looks for the prostate cancer-specific DD3 gene, used to help guide the decision for a repeat biopsy.

penile (adj.): relating to the penis.

penile implants: bendable, inflatable, or mechanical prostheses that enable a man with ED to have erections sufficient for penetration.

perforation: puncture.

perineum: the area between the scrotum and rectum.

perineural invasion: a term meaning that prostate cancer has been found in the spaces around the nerves near the edge of the prostate, found on biopsy. Because cancer that has penetrated the capsule can still be cured, perineural invasion has no long-term impact on a man's prognosis.

peripheral zone: the largest part of the prostate and the area where most prostate cancer occurs.

periprostatic tissue: tissue just outside the prostate.

Peyronie's disease: a disorder of the connective tissue within the penis that can cause curvature during erection.

PHI (prostate health index): a "second-line" blood test that combines total PSA and free PSA with another form of PSA, pro-PSA; this test can help predict who is likely to have significant prostate cancer on biopsy.

phosphodiesterase inhibitors: drugs such as sildenafil (Viagra) that can help facilitate an erection.

phytoestrogens: estrogens derived from plants. The prefix *phyto* means "coming from plants."

PIN: prostatic intraepithelial neoplasia; abnormal cells, found in a needle biopsy, that are strongly linked to prostate cancer.

placebo: a "sugar pill" often taken by participants in a medical study. Patients taking a placebo are compared with patients taking actual medications.

placebo effect: a phenomenon that happens often in medical studies, in which patients taking a placebo have an inexplicable improvement in symptoms.

poly ADP-ribose polymerase (PARP) inhibitors: new drugs used to treat advanced prostate cancer that work especially well in men with mutated DNA damage repair genes, such as BRCA1/2.

pressure-flow studies: tests to monitor bladder pressure changes as a man urinates.

proliferation: spread or growth.

prostate: a muscular, walnut-shaped gland about an inch and a half long that sits directly under the bladder. Its main function is to make part of the fluid for semen.

prostatectomy: an operation to remove all or part of the prostate.

prostate-specific antigen: see *PSA.*

prostatic (adj.): relating to the prostate.

prostatic abscess: localized accumulation of pus, like a pimple, under pressure in the prostate.

prostatic calculi: the prostate's version of gallstones or kidney stones. They're usually tiny and harmless. But when they get infected, as they often do in men with chronic bacterial prostatitis, they can cause an infection to persist and symptoms of urinary tract infections and prostatitis to return again and again.

prostatic urethra: the part of the urethra that runs through the prostate.

prostatitis: inflammation of the prostate.

prosthesis: an artificial replacement for part of the body that is either missing or not functioning properly.

proton-beam radiation: an approach to external-beam radiation therapy that uses charged particles instead of electromagnetic waves. The proton beam shoots in a straight line, but it can be stopped abruptly—for example, at the delicate rectal wall, just on the other side of the prostate, so the fragile tissue in the rectum can be spared.

PSA: prostate-specific antigen, an enzyme made by the prostate. Levels of PSA can be checked through a simple blood test; elevated amounts of PSA in the blood can signal prostate cancer.

PSA density: the blood PSA score divided by the volume of the prostate, as determined by transrectal ultrasound.

PSA velocity: PSA's rate of change from year to year.

PSMA: prostate-specific membrane antigen, a protein that is made on the surface of prostate cells.

PSMA PET: an imaging technique that targets PSMA and can spot extremely small areas of prostate cancer.

psychogenic erectile dysfunction: erection problems that are psychological, not physiological, in nature. Doctors making this ruling if a man can't produce an erection during sexual activity but has several a night while he sleeps.

pulmonary embolus: a blood clot in the lungs, a potential complication of radical prostatectomy. This is extremely serious and can be fatal.

pulsed Doppler ultrasound: a test that uses high-resolution ultrasound to evaluate the arteries' blood supply to the penis.

quality of life: basically, this means how good a patient thinks life is. When quality of life is excellent, a patient is relatively untroubled by symptoms or pain. When it is poor, pain or symptoms have interfered with a man's ability to function, to pursue his daily activities, and to enjoy his life.

radiation "seeds": see *brachytherapy.*

radiation therapy: see *external-beam radiation therapy* and *brachytherapy.*

radical prostatectomy: the operation to remove the prostate, and the gold standard for curing localized prostate cancer.

radionuclide scintigraphy: see *bone scan.*

radium 223 (Xofigo): a radiopharmaceutical drug used to treat metastasized cancer and pain in the bone.

randomize (verb): doctors use this verb when discussing medical studies in which some men are assigned one treatment or another at random.

receptors: highly specific "locks" in cells that are opened, or activated, only by certain hormones or chemical signals, which act as "keys."

regeneration: regrowth.

resect (verb): to cut out; to remove surgically.

resectoscope: an instrument used in the TUR procedure. Threaded through the penis, it shines a light that allows surgeons to view the prostate as they chip away at excess tissue.

retreatment: a repeat procedure to treat the same initial problem.

retrograde ejaculation: see *dry ejaculation.*

retropubic (adj.): behind the pubic bone; a surgical approach. In retropubic prostatectomy, the surgeon makes an incision in the lower abdomen, separates the abdominal muscles, and moves the bladder aside, unopened, to reach the prostate directly (as opposed to the suprapubic approach, in which the prostate is reached by cutting through the bladder).

robotic radical prostatectomy: also called robotically assisted radical prostatectomy; this technique is performed laparoscopically, using instruments designed to mimic the movement of human hands, wrists, and fingers. This allows the surgeon a greater range of motion and more precision.

salvage therapy: a medical term for "Plan B." It is another form of treatment given because the first form of treatment the patient underwent was not successful in curing the problem. In prostate cancer, this is mainly the use of radiation therapy, cryoablation, or hormonal therapy in men who develop a rising PSA level after surgery or radiation therapy for localized disease.

selenium: a mineral found in fruits and vegetables, meats, and fish that may help prevent prostate cancer.

semen: the fluid that transports sperm.

seminal vesicles: glands that, like the prostate, are sex accessory glands. Fluid secreted by these glands is critical for ensuring the proper consistency of semen.

sex accessory tissues: glands such as the prostate, seminal vesicles, and Cowper's glands, which produce secretions that become part of the fluid in semen.

sinusoids: spongy chambers within the penis that become engorged with blood during an erection.

small-cell carcinoma: a variety of prostate cancer. Cells in these tumors have a makeup similar to that of other small-cell cancers (of the lung, for example), and they respond to the same kinds of chemotherapy drugs used to treat those tumors.

spinal anesthesia: a shot of local anesthetic delivered into the small of the back through the dura, the membrane lining the spinal cord, and into the spinal fluid. Within minutes, the patient feels numb, relaxed, and heavy from the waist down.

spinal cord compression: a very serious problem in men with metastatic prostate cancer. This happens when cancer eats away at the spine, causing part of the spinal column to collapse, trapping and sometimes crushing nearby nerves.

spot radiation: localized external-beam radiation treatment targeted at one or several painful bone metastases. It can ease pain dramatically in these sites.

stage of prostate cancer: the extent of the disease—how big it is and how far it has spread. The stage of prostate cancer has a major role in determining what treatment a man should receive. See also *clinical stage of prostate cancer* and *pathologic stage of prostate cancer.*

staging pelvic lymphadenectomy: dissection of the pelvic lymph nodes to see whether they contain prostate cancer. This procedure is generally performed just before a radical prostatectomy.

statins: drugs that lower cholesterol and reduce the risk of a heart attack or stroke.

stent: a tube implanted and left in place to hold open a space that would otherwise collapse or be compressed.

step-up hormonal therapy: a gradual approach to hormonal therapy. The idea here is to start modulating the male hormones with agents that have the fewest side effects, and then to escalate as needed if the disease progresses.

stereotactic ablative radiotherapy (SABR) or stereotactic body radiation therapy (SBRT): an ultra-short, high-dose form of radiation therapy.

stress incontinence: condition in which urine leaks during certain activities, such as running or playing golf.

stricture: a blockage caused by scar tissue.

stromal cells: cells found in the prostate's smooth muscle tissue, which contract automatically to launch secretions into the urethra.

strontium-89: a highly effective radioactive substance, injected into the body, that is specially tailored to treat bone pain in cancer patients.

subcapsular orchiectomy: a cosmetic approach to orchiectomy. In

this operation, a surgeon opens the lining of the testicles and empties the contents of each one. The lining is closed again, and this
empty shell is placed back inside the scrotum—so nothing looks
different; in other words, no one can tell from outward appearance
that there's nothing inside the testicles.

suprapubic (adj.): above the pubic bone; a surgical approach to the
prostate.

surgical margins: the edges of removed tissues. These are assessed
when pathologists look at the edges of tissue that has been cut out
during surgery. If no cancer appears on these edges, the margins
are said to be clear, or negative. If this is the case, it is likely that
all the cancerous tissue was removed. If the margin is positive, the
surgeon might not have been able to cut out all the cancer.

sutures: stitches used to close an incision.

template: a highly sophisticated map of the prostate that helps doctors know exactly where to insert radioactive seeds.

testes or testicles: housed in the scrotum, these are a man's reproductive organs and the main source of the male hormone testosterone
and of sperm.

testosterone: the male hormone, or androgen, which is important
to the prostate and is essential for sex drive and fertility. It is also
responsible for such "manly" characteristics as postpuberty body
hair and the deepening of the voice. Lowering testosterone levels is
a major goal of hormonal therapy to treat prostate cancer.

thermal ablation: using heat to destroy tissue.

three-dimensional conformal radiation: approach to external-beam
radiation in which many X-ray beams, shaped to fit the target area,
are focused on the prostate, delivering a homogenous, high dose of
radiation.

total androgen blockade, or ablation: a form of hormonal therapy
to treat prostate cancer. The theory here is that even low levels of
testosterone and DHT, engendered by the adrenal androgens, can
stimulate cancer in the prostate and must be stopped. This can be
accomplished by combining whatever achieves a castrate level of
testosterone—surgical castration, estrogens, or an LHRH agonist—
with an antiandrogen.

transabdominal (adj.): through the abdomen.

transition zone: the innermost ring of the prostate; it is tissue that
surrounds the urethra. This is the sole site affected by BPH.

transperineal (adj.): through the perineum.

transrectal (adj.): through the rectum.

treatment-planning CT scan: CT images that show the physical terrain of the target area—the prostate and surrounding organs—
before radiation treatment.

trilobar enlargement: a type of BPH involving three (two lateral and one middle) lobes, in which obstruction can occur in the bladder neck as well as the urethra.

tumor suppressor gene: a gene that acts as a brake to prevent the out-of-control cell growth of cancer.

TUR: abbreviation for transurethral resection of the prostate, the gold standard operation to treat symptoms of BPH. It does not require an incision; instead, prostate tissue is reached, chipped away, and removed in tiny fragments through the urethra.

ultrasound: a painless, noninvasive way of imaging that creates a picture with high-frequency sound waves, like sonar on a submarine. It may be done either from outside, through the abdomen, or transrectally, via a wand inserted in the rectum. Transrectal ultrasound can determine the size of the prostate and direct the needle used for biopsies.

ureters: muscular, one-way channels that work like toothpaste tubes, squeezing urine out of the kidneys and onward toward the bladder.

urethra: a tube that, like the prostate, is involved in both the urinary tract and reproductive systems. It serves as a conduit not only for urine but also for secretions from the ejaculatory ducts and the prostate.

urethral sphincter: the muscle responsible for urinary control.

urethral stricture: scar tissue that blocks the urethra.

urge, or urgency, incontinence: a condition in which a man knows he has to go to the bathroom, but some urine leaks as he's trying to get there.

urinalysis: microscopic and chemical analysis of urine.

urinary retention: condition in which the bladder stays completely or partially full. Acute urinary retention means someone can no longer urinate. This is a very serious condition that requires immediate treatment.

urodynamic studies: tests that measure urinary flow, pressure, and volume to find out whether urinary trouble is caused by BPH or a problem with the bladder.

uroflowmetry: a test to measure the amount of urine a man passes and the speed of his urinary stream.

urologist: a physician who specializes in the diagnosis and medical and surgical treatment of problems in the urinary tract and male reproductive systems.

USPSTF (U.S. Preventive Services Task Force): a health policy-setting group that in 2012 recommended against routine screening for prostate cancer in men of average risk and in 2017, after a backlash and many men were diagnosed with cancer at a later stage that was more difficult to cure, changed its recommendation.

UTI: urinary tract infection; the presence of bacteria in the urine, sometimes associated with fever.

vacuum erection device: an apparatus that creates suction using an airtight tube, which is placed temporarily around the penis. An attached pump withdraws air, creating reduced atmospheric pressure—a vacuum—around the penis, causing it to become engorged with blood. The penis becomes erect. Then a constricting ring similar to a rubber band keeps the blood trapped in the penis so the erection can be sustained.

vascular (adj.): involving blood vessels.

vas deferens: one of the two hard, muscular cords that wind their way from the epididymis to the base of the prostate, where they meet with the duct of the seminal vesicle to form the ejaculatory duct.

vasectomy: a surgical procedure that is a form of male contraception. When the vas deferens is cut, sperm cannot exit the penis through ejaculation and instead are reabsorbed into the body.

vasodilators: drugs that open up blood vessels, making a wider channel for blood to go through. In the penis, they also cause the smooth muscle tissue to relax and the veins to close; some vasodilators, injected in tiny amounts in the penis, are used to produce erections.

venous (adj.): relating to the veins.

venous leak: a common cause of erectile dysfunction. Even though the arteries fill the penis with blood, producing a partial erection, the veins don't clamp down to keep this blood trapped inside the penis, so a full erection can't be achieved.

vitamin E: an antioxidant.

wide excision: during a radical prostatectomy, this means that a surgeon cuts out as much tissue as possible surrounding the prostate in an aggressive attempt to remove every bit of cancer.

X-ray therapy: see *external-beam radiation therapy.*

zones of the prostate: there are five distinct regions of the prostate. The two most commonly referred to are the transition zone and the peripheral zone.

Where to Get Help

You're not alone: there are many sources of good information available to help you. Here are a few of them.

American Cancer Society
250 Williams Street NW
Atlanta, GA 30303
(800) 227-2345
www.cancer.org/cancer/prostate-cancer.html
This national community-based organization provides comprehensive information and resources, referrals to treatment centers, and free publications.

American Urological Association, Urology Care Foundation
1000 Corporate Boulevard
Linthicum, MD 21090
(800) 828-7866
(410) 689-3700
www.urologyhealth.org
This foundation supports research and provides educational materials on prostate cancer, erectile dysfunction, and other urologic conditions.

The Brady Urological Institute
The Johns Hopkins Hospital
600 North Wolfe Street
Baltimore, MD 21287
(410) 955-6100
http://urology.jhu.edu
This website has many articles about the latest research and treatment in prostate cancer at Johns Hopkins.

National Association for Continence
PO Box 1019
Charleston, SC 29402
(800) BLADDER
www.nafc.org

This is a nonprofit organization dedicated to improving the lives of people with incontinence. It offers educational resources and programs.

National Cancer Institute Cancer Information Service
BG 9609 MSC 9760
9609 Medical Center Drive
Bethesda, MD 20892-9760
(800) 4-CANCER
www.cancer.gov
This is a national clearinghouse with an extensive health information database and educational materials, including information about clinical trials.

National Hospice and Palliative Care Organization (NHPCO)
1731 King Street
Alexandria, VA 22314
(703) 837-1500
www.nhpco.org
The goal of NHPCO is to help patients "carry on an alert, pain-free life and to manage other symptoms," so their days "may be spent with dignity and quality at home or in a homelike setting."

National Library of Medicine
www.nlm.nih.gov
This website allows you to gain access to millions of scientific publications and abstracts.

The Prostate Cancer Foundation
1250 Fourth Street
Santa Monica, CA 90401
(800) 757-2873
www.pcf.org
The Prostate Cancer Foundation's mission is to fund the cure for prostate cancer by supporting research that will rapidly translate into treatments. Its website has information on diagnosis and treatment, clinical trials, and stories for patients and family members. In an effort to "crowd-fund" the cure, the PCF has also launched Many vs. Cancer, a movement to end prostate cancer.

Us TOO International
2720 S. River Road, Suite 112
Des Plaines, IL 60018-4106
(630) 795-1002
Helpline: (800) 808-7866 (800-80-US-TOO)
www.ustoo.org
Us TOO International provides educational materials and resources, and serves as a community resource with more than 200 volunteer-led support groups.

Index